Kinanthropometry IV

Other titles from E & FN Spon

Biomechanics and Medicine in Swimming
Edited by D. Maclaren, T. Reilly and A. Lees

Intermittent High Intensity Exercise
Edited by D.A.D. Macleod, R.J. Maughan, C. Williams, C.R. Madeley, J.C.M. Sharp, R.W. Mutton and J. Graham

Foods, Nutrition and Sports Performance
Edited by C. Williams and J.T. Devlin

Physiology of Sports
Edited by T. Reilly, M. Secher, P. Snell and C. Williams

Science and Football
Edited by T. Reilly, K. Davids, W.J. Murphy and A. Lees

Science and Football II
Edited by T. Reilly, J. Clarys and A. Stibbe

Drugs in Sport
Edited by D. Mottram

Sport and Physical Activity
Edited by T. Williams, L. Almond and A. Sparkes

Science and Golf
Edited by A. Cochran

Advanced Materials in Sports Equipment
K. Easterling

Journal of Sports Sciences

For more information about these and other titles published by us, please contact: The Promotion Department, E & F N Spon, 2–6 Boundary Row, London SE1 8HN. Telephone: 071 522 9966.

Kinanthropometry IV

Edited by

William Duquet
Institute of Physical Education and Physiotherapy
Vrije Universiteit Brussel
Belgium

and

James A.P. Day
Department of Physical Education
University of Lethbridge
Canada

Proceedings of the International Congress on Youth, Leisure and Physical Activity and Kinanthropometry IV
Vrije Universiteit Brussel, Belgium 1990

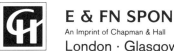

E & FN SPON
An Imprint of Chapman & Hall
London · Glasgow · New York · Tokyo · Melbourne · Madras

Published by E & FN Spon, an imprint of Chapman & Hall, 2–6 Boundary Row, London SE1 8HN, UK

Chapman & Hall, 2–6 Boundary Row, London SE1 8HN, UK

Blackie Academic & Professional, Wester Cleddens Road, Bishopbriggs, Glasgow G64 2NZ, UK

Chapman & Hall Inc., One Penn Plaza, 41st Floor, New York, NY 10119, USA

Chapman & Hall Japan, Thomaon Publishing Japan, Hirakawacho Nemoto Building, 6F, 1-7-11 Hirakawa-cho, Chiyoda-ku, Tokyo 102, Japan

Chapman & Hall Australia, Thomas Nelson Australia, 102 Dodds Street, South Melbourne, Victoria 3205, Australia

Chapman & Hall India, R. Seshadri, 32 Second Main Road, CIT East, Madras 600 035, India

First edition 1993

© William Duquet and James A.P. Day

Printed in Great Britain by St Edmundsbury Press Ltd, Bury St Edmunds, Suffolk

ISBN 0 419 16770 6

A catalogue record for this book is available from the British Library

Library of Congress Cataloging-in-Publication data available

Printed on permanent acid-free text paper, manufactured in accordance with ANSI/NISO Z39.48-1992 and ANSI/NISO Z39.48-1984 (Permanence of Paper).   [Paper = Magnum, 70 gsm]

Printed on permanent acid-free text paper, manufactured in accordance with ANSI/NISO Z39.48-1992 and ANSI/NISO Z39.48-1984 (Permanence of Paper).   [Paper = Magnum, 70 gsm]

In memory of Jan Broekhoff

Contents

Preface

These proceedings offer a selection of the contributions to the Kinanthropometry sessions of the International Congress on Youth, Leisure and Physical Activity and Kinanthropometry IV, held at the Vrije Universiteit Brussel from 21–25 May 1990.

The editors wish to express their sincere thanks to the organizing committee and its president L. Bollaert. The scientific committee, chaired by M. Hebbelinck, consisted for the area of Kinanthropometric aspects of J. Borms, G. Beunen, J.E.L. Carter, J.P. Clarijs, J.A.P. Day, W. Duquet, R. Hauspie and M. Hebbelinck. Our sincere gratitude also goes to the members of the reviewing board, who are listed separately, and to the staff of the Department of Biometry and Biomechanics of the V.U.B., in particular Mr. Freddy Witpas, for his efficient and continuous logistic collaboration throughout the whole editing process.

Our appreciation also goes to the following ministries, industries and other maecenas: Ministry of the Flemish Community (BLOSO, Public Health and International Cooperation), Belgian National Research Fund (NFWO), Vrije Universiteit Brussel, Coca-Cola, Generale Bank, Biblo Editions, WESCO, Province of Brabant, and Upjohn.

W. Duquet
J.A.P. Day

Reviewers

G. Beunen (Katholieke Universiteit Leuven)
J. Borms (Vrije Universiteit Brussel)
J.E.L. Carter (San Diego State University)
J.P. Clarijs (Vrije Universiteit Brussel)
J.-P. Cuerrier (Université de Sherbrooke, Québec)
J.A.P. Day (University of Lethbridge, Alberta)
K. De Martelaere (Vrije Universiteit Brussel)
K. De Meirleir (Vrije Universiteit Brussel)
W. Duquet (Vrije Universiteit Brussel)
R. Hauspie (Vrije Universiteit Brussel)
M. Hawes (University of Calgary, Alberta)
M. Hebbelinck (Vrije Universiteit Brussel)
R.M. Malina (University of Texas, Austin)
A. Martin (University of British Columbia, Vancouver)
T. Reilly (Liverpool John Moores University)
B. Van Gheluwe (Vrije Universiteit Brussel)
L. Van Puymbroeck (Vrije Universiteit Brussel)

MONKEY BUSINESS : EVOLUTION, CULTURE, AND YOUTH SPORT

J. BROEKHOFF
University of Oregon, Eugene, Oregon, USA

Keywords: Youth sport, Culture, Education, Evolution, Genetics, Selection, Training, Somatotype.

1 Introduction

It seems only fitting at an international congress on "Youth, Leisure and Physical Activity" that we as kinanthropometrists reflect on our role as scientists in the area of highly competitive sports for children and youth. To become successful in a sport, children often have to participate in years of intensive training. In certain sports such as gymnastics and figure skating it is not uncommon for boys and girls to spend ten or more years in concentrated training before they have even reached puberty. Only a very small percentage of these young athletes reach the top as many drop out somewhere along the arduous road. It is not surprising that the way to success in sport is often described in Darwinian terms as a "survival of the fittest." The hierarchy in an American gymnastics team, for example, has been likened to a "pecking order" (Mounts 1989) and a story about a family with unusually talented, athletic offspring was cleverly titled "Designer Genes" (Cazaneuve 1990).

The longer period of training in many sports is necessitated by the ever-increasing levels of endurance, strength, skill and sophistication demanded by the final event. The top gymnast of ten years ago would be ill-prepared to compete at a regional meet now and the record times in swimming or track, once set in the Olympic Games, are routinely broken in High School competition. At the same time, the rewards of becoming a super athlete in terms of crowd adulation and financial security have grown dramatically for many sports. Small wonder, then, that sport scientists have turned attention to the discovery and identification of children with special talents for some branch of sport. This "search for sporting excellence" (Fisher 1990), has become better organized and more systematic in recent times, not least because entire nations consider sporting talent as an important resource (Anthony 1985). The aim of sport scientists in this *selection* process is to predict which young athletes are most likely to emerge from years of training as the champions of the future (Hebbelinck 1988).

Notwithstanding the attempts by scientists to identify talent at a very young age, the entire process of producing champion athletes, especially

1

in countries like the United States, shows some interesting parallels with Darwin's process of *natural selection*. One could argue that, in a fairly haphazzard way, thousands of children are set on a road which leads to success for only the very few who possess the right genome. For sport scientists several important questions arise: To what extent can prolonged and intensive training modify or compensate for imperfections in the genome? Given the extreme specializations in some sport events, is it realistic to say that hard training will overcome even a slight drop-off in talent? A much harder question, of course, is whether the means justify the ends. Is the quest for ever-higher physical performance warranted in view of the increasing sacrifices in time and exertion by children during a crucial period of their growth and development?

2 Types of Selection

Charles Darwin used the principle of *natural selection* to account for the diversification of living forms. By their ability to adapt to changing environments certain organisms survived and their offspring, inheriting the traits that enabled their forbears to adapt, continued to thrive. Organisms that failed to adapt became extinct. Darwin's theory of evolution under the principle of natural selection has often been used to imply a law of progression. Spencer's catch phrase "survival of the fittest", intimated that the fittest were also the most advanced on a general scale of progress. As Gould (1977) indicates, however, "natural selection is a theory of *local* adaptation to changing environments. It proposes no perfecting principles, no guarantee of general improvement". Adaptations to environmental change are irreversible and the course of evolution is indeterminate. The theory of evolution, therefore, is retrodictive rather than predictive (Ingold 1986). Those, who use the theory of evolution to proclaim homo sapiens as the culmination of necessary progress are guilty of what Mandelbaum calls the 'retrospective fallacy': "the tendency to view earlier events as though they were controlled by their subsequent outcomes, when at the time of their occurrence any number of other outcomes might have been equally probable" (Ingold, p.15).

It is not difficult to see how a theory about local adaptation to a changing environment could be applied to sport as part of a cultural environment. Successful athletes are then seen as the product of a relatively long period of adaptation to the specific demands of a sport event. They are the survivors among large masses of children who, for a number of reasons, tried but failed to adjust to training and competition. To be sure, dropping out of sport hardly leads to literal extinction as it did for non-adapting species in Darwin's theory. The time scale of selection in sport, moreover, is but an instant compared to the scale of evolutionary change and the adaptation process usually stops short of Darwin's crucial concept of selective breeding. The idea of the selective breeding of humans in the realm of sport is not entirely novel, however, and we intend to return to it later.

As we mentioned earlier, changes in the natural environment and resultant variations under the mechanism of natural selection do not hold some innate promise of progress in nature. As Ingold (p.17) notes: "If, in certain lines, progress has taken place, *its cause must be found in the circumstances, not in the mechanism.*" Here is a very important difference between selection in sport and natural selection, as changes in a cultural environment, at least in principle, are subject to human intervention. Whereas the theory of evolution is retrodictive, selection in a cultural environment opens possibilities for prediction. Interestingly, Darwin gained valuable insight about the process of natural selection by observing plants and animals under domestication. The first chapter of "The Origin of Species" is concerned with variation under domestication and in it Darwin (1859) discusses how animal breeders achieve astonishing results in a relatively short time-span through conscious or *artificial selection*. "One of the most remarkable features in our domestic races," he comments, "is that we see in them adaptation, not indeed to the animal's or plant's own good, but to man's use or fancy" (Darwin, p. 47).

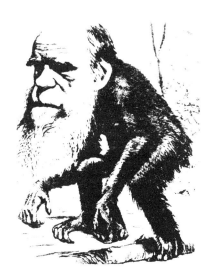

Darwin's quote gives ample reason for thought. If by analogy to *artificial selection*, conscious selection in sport is indeed not to the good of children athletes, but to the use or fancy of an adult society, then sport scientists have to face an ethical dilemma. The literature on talent identification too often avoids ethical questions. One might agree with Wolanski (1984, p.5) when he pleads, in the foreword to a book on the genetics of psychomotor traits in man, that individuals, according to their aspirations and dispositions, should find an appropriate place in society through proper occupational selection. It is less reassuring when he continues to say that "it is also important for the society, community and nation to appropriately utilize the potential capacity contained in the gene pool of the population and in the cultural traditions of ethnic groups." According to Wolanski, a *pre*selection of children for a particular sport branch should be made as early as 4 to 6 years of age and should be based on a number of psychomotor traits. Final selection then occurs through "spontaneous" attrition, as the less talented or less persistent children drop out. Given this scenario and others like it, a third type of selection, the search for sporting excellence and talent in young children may well develop into a process of *unnatural selection*.

3 The Secular Trend

Conscious selection and its power of prediction depend very much on the ability to assess the importance of inherited traits in their interrelatedness with environmental factors such as physical training. A crucial question, in this context, is whether environmental factors can significantly alter bodily form and function beyond reasonable genotypical constraints. In Darwin's time, it was generally agreed that human beings had freed themselves from the direct influence of natural selection on bodily form through their ability to adapt to the environment through culture. A.R. Wallace postulated that, henceforth, human evolution would be a matter of the mind or the intellect and not of bodily form (Ingold, p.50). In this respect, it is interesting to consider the secular changes in maturation and growth that started in the mid-eighteenth century, a trend that was largely limited to Europe, Australia, Canada, the United States, and Japan (Malina 1983a).

The secular trend is well documented (Himes 1979; Malina 1979; Roche 1979). From 1830 to 1960, the average age at menarche decreased at a rate of 4 months per decade in Europe. Over the same time period increases in weight and stature were observed with each successive generation. These increases were small at birth and most pronounced in late childhood and mid-adolescence. From 1860 to 1960, for example, the increase in stature per decade was 1.9 cm in late childhood and mid-adolescence, but only .6 cm for adults (Malina 1983a). A recent study of the secular shift in the growth of Japanese children indicates that the secular trend toward earlier menarche was largely a reflection of the secular change in the general tempo of physical growth. Both mean height and weight varied significantly at the age of menarche, but the percentage of mean height achieved at the time of menarche remained relatively stable at 95% (Tsuzaki et al. 1989). In recent decades, the trend of accelerated maturation and increase in stature appears to have slowed down in many countries or stopped altogether (cf. Chinn et al. 1989; Richter and Kern 1987; Roche 1979; Wellens et al. 1990).

Similar to the theories and explanations of evolution under the process of natural selection, the explanations for the secular trend are all retrodictive and, therefore, to a large extent speculative. As Roche (1979) has pointed out, secular trends by nature are caused almost entirely by environmental factors. The most obvious environmental causes for the trend are seen in a general improvement in living and working conditions that followed the industrial revolution: better nutrition, medical care, socio-economic conditions and the like. Certain environmental factors that are known to influence growth tempo are family size, climate, altitude, and urbanization. Children from smaller families, for instance, mature earlier and are taller than children from large families (Malina 1979). Urban children also tend to mature earlier than their rural counterparts. This may have inspired Adams (1981) to propose his stimulation-stress factor hypothesis (SSF). This multiple factor includes stresses brought about by crowding, handling, noise, light, and smell. There is little scientific evidence, however, that these sensory stimuli which can be both pleasant or unpleasant accelerate human growth. The various environmental explanations of the secular trend are not mutually exclusive and while no single one offers a necessary and sufficient cause, together they make at least for a plausible conjecture.

Genetic explanations for the secular trend are more tendentious. Some have proposed a theory of genetic drift caused by such factors as increased outbreeding, migration, and interclass mobility. As Malina (1979) indicated, it would be very hard indeed to explain secular changes on various continents by a systematic genetic shift. Natural selection and heterosis have also been rejected as likely causes. For one thing, there is no evidence that tall couples produce more offspring than short people. Chiarelli (1977) noted the fact that Italians born during the two world wars did not show a secular trend in stature. The same temporary cessation of the trend was observed for the Japanese and a number of other countries during the Second World War (Tanner 1978). He speculated that the shortage of food during the time of conception was especially hard on women with a linear, ectomorphic physique. These women could not maintain the necessary amount of fat for pregnancy and three months of lactation, postulated by the critical weight theory (Frisch 1975). Endomorphic women would have less difficulty maintaining the necessary fat percentage in times of curtailed food supplies and thus were likely to produce more children, of shorter stature, than ectomorphic women. The theory assumes that the average adult stature of children born of endomorphic mothers is smaller than the adult height of children by ectomorphic mothers, for which there is no conclusive evidence. Clearly, interruptions of the secular trend during times of food shortage can easier be explained by environmental factors.

4 Delayed Maturation

The presumed influence of environmental factors on the secular trend of accelerated growth has an interesting, but reverse, parallel in the domain of youth sport. It is well known that a high percentage of girls and women who engage in highly competitive sport, especially in gymnastics, figure skating, diving, and long distance running, experience secondary or primary amenorrhoea and may show a significant delay in menarche (Malina et al. 1978; Dale et al. 1979; Frisch et al. 1981). The same phenomena have been observed in ballet dancers (Frisch et al. 1980; Warren 1980). An explanation for these disruptions in reproductive ability was originally provided by Frisch and Revelle (1971) who stated their so-called "critical weight hypothesis." The researchers observed that at the time of menarche body weight was significantly less variable than stature and established a "critical" weight required for the onset of menstruation. The hypothesis received a lot of criticism (Trussel 1980; Malina 1983b; Tsuzaki 1989) but has been maintained albeit with a number of modifications. Frisch (1987) now considers that a particular ratio of fat to lean mass (approximately 17%) is normally necessary for menarche and for the maintenance of female reproductive functions (approximately 22%).

The critical fat hypothesis has attractive features in explaining anovulatory menstrual cycles and the incidence of secondary amenorrhoea in well-trained athletes and women who diet excessively. In the case of secondary amenorrhoea there is ample anecdotal evidence that menses are restored through a forced or voluntary cessation of training. Frisch also considered primary amenorrhoea and what she referred to as delayed menarche in female athletes, the result of a decreased body fat percentage caused by intense prepubertal training. She reported a positive relationship between the number of years of intensive training before puberty and the age at menarche (Frisch 1981). The relatively late age at menarche of many athletes, according to Frisch, can be explained largely by the environmental factor of intensive physical training: the earlier the training begins the later menarche tends to occur. Similar findings were reported by the East German researcher Marker (1981). Figure skaters, gymnasts, and divers who had the longest prepubertal training periods (an average of 7 to 10 years) were significantly older than volleyball players, handball players, and canoeists (average prepubertal training from 1 to 2 years) at the time of menarche.

More recently, researchers have become more attentive to the genetic factors that may play a role in the late maturation of certain groups of athletes. Stager and Hatler (1988) studied groups of female competitive swimmers and control subjects, who were paired with their sisters. On the basis of questionnaires it was determined that the athletes (14.3 yrs.) were significantly older at the time of menarche than their sisters (13.7 yrs.), who were, in turn, significantly older than the control subjects (12.9 yrs.) and their siblings (13.0 yrs.). The interpretation of the findings was complicated by the fact that a much greater percentage (75%) of the athletes' sisters participated in sport than the sisters of the controls (26%). Although the authors did not rule out the role of intense prepubertal activity, they also saw support for the importance of inherited characteristics in the regulation of the rate of maturation. There is no doubt that the study of the maturational patterns of athletes can benefit greatly by including familial information.

Theintz et al. (1989) emphasized the importance of familial data in their longitudinal growth study of young elite female gymnasts, moderately trained swimmers, and sedentary school girls. At the beginning of the study, parental data on recalled pubertal growth and pubertal maturation for the three groups were contrasted. Parents of gymnasts were significantly lighter and shorter than the parents of the swimmers and the control subjects. Recalled menarche in the mothers of the gymnasts occurred significantly later than in the other mothers. The young gymnasts, predictably, were lighter and shorter for age than swimmers and controls. Their skeletal age (11.0 ± 1.3 yrs.) lagged well behind their chronological age (12.6 ± 1.2 yrs.). On the basis of hereditary factors, therefore, one would not expect the target height of the gymnasts to be the same as that of the other girls. After at least 5 years of training of progressive intensity, the relatively short stature of the gymnasts at 12.6 years was still appropriate considering parental heights. The authors concluded that knowledge of patterns of parental development is essential when studying the potential long-term effects of physical activity on growth.

5 Late Maturation

The hypothesis that menarche in elite athletes is delayed because of prolonged training of high intensity was questioned, among others, by Malina (1983). He indicated that late maturing girls share a number of physical characteristics, such as a more ectomorphic physique and less weight for height, which may predispose them to athletic success in selected sports. To use Wolanski's concept of "spontaneous selection," one could argue that in gymnastics, figure skating, and ballet, late maturing girls are "selected out" over a long period of hard training because they possess the physical traits best suited to the demands of the athletic events. The studies by Stager and Theintz, cited above, certainly corroborate the hypothesis that the pattern of late maturation among certain groups of female athletes is just that, and not one of delayed maturation.

One of the weaknesses of the studies that reported a positive relationship between the number of years of training before puberty and age at menarche is their quasi-experimental design. In a Monte Carlo experiment, Stager et al. (1990) proposed that these reported relationships between early training history and age of menarche may be an artifact of the way researchers have defined the population from which they derived their samples. To test this proposition, the authors created a data set for 30,000 "athletes" who were randomly assigned an age at which they started training (AIT) and an age at menarche (AOM). As expected, there was no relationship between between AIT and AOM for the entire population (r= -.062). The researchers next formed two subgroups: one in which the athletes began training before menarche (PRE) and one in which the athletes started training after menarche (POST). Statistical analysis of the subgroup data indicated that the age at menarche for the POST group (11.69 $\pm$ 1.38) was significantly lower than that of the PRE group (13.91 $\pm$ 2.08). In spite of the absence of a correlation between AIT and AOM in the total population, the authors found significant relationships between these two variables in the subgroups: r=.454 for PRE and r=.412 for POST. Stager at al. concluded that defining the subgroups by AIT created biased samples of the population and produced spurious results of the same magnitude reported in the literature.

To make informed decisions about the issue of "delayed" versus "late" maturation is of great importance to prepubertal athletes and their parents. There is little doubt that excessive weight loss, caused by extensive training, could result in secondary and primary amenorrhoea, a shortened luteal phase or anoveal menstrual cycles (Frisch 1987). The claim that a normal maturational pattern could be delayed significantly by long-term, progressive training is on much more dubious ground. More likely, the extremely high demands, in terms of strength, skill, and endurance, of certain sports necessitate ever longer periods of preparation and require increasing specialization of bodily form. In a very real sense there is a "natural" or "spontaneous" selection at work that favors certain physique types and discards others. Some of the findings of our own longitudinal study of elite gymnasts appear to corroborate that view.

8

6 Physique Type

Tanner (1964) once commented that the Olympic Games are largely a festival of individuals with physiques that occupy the north-eastern parts of the somatotype distribution on a somatochart. The north-eastern sector of such a somatochart is populated with persons who have a high degree of mesomorphy combined with some ectomorphic traits, but with low endomorphy. In certain sports and events such as weight lifting, shot putting, and discus throwing, physique types may move to the north-west as the endomorphic component increases. Even within the confines of the mostly mesomorphic, athletic physiques finer distinctions can be made. It does not take a somatotype expert, for instance, to recognize the difference between the physique types of a long distance runner and a sprinter. Researchers have demonstrated that in many sports, for both men and women, competition at the elite level requires a body form and structure that is attuned to the activity within fairly specific boundaries (cf. Carter 1981, 1984; Carter et al. 1982; Tanner 1964). The further refinement and increased sophistication of sport skills in recent decades have only accented the need for morphological specificity. In gymnastics, for example, the average height of the elite gymnasts has decreased over time, especially for females.

There has been considerable debate over the years about the degree to which exercise and physical activity can modify the shape and structure of the human body. Older theories (Sheldon et al. 1940; Sheldon 1953) saw the somatotype as a genotype that could only be altered under extreme conditions of malnutrition or chronic disease. Although modern theorists consider the somatotype to be a phenotype, most would agree with Carter (1978) that "the influence of physical training upon physique appears to be small compared with the range of genetically determined variation in structure." For the prediction of athletic success, therefore, an individual's somatotype is of great importance. In our longitudinal study of young elite gymnasts (Broekhoff et al 1986; Nadgir 1987), somatotype components were consistently among the variables that discriminated between the gymnasts (average age of 12.7 years) and age-matched controls. The former were significantly less endomorphic and more mesomorphic than the latter. Equally important, group measures of somatotype dispersion (Carter et al. 1983) showed considerably less variability in physique type among male and female gymnasts than among the controls.

The prediction of the adult somatotype from a child's known physique type at any age before the beginning of the pubescent growth spurt always contains a significant error component. As Tanner (1973) indicated there appears to be a considerable independence between the factors controlling growth before puberty and those controlling the magnitude of the growth spurt. Often the adult somatotype is masked somewhat by age-specific

9

growth gradients that lend a particular *gestalt* to a developmental period (Zeller 1964). The period preceding the start of the pubescent growth spurt, which roughly coincides with the elementary school years, is marked by growth in a linear direction creating a more ectomorphic *gestalt*. During the second half of the pubescent spurt the direction of growth changes to emphasize increases in antero-posterior and lateral dimensions. For females this usually means an accelerated broadening of the hips and an increase in subcutaneous fat tissue. Males see a broadening of the shoulders and experience accelerated muscular development. The extent to which the events of puberty modify an individual's prepubertal physique is never totally predictable. This poses a serious problem for those who are looking for ideal physique types among children of a tender age.

The female gymnasts in our growth study (Nadgir 1987) conformed to the stereotypical image of the sport: they were smaller, less ponderous, and had higher body density than the controls. They also had relatively broad shoulders, narrower hips, long trunks, and short limbs. As a group, these girls also showed the late maturation pattern reported for gymnasts elsewhere in the literature (Broekhoff et al. 1989). Somatotypically, late maturation is often linked to an ectomorphic physique with its proportionally long arms and legs. Female gymnasts, with their relatively short arms and legs, may very well be a subset of a late maturing population with inherited structural traits that differ from those within the mainstream of late maturers. The average somatotype of the young gymnasts (N=46) was 2.2-4.1-3.1 which was very close to the physique type of 15 Olympic gymnasts (2.1-3.7-3.4) reported by Carter (1984). When the 46 gymnasts were divided into a younger (8 to 13 yrs) and an older group (13-18 yrs), the average somatotypes did not differ significantly. The older gymnasts (2.4-4.1-2.8) were slightly more endomorphic and less ectomorphic than the younger girls (2.0-4.1-3.4).

It is clear that a prepubertal physique type with above average mesomorphy is an advantage to female gymnasts. In the main, the older girls in our sample retained that somatotype throughout puberty and showed significantly greater shoulder width than their controls (Nadgir, p.83). How the younger gymnasts will be affected by the pubescent growth spurt, only time can tell. Undoubtedly there will be a continued selection process predicated on the physical changes of the pubescent period. The uncertainties created by the physical changes during puberty may well be responsible for the trend in female gymnastics to create champions at an earlier and earlier age. The consequence of this has been that serious training in the sport must start well before puberty, often as early as five or six years of age.

For male gymnasts the situation is somewhat different as the ideal physique is only established after the pubescent growth spurt. Before adolescence, male gymnasts have many of the physical characteristics of their female counterparts, but in comparison to mature gymnasts they still lack in muscular development. Our sample of male gymnasts (N=34), for example, had an average somatotype of 1.5-4.6-3.8 which was significantly less mesomorphic and more ectomorphic than a comparative group of 11 Olympic gymnasts (1.4-5.5-2.5). The dispersion of somatotypes in the two groups was very similar and, as mentioned earlier, much smaller than that of the control group. At an average age of 12.5 years, the great majority of the young gymnasts still had to experience peak velocity in muscular strength. For many boys an accelerated linear growth during the first phase of the adolescent growth spurt is not always followed by sufficient broadening out and muscular development. Several boys in our study, who were in youth selection teams before they started their pubescent growth spurt, dropped out of gymnastics for that reason. Their post-pubertal bodies were no longer ideal for performing intricate skills requiring precise timing and great muscular strength.

In gymnastics, having an ideal somatotype, desirable body proportions and height are by no means the only prerequisites for success. Perhaps, though, it is easier to accept that these morphological traits are determined largely by genetics, but that factors related to the learning of motor skills are more amenable to change by environmental manipulation. Even here, though, one needs to proceed with caution. Two investigations with 14 of the female gymnasts in our study (Debu et al. 1987; Debu and Woollacott 1988) analyzed response latencies of eight muscles at the leg, trunk, and neck levels during stance perturbations. The authors unexpectedly found that the response latencies of the neck muscles, especially during backward perturbance, were significantly longer in the older gymnasts (11 to 16 yrs) than in the control subjects. These differences were not observed for the younger gymnasts (7 to 10 yrs) and their controls. The researchers interpreted the longer response latencies as an uncoupling of the neck muscles from the response radiating in the lower half of the body, thus enabling the gymnasts to collect information about their spatial position without interfering with the response in the lower part of the body. Since the response latencies of the younger gymnasts and their controls did not differ, the authors attributed the differences between the older subjects to the effect of gymnastics training.

It is attractive to attach developmental significance to the differences between the older gymnasts and their controls. The researchers proposed that, with increasing exposure to gymnastics, the mechanism used to stabilize the head became relatively independent from the mechanism used to stabilize the center of mass. It certainly is not unreasonable to assume that certain synergies are flexible enough to adapt to changing conditions of the environment, especially to those created by years of repetitive training. Nevertheless, there is an alternative explanation that is more in line with the heriditability of psychomotor traits. Since the older subjects formed a cross-sectional sample, it is impossible to rule out the possibility that the gymnasts already possessed longer latencies than the controls at the time they started their gymnastics training. The fact that no differences were observed between the younger groups can only be considered as presumptive evidence of a training effect. Many of the older gymnasts, moreover, were recruited nationwide and lived in a special dormatory, whereas the younger children were predominantly from the hometown. It would be hard to argue, therefore, that the younger and older subjects were drawn from similar populations.

7 Spontaneous Selection and Education

Although many teachers and coaches have developed reasonable skills in identifying athletic talent in young athletes, when it comes to differentiating between the very good and the very best, a lot of guesswork is involved. In spite of the best intentions, sport scientists have done but little to take the guesswork out of the selection process. Considering the multitude of factors that have to coalesce in the making of a champion athlete, this is not at all surprising. Scientists can make fairly accurate predictions of adult height and give adequate projections of a person's future somatotype, yet it is clear that such estimates are in no way definitive of what it is that makes for an elite athlete. In the present state of affairs, and in most sports that require exceptional levels of skill and coordination, athletic talent rises to the top after a "weeding-out" process of years and years of intense physical and mental training. At this time there seems to be no alternative to this process of "spontaneous selection" that shows so many similarities with Darwin's principle of natural selection.

In the sections above we have made a strong case for the role that hereditary traits play in the process of "spontaneous selection." Future studies with more emphasis on the characteristics of the grandparents, parents, and siblings of athletes will undoubtedly reinforce the importance of the genome. It is unlikely, however, that Darwin's "artificial selection" through selected breeding, in some "Brave New World," will be attempted in the search for champion athletes. For one thing the "incubation" period is much too long and the entire process too cumbersome and fallible to show much promise. Tinkering with the human genome in the embryonic stages holds more promise once we have become adept in mapping the pages of the 23 books of genetic material. But what remains of sport when in a future world sets of "designer genes" are pitted against each other? Not an entirely irrelevant question for today's world of sport in which anabolic steroids and blood doping represent not so much a difference in kind as in degree.

Adaptation under natural selection has led to many forms of movement that are pleasing to human beings. We delight in the effortless grace with

12

which monkeys in a zoo swing from branch to branch in a game of tag. Large audiences in gymnasia and sporthalls also delight in the skills of gymnasts who move around uneven parallel bars with breathtaking audacity. The effortlessness that comes natural to monkeys, takes gymnasts six to ten years of training to hone and perfect. The movements of monkeys stand at the end of an evolutionary process prodded by changes in a natural environment, the gymnasts' moves stand at the end of an adaptation process to a cultural fashion. Sport scientists are understandably intrigued with predicting which young children will eventually reach the perfection of the champion gymnast, diver, or figure skater. But perhaps it has become time to ask questions about the educational implications of asking young children to dedicate themselves to distant ends that become increasingly impossible to reach for all but the exceptionally talented.

At first face, questions about the meaning of elite sport for young children appear to touch mainly philosophical problems. It puts into question certain aspects of sport as part of a cultural environment. From that angle, the answers are by no means unambiguous. Kinanthropometrists can remain on stabler ground by conducting more studies of the effect of long-term, intensive training on the growth and development of young children. Who are the children who persevere in spite of inevitable injuries, what or who motivates them? What are the developmental costs for sport prodigies in later life? Are they the priviledged youths who in ancient times roamed the gymnasia of ancient Greece or are they the child laborers of the late twentieth century?

8 References

Adams, J.F. (1981) Earlier menarche, greater height and weight: A stimulation stress factor hypothesis. **Gen. Psych. Monographs**, 104 (1), 3-22.

Anthony, M. (1985) The farming of Soviet children. **Sports Fitness**, 1 (6), 68-72.

Broekhoff, J. Nadgir, A.K. and Pieter, W. (1986) Morphological differences between young gymnasts and non-athletes matched for age and gender, in **Kinanthropometry III** (eds T. Reilly, J. Watkins and J. Borms), E. & F.N. Spon, London, pp. 204-210.

Broekhoff, J. Nadgir, A.K. and Pieter, W. (1989) Self-assessment of maturity by female adolescent gymnasts. Paper presented at the World Congress of AIESEP, Jyvaskyla, Finland.

Carter, J.E.L. (1978) Prediction of outstanding athletic ability : The structural perspective, in **The International Congress of Activity Sciences: Exercise Physiology** (eds F. Landry and W.A.R. Orban), Symposia Specialists, Miami, Fla., pp. 29-42.

Carter, J.E.L. (1980) **The Heath-Carter Somatotype Method**. San Diego State University, San Diego, California.

Carter, J.E.L. (1981) Somatotypes of female athletes, in **The Female Athlete: A Socio-Psychological and Kinanthropometric Approach** (eds J. Borms, M. Hebbelinck and A. Venerando), Karger, Basel, pp. 85-116.

Carter, J.E.L. (1984) Somatotypes of Olympic athletes from 1948 to 1976, in **Physical Structure of Olympic Athletes, Part II** (ed J.E.L. Carter), Medicine Sport Sci., 18, Karger, Basel, pp. 80-109.

Carter, J.E.L. Aubry, S.P. and Sleet, D.A. (1982) Somatotypes of Montreal Olympic athletes, in **Physical Structure of Olympic Athletes, Part I** (ed J.E.L. Carter), Medicine Sport Sci., 16, Karger, Basel, pp. 53-80.

Cazaneuve, B. (1990) Designer genes : The Mills family is America's first family in spinning, speeding and soaring. **The Olympian**, 16 (7), 10-14.

Chiarelli, B. (1977) On the secular trend of stature : A body constitution interpretation. **Current Anthropol.** , 18 (3), 524-526.

Chinn, S. Rona, R.J. and Price, C.E. (1989) The secular trend of primary school children in England and Scotland 1972-79 and 1979-86. **Ann. Hum. Biol.** , 16 (5), 387-395.

Dale, D. Gerlach, D.H. and Wilhite, A.L. (1979) Menstrual disfunction in distance runners. **Obstet. Gynecol.** , 54, 47-53.

Darwin, C. (1859) **The Origin of Species**. A mentor book, New American Library, New York, 1958.

Debu, B. and Woollacott, M. (1988) Effects of gymnastics training on postural responses to stance perturbations. **J. Mot. Behavior**, 20 (3), 273-300.

Debu, B. Woollacott, M. and Mowatt, M. (1987) Development of postural control in children: Effects of gymnastics training, in **Advances in Motor Development Research, 1** (eds J.E. Clark and J.H. Humphrey), AMS Press Inc., New York, pp. 41-69.

Fisher, R.J. and Borms, J. (1990) **The Search for Sporting Excellence**. ICSSPE Sport Science Studies 3, Verlag Karl Hofmann, Schorndorf, Federal Republic of Germany.

Frisch, R.E. (1975) Critical weight at menarche. **Am. J. Dis. Child.**, 129, 258-259.

Frisch, R.E. (1987) Body fat, menarche, fitness and fertility. **Hum. Reprod.**, 2 (6), 521-533.

Frisch, R.E. and Revelle, R. (1971) Height and weight at menarche and a hypothesis of menarche. **Arch. Dis. Child**, 46, 695-701.

Frisch, R.E. et al. (1981) Delayed menarche and amenorrhoea of college athletes in relation to the onset of training. **J. Am. Med. Assoc.**, 246, 1559-1563.

Frisch, R.E. Wyshak, G. and Vincent, L. (1980) Delayed menarche and amenorrhoea of ballet dancers. **New Engl. J. Med.**, 303, 17-19.

Gould, S.J. (1977) **Ever Since Darwin: Reflections in Natural History**. W.W. Norton, New York.

Hebbelinck, M. (1988) Talent identification and development in sport: kinanthropometric issues, in **New Horizons of Human Movement,** Seoul Olympic Scientific Congress Organizing Committee, Seoul, pp. 22-33.

Ingold, T. (1986) **Evolution and Social Life**. Cambridge University Press, Cambridge.

Malina, R.M. (1979) Secular changes in size and maturity : Causes and Effects, in **Monogr. Soc. Res. Child.**, 44 (3-4), pp. 59-102.

Malina, R.M. (1983a) Secular changes in growth, maturation, and physical performance, **Exercise and Science Review**, pp. 204-255.

Malina, R.M. (1983b) Menarche in athletes : a synthesis and hypothesis. **Ann. Hum. Biol.**, 1, 1-24.

Malina, R.M. et al. (1978) Age at menarche and selected menstrual characteristics in athletes at different competitive levels and in different sports. **Med. Sci. Sports**, 3, 218-222.

Märker, K. (1981) Influence of athletic training on the maturity process of girls, in **The Female Athlete** (eds J. Borms, M. Hebbelinck and A. Venerando), S. Karger, Basel, pp. 117-126.

Mounts, K. (1989) The pecking order. **The Olympian**, 15 (9), 33-35.

Nadgir, A.K. (1987) **A morphological study of young male and female competitive gymnasts**. Microfiche Doct. Diss., Microform Publications, Eugene, Oregon.

Richter, J. and Kern, G. (1987) Secular changes in the development of children born in Goerlitz, German Democratic Republic, 1956 to 1967. **Hum. Biol.**, 59 (2), 345-355.

Roche, A.F. (1979) Secular trends in stature, weight and maturation, in **Monogr. Soc. Res. Child.**, 44 (3-4), pp. 3-27.

Sheldon, W.H. (1951) **Atlas of Men: A Guide for Somatotyping the Adult Male at All Ages**. Gramercy Publishing Company, New York.

Sheldon, W.H. Stevens, S.S. and Tucker, W.B. (1945) **The Varieties of Human Physique**. Harper and Brothers, New York.

Stager, J. M. and Hatler, L.K. (1988) Menarche in athletes : The influence of genetics and prepubertal training. **Med. Sci. Sports Exer.**, 20 (4), 369-373.

Stager, J.M. Wigglesworth, J.K. and Hatler, L.K. (1990) Interpreting the relationship between age of menarche and prepubertal training. **Med. Sci. Sports Exer.**, 22 (1), 54-59.

Tanner, J.M. (1964) **The Physique of Olympic Athletes**. George Allan & Unwin, London.

Tanner, J.M. (1973) **Growth at Adolescence**. Blackwell Sci. Publ., London, 2nd ed., pp. 91.

Tanner, J.M. (1978) **Foetus into Man**. Harvard University Press, Cambridge, Mass.

Theintz, G.E. et al. (1989) Growth and pubertal development of young female gymnasts and swimmers : A correlation with parental data. **Int. J. Sports Med.**, 10, 87-91.

Trussel, J. (1980) Statistical flaws in evidence for the Frisch hypothesis that fatness triggers menarche. **Hum. Biol.**, 52, 711-720.

Tsuzaki, S. et al. (1989) Lack of linkage between height and weight and age at menarche during the secular shift in growth of Japanese children. **Ann. Hum. Biol.**, 16 (5), 429-436.

Warren, M.P. (1980) The effects of exercise on pubertal progression and reproductive functions in girls. **J. Clin. Endocrinol. Metab.**, 51, 1150-1157.

Wellens, R. et al. (1990) Age at menarche in Flemish girls : current status and secular change in the 20th century. **Ann. Hum. Biol.** 17 (2), 145-152.

Wolanski, N. and Siniarski, A. (1984) **Genetics of Psychomotor Traits in Man**. Int. Soc. of Sport Genetics and Somatology, Warsaw.

Zeller, W. (1964) **Konstitution und Entwicklung**. Verlag für Psychologie, Dr. C.J. Högrefe, Göttingen.

Part One

Body Composition and Growth

1

REGIONAL ADIPOSITY AND THE SEX HORMONES

A.D. MARTIN and M. DANIEL
The University of Manitoba, Winnipeg, Canada

Keywords: Adiposity, Sex hormones, Obesity, Body fat, Somatotypes, Fat patterning.

1 Introduction

The health hazards of obesity are well known, but the relationship between fatness and morbidity is not simple. Certainly, fatter people have a greater incidence of cardiovascular disease, but there is also an optimal level of fatness below which cardiovascular disease incidence rises. Also, investigation of sex differences reveals a paradox: women are considerably fatter than men, yet experience far less of the morbidity and mortality associated with obesity than men do. Vague was the first to attribute this to sexual dimorphism in adipose tissue patterning, distinguishing the female, *gynoid* distribution, characterised by hip and gluteal fat, from the male or *android* distribution, characterised by abdominal fatness (Vague 1956). Since then a large body of research has examined the relationship between adipose tissue distribution and health. A primary step was the selection of quantitative measures of adipose tissue distribution. Though skinfold ratios are sometimes used, the ratio of waist circumference to hip circumference (WHR) has become by far the the most common index. Despite the fact that these circumferences include bone, muscle and organs as well as adipose tissue, WHR is a stronger risk factor than obesity alone for cardiovascular disease, hypertension, stroke, hyperlipidemia, hyperinsulinemia, glucose intolerance and diabetes. Several mechanisms have been suggested, some that regard the relationship between abdominal adipose tissue and health risk as causative, others that see increased abdominal deposition of fat as the result of other factors which influence cadiovascular risk separately. Nonetheless, it is now clear that all adipose tissue is not the same: the metabolic characteristics of adipocytes, particularly their response to certain hormones, differ at different sites in the body.

The obvious sex differences in adipose tissue patterning suggest that the sex steroids play an important role. As yet, this has not been proved, but the circumstantial evidence is considerable. In this paper we examine evidence relating to the hypothesis that it is the androgen/estrogen balance that regulates adipose tissue patterning in the body.

2 Adipose Tissue Morphology Through the Lifespan

At birth, girls have slightly more fat than boys, but no difference in patterning is apparent (Poissonnet et al. 1984). Girls retain their fatter levels as skinfold thicknesses decrease in both sexes between 9 months and 7 years. They then rise, and the values in females diverge further from the boys at about 8 years, until the marked differences seen in early adulthood are reached (Fig. 1).

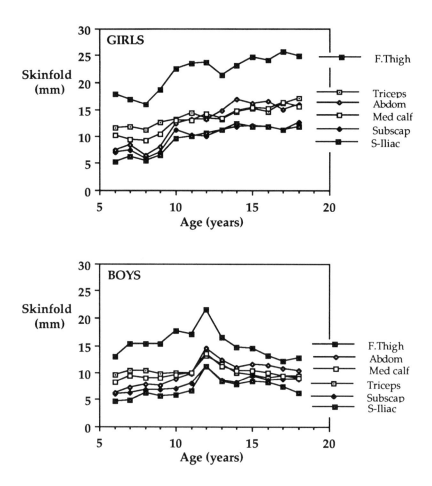

Fig. 1. Age changes in skinfold thickness at six sites. Cross-sectional data, adapted from Ross and Marfell-Jones (1982).

The only anomaly in this pattern occurs at age eleven when boys' skinfolds all show a rapid jump giving them levels of subcutaneous fat that are similar to girls at about age twelve. The boys' skinfolds decline rapidly thereafter and continue to diverge from those of the girls until adulthood. While the decline of fatness in boys can be readily attributed to the pubertal increase in testosterone, the cause of the temporary rise in fatness before puberty has not been clarified, though it is most probably associated with a relative estrogen excess. Changes in adipose tissue patterning are difficult to assess as almost nothing is known about internal fat deposition during growth because, prior to the very recent use of magnetic resonance imaging no safe imaging techniques were available. Changes in body density during growth give little insight into internal fat deposition because of the confounding effect of rapid growth of the lean tissues. Perhaps the clearest demonstration of sexual dimorphism in adipose tissue patterning is seen in the waist girth-to-upper thigh girth ratio (Fig. 2). While this ratio declines with age in both sexes, girls show a consistently faster decline than boys, leading to the android/gynoid distinction in early adulthood. This graph almost certainly underestimates the trend since thigh muscle girth in the boys is increasing much more rapidly than in the girls. Other studies confirm that puberty results in a more generalised distribution in girls, with a tendency toward the periphery, in contrast to boys, who tend to localize fat centrally (Baumgartner et al. 1987; Baumgartner et al. 1986; Harsha et al. 1980; Mueller 1982; Rolland-Cachera et al. 1989).

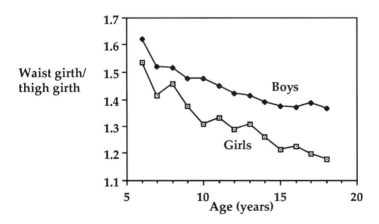

Fig. 2. Age changes in waist-to-thigh girth ratio in boys and girls. Cross-sectional data, adapted from Ross and Marfell-Jones (1982).

Patterning changes through adulthood are clearer. In men, increasing age brings about more centralised adiposity (increasing WHR), due mostly to increasing intra-abdominal deposition. Women in their reproductive years tend to accumulate fat as they age, but still retain the gynoid pattern. However, as Vague has pointed out, sexual dimorphism is much less marked in the later years of life (Vague 1956). The shift towards the android pattern in women occurs after menopause, but some studies fail to demonstrate this difference between pre- and post menopausal women. A confounding factor here is that WHR increases, not just through menopause, but also with increasing levels of adiposity (Fig. 3). Though far from conclusive, the observed age changes suggest that the hormonal shifts coinciding with puberty and menopause are connected to the pattern of adipose tissue distribution in females.

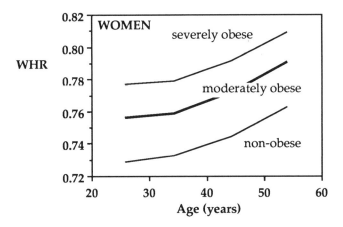

Fig. 3. Changes in waist-to-hip girth ratio with age in women. Adapted from Lanska et al. (1985).

3 Endocrine Changes

As the adolescent growth spurt begins and height velocity increases, estrogen levels rise, though in an erratic and sometimes cyclic pattern until menarche, then begin to fluctuate regularly with the menstrual cycle (Enriori et al. 1984; Tanner 1978). Thus the pubertal rise in estrogens precedes menarche. However, because of the limited data on hormone levels in children the relationship between hormones and adiposity is not clear. It was thought that a certain degree of fatness was necessary for menarche to occur; fat was seen as the determinant of menarcheal timing

(Frisch 1976; Frisch et al. 1974). This "critical fat hypothesis" was in accordance with earlier evidence that fatter girls generally attain menarche at an earlier age than lean girls (Garn et al. 1959). These observations were valid (Garn 1986), and this phenomenon is still notable today (Frisancho et al. 1982). However, there is no critical threshold level of either fatness or weight with respect to menarche (Garn et al. 1983).

What appears "critical" is the duration and level of estrogen exposure in those whose menarche occurs early. A recent investigation has shown significant inverse relationships between age at menarche and levels of estrone and estradiol, the conclusion being that women whose menarche occurred early produced larger amounts of estrogens than other women (MacMahon et al. 1982). This same study also showed that women who experience early menarche continue to produce larger amounts of estrogens beyond the immediate peri-menarcheal years up to the age of 39 years, the age limit of the study (MacMahon et al. 1982). Thus, since recent studies suggest that it is actually maturational timing which has a greater immediate and long-term effect on levels of fatness than levels of fatness have on maturational timing (Garn 1986; Garn et al. 1986), it may very well be that it is the duration and level of exposure to estrogens during the peri-menarcheal period which determines both menarcheal timing and adiposity. However, it will require longitudinal observation to confirm this.

Apart from menarche, estrogens are associated with adiposity in other ways. Estradiol and percent body fat are significantly correlated in both young women (Rice 1988) and postmenopausal women (Jensen et al. 1985; Vermeulen et al. 1978, 1979). There are close relationships between excessive body weight and metabolic transformation of androstenedione to estrone (MacDonald et al. 1978), and the association of obesity with increased estrone production has been noted in young and older women as well as in men (Kirschner et al. 1981). In postmenopausal women, ovarian estrogen production ceases almost completely, although androgens may continue to be produced by the ovaries (Greenblatt et al. 1976; Judd et al. 1974). Levels of plasma estradiol and estrone are lower than those observed at the follicular phase of the normal menstrual cycle in young women (Samoljik et al. 1977), and the estrone to estradiol ratio is greater than two (Judd et al. 1974; Samoljik et al. 1977; Vermeulen et al. 1978), as in men (Samoljik et al. 1977). In the follicular phase of normal young women, this ratio is close to unity (Samoljik et al. 1977; Santen et al. 1978). After menopause, serum concentrations of both estrone and estradiol change little with age (Jensen et al. 1985).

Thus, the female sex hormones display a strong relationship to adiposity throughout the reproductive years, and beyond. It appears that adiposity is an aspect of sexual dimorphism which is initiated by the sex hormones during puberty, and maintained by the sex hormones throughout the reproductive years by central (ovarian) and peripheral (adipose tissue aromatization) mechanisms. However, beyond general correlations with regional adiposity, the involvement of sex hormones in establishing morphological variations in tissue storage and mobilization of fat remains to be considered.

4 Androgen/Estrogen Balance

Much evidence supports the idea that body fat morphology is more a function of the androgenic/estrogenic balance than of estrogens alone. The onset of androgen secretion in the pubertal male or the administration of exogenous testosterone to the hypogonadal male is accompanied by a change in fat distribution towards the android type (Vague et al. 1974). Android distribution in women is common throughout the postmenopausal years, a time of androgen excess due to an increase in free testosterone and the decrease in circulating estrogens. High-dose postmenopausal estrogen therapy counteracts the increased fat mass common to the postmenopausal state (Jensen et al. 1986), and postmenopausal women on estrogen replacement therapy display less android distribution of fat (Seidell et al. 1989). In keeping with estrogenic dominance, most non-obese premenopausal women are of the gynoid body type. This appears to be specifically due to high levels of circulating estradiol; supporting this is the fact that in men, gynoid adiposity is associated with increased levels of plasma estradiol (Sparrow et al. 1980), and shifts toward gynoid body fat distribution can be experimentally induced in males by treatment with estrogens (Lafontan et al. 1985).

Additional evidence in support of the relative androgenic/estrogenic balance perspective comes from study of transsexuals, who generally undergo endocrine therapy to provide masculinization or feminization of body shape and subcutaneous adipose tissue. While administration of sex hormones does in fact achieve these goals, the resulting changes in adiposity have rarely been quantified (Prior et al. 1989). Case histories demonstrate the effects of androgens and estrogens on deltoid and trochanter adipocytes in two transsexuals who were measured before and after long-term sex steroid treatment. A female-to-male transsexual given androgen treatment for 45 months, displayed an "important" decrease of % body fat, a similar decrease in trochanter adipocyte number, a "lesser" decrease of deltoid adipocyte number, a "strong" increase of deltoid adipocyte volume and a decrease of trochanter adipocyte volume (Vague et al. 1984). A male-to-female transsexual given supra-physiologic doses of estrogens over 34 months displayed no change in % body fat, a "moderate" increase of both deltoid adipocyte number and trochanter adipocyte number, an important increase of trochanter adipocyte volume and a "dramatic" decrease of deltoid adipocyte volume (Vague et al. 1984). These results demonstrate for the first time the opposite effects of estrogens on deltoid and trochanter adipocytes in humans and vividly illustrate the effects of shifts in relative androgenic/estrogenic balance.

Simply because regional changes in adipose tissue distribution correspond in time with changes in serum levels of reproductive hormones, does not prove a causal relationship. Adipose sites that differ in their growth or decline must also show specific differences in the metabolism of adipocytes, and differences in the size or number of cells.

5 Cellular and Metabolic Characteristics of Adipocytes

5.1 Adipocyte Size and Number

The link between body fat distribution and the sex hormones must involve regional differences in the cellular characteristics of adipocytes. In men, android body fat is associated with an increased size of abdominal adipocytes (Ashwell et al. 1978; Kissebah et al. 1982) and a greater percentage of this is located internally (Ashwell et al. 1985; Grauer et al. 1984). Men also have larger omental and mesenteric fat cells than premenopausal women, in whom omental fat cell size has been found to be the smallest (Fried et al. 1987). Premenopausal women are generally of gynoid distribution and consistently display greater size of gluteal and femoral adipocytes (Fried et al. 1987; Rebuffé-Scrive et al. 1985). There may also be a greater number of fat cells in these regions (Lanska et al. 1985; Vansant et al. 1988). Gluteal-femoral fat cell hypertrophy, such that these fat cells are larger than those in the abdominal region, characterizes premenopausal women; this difference disappears with menopause due to the increased size of abdominal adipocytes which occurs with menopause (Rebuffé-Scrive et al. 1985). Women of android distribution have significantly larger abdominal adipocytes than women of gynoid distribution (Evans et al. 1983; Hartz et al. 1987; Vansant et al. 1988) just as men do. Men and women of android body fat distribution are said to display abdominal adipocyte hypertrophy (Lanska et al., 1985). There are thus two fat depots of special importance, one located in the abdominal region and the other located in the gluteal-femoral region, and two mechanisms which can influence adipose tissue thickness, adipocyte hyperplasia and adipocyte hypertrophy. It is interesting to note that abdominal, but not femoral, adipocyte volume has been shown to correlate with relative androgenic/estrogenic activity (Evans et al. 1983). Regional differences in fat cell size are accompanied by metabolic differences, and the sex hormones are involved in mediating these differences. The regional characteristics of adipocytes are summarised in Table 1.

25

Table 1. Regional Characteristics of Adipocytes in Men and Pre- and Postmenopausal Women

Adipocyte region	Cellular characteristics	Pre-menopause (Gynoid)	Post-menopause (Android)	Men (Android)
Abdominal	normal	*		
	enlarged		*	*
Gluteal-femoral	normal			*
	enlarged	*	*	
	hyperplasia	*	*	

5.2 Adipocyte Metabolism

The main function of adipose tissue is to store triglyceride during periods of affluence and to release the stored lipids as fatty acids when needed. Lipogenesis involves the hydrolysis of blood triglycerides, controlled by the rate-limiting enzyme lipoprotein lipase (LPL), and the resynthesis into adipose triglycerides. Lipolysis, the release of fatty acids from adipose tissue, is accomplished by the action of hormone-sensitive lipase. Lipogenesis and lipolysis display sex and regional differences. Both aspects of adipocyte metabolism as well as the direct effect of estrogens on these processes have been studied.

5.2.1 Lipolysis

Investigations of regional adipocyte metabolism in humans have shown that the larger size of abdominal adipocytes is associated with a greater rate of lipolysis *in vitro* (Arner et al. 1981; Kissebah et al.,1982; Smith et al. 1979). Abdominal fat cells also show a diminished sensitivity to the anti-lipolytic action of insulin (Bolinder et al. 1983). Omental adipocytes have been found to be more sensitive to lipolytic agents than subcutaneous fat cells, and are associated with lower activities of LPL than the latter (Lithell et al. 1978; Smith 1985). Such studies help to explain the high frequency of impaired glucose tolerance found in upper body (android) obesity; it may be that an increased or greater rate of free fatty acid release *in vivo* could inhibit glucose uptake by peripheral tissues, thus contributing to insulin resistance (Evans et al. 1988).

Regarding catecholamines, adipocytes in the abdominal subcutaneous regions have been found to be more responsive than those of femoral regions to norepinephrine, and norepinephrine has been found to be more lipolytic than epinephrine (Lafontan et al. 1985). The femoral subcutaneous regions are particularly insensitive to epinephrine-stimulated lipolysis *in vivo* (Lafontan et al. 1979), and differences in epinephrine-stimulated adenylate cyclase activities in adipocytes withdrawn from various regions have been demonstrated *in vitro* (Kather et al. 1977). Furthermore, there appear to be both sex and regional differences in the distribution of activity of adipocyte adenylate cyclase (Kather et al. 1977) and, since human adipocytes possess both ß- and α_2-adrenoreceptors coupled respectively in a positive and negative fashion to plasma membrane adenylate cyclase, adenylate cyclase activity is of prime importance in controlling the lipolytic activity of adipocytes (via cyclic-AMP production) through protein-kinase and hormone-sensitive lipase activation (Lafontan et al. 1985).

Human evidence regarding the direct effects of estrogens on adipocyte lipolysis is lacking, though in rats, various adipose tissues have unequivocally been found to be estrogen target tissues (Gray et al. 1981; Wade et al. 1978). Estrogens increase *in vitro* catecholamine-stimulated lipolysis in adipocytes by enhancing hormone-sensitive lipase activity (Wade et al. 1985). The strong regulatory effects of estradiol on enzyme activities in rat adipose tissue are mediated in turn by cyclic-AMP (Tomita et al. 1984), as in humans, which is thought to be the likely mechanism whereby the estrogens promote lipolysis in rat fat cells (Pasquier et al. 1988).

5.2.2 Lipogenesis

It appears that the sex hormones also account for sex and regional differences in LPL regulation, and therefore lipogenesis. Convincing evidence has been found mainly in the rat. Estradiol has been found to reduce LPL activity in both intact and gonadectomized animals (Dark et al. 1984; Gray et al. 1980; Hamosh et al. 1975; Steingrimsdottir et al. 1980; Wade et al. 1985; Wilson et al. 1976) as well as influencing hormone-sensitive lipase (Krakower et al. 1988) while progestin, only affecting female adipose tissue (Gray et al. 1980), counteracts the estrogen effects on LPL (Gray et al. 1980; Steingrimsdottir et al. 1980). Androgen inhibition of adipose tissue LPL appears to result from estradiol formed by aromatization rather than from a direct effect (Gray et al. 1979).

In humans, available data regarding sex steroid effects on adipose tissue and plasma LPL activity are contradictory. However, endogenous sex steroid levels have only been measured in a few investigations; most studies have utilized exogenous sex steroids and have looked specifically at their effect on postheparin plasma LPL. A recent investigation of *endogenous* sex steroid levels and their relationship with LPL activity in obese pre- and post-menopausal women found estradiol to be a major negative regulator of fasting adipose tissue LPL, independent of degree of obesity (Per-Henrick et al. 1988). This work supports previous animal

27

research. The obvious implication is that estradiol, the dominant estrogen in premenopausal women, would limit lipogenesis due to its effect on LPL, while in postmenopausal women the lack of estradiol would theoretically allow lipogenesis, given the lack of inhibition of LPL.

A key question concerns the degree to which variations in LPL activity affect sex and regional differences in adiposity. There have been some studies in this area. Two investigations have compared subcutaneous fat deposits of moderately obese women and found higher activities of LPL in the gluteal and femoral regions than in the abdominal or triceps region in parallel to the cell size differences (Bosello et al. 1984; Lithell et al. 1978). Similar results have been observed recently in lean women (Rebuffé-Scrive et al. 1985), and a study of morbidly obese men and women also found that fat cell size and LPL activity were higher in the femoral region than in abdominal and gluteal subcutaneous deposits in women, with men showing less marked regional variations (Fried et al. 1987). Other studies have reported higher adipose tissue LPL activity in the gluteal region of females compared to males (Björntorp et al. 1975; Taskinen et al. 1980, 1981); however, none of these latter investigations considered regional differences in LPL activity between the sexes.

The role of estrogens in mediating the interplay between lipolysis and lipogenesis as related to regional differences in adipocyte metabolism is illustrated by differences which occur with alterations of reproductive status.

There have been several investigations of regional adipose tissue metabolism in women which have controlled reproductive status. In both pregnant and nonpregnant women, lipid assimilation was favoured in the femoral depot over the abdominal depot due to elevated LPL activity in the femoral depot, and lipolysis was significantly less in the femoral region (Rebuffé-Scrive et al. 1985). These results are in keeping with previous results reported for nonpregnant women. However, during lactation and late pregnancy, basal lipolysis increased significantly in the femoral region, and LPL activity decreased significantly (Rebuffé-Scrive et al. 1985; Smith 1985). There was, in fact, no difference between the lipolytic rate of the abdominal and femoral regions during lactation, and the decreased femoral LPL activity acted synergistically to increase lipid mobilization from this depot considerably during lactation (Rebuffé-Scrive et al. 1985). Thus, the previous pattern favoring triglyceride accumulation in the femoral adipocytes in nonpregnant and pregnant women becomes changed so that this depot can be effectively utilized. It is therefore possible that femoral adipose tissue may serve as an important source of energy supply during lactation. This possibility is supported by the characteristic preponderance of the femoral fat depots in women and by the contrasting fact that men usually only have a small femoral fat depot (Krotkiewski et al. 1983; Sjöström et al. 1972).

While the foregoing discussion provides metabolic evidence for sex, age and regional differences in adipose tissue distribution, it does not openly indicate the role of the sex hormones. The characteristic metabolic features of the femoral region might be due to either inherent characteristics of the adipocytes in this region, or to the specific effects of female sex hormones in this region, or both. A study of femoral, mammary and abdominal adipocyte metabolism in pre and post menopausal women provides a clearer look at the role of the female sex hormones. In premenopausal women femoral adipocytes were characterized by a higher LPL activity than abdominal or mammary adipocytes, while lipolytic responsiveness and sensitivity in the latter two was higher than in femoral tissue (Rebuffé-Scrive et al. 1986). In postmenopausal women no differences were found among the three regions; consequently, menopause seems to be associated with a decrease of not only the elevated LPL activity of femoral adipocytes, but also the high lipolytic response in abdominal and mammary adipose tissue (Rebuffé-Scrive et al. 1986). It appears, therefore, that female sex hormones increase LPL activity in femoral adipocytes, causing them to become enlarged, and also stimulate lipolysis in abdominal and mammary adipocytes. These results, summarised in Table 2, support the

Table 2. Relative Lipolytic Enzyme Activity and Relative Lipoprotein Lipase (LPL) Activity According to Adipocyte Region.

Relative Lipolytic Enzyme Activity According to Adipocyte Region

Region	Pre-menopause	Pregnancy	Lactation	Post-menopause	Men
Abdominal	normal	normal	normal	high	high
Gluteo-femoral	low	low	high	normal	normal

Relative Lipoprotein Lipase Activity According to Adipocyte Region

Region	Pre-menopause	Pregnancy	Lactation	Post-menopause	Men
Abdominal	normal	normal	normal	normal	normal
Gluteo-femoral	high	high	low	low	low

hypothesis that the secondary sex characteristics of female adipose tissue distribution might be caused by regionally specific effects of sex steroid hormones on adipocyte metabolism (Rebuffé-Scrive et al. 1986).

Evidence of the direct role of the sex hormones in regional fat cell metabolism is provided by a study of middle-aged men and postmenopausal women who underwent sex hormone treatment. Before hormone treatment both fat cell size and LPL activity were found to be similar in subcutaneous abdominal and femoral regions in postmenopausal women (Rebuffé-Scrive et al. 1987), and this clearly differs from the previously noted characteristics of young women. The difference appears to be due to hormonal status, because estrogen and progestin administration to the postmenopausal women significantly enhanced femoral, but not abdominal, adipocyte LPL activity (Rebuffé-Scrive et al. 1987) The role of female sex hormones in lipid accumulation and enlargement of the femoral depot is further illustrated by the observation that estrogen administration to males with prostate carcinoma leads to an enlargement of both the femoral cells (Krotkiewski et al. 1978) and gluteal fat cells (Bani-Sacchi et al. 1987). Treatment of the middle-aged men with testosterone increased basal lipolysis in the abdominal cells, suggesting a potential regulatory role of male sex hormones on abdominal adipocyte lipolysis; no effect on lipolysis in postmenopausal women was noted with female sex hormone treatment (Rebuffé-Scrive et al. 1987).

There thus appears to be considerable evidence for the influence of the sex steroids in establishing sex and age dependent variations in regional adipocyte metabolism. In particular, it appears that LPL is regulated by the sex hormones, especially in the femoral region. Female sex hormones increase, while testosterone seems to inhibit, LPL activity (Rebuffé-Scrive et al. 1985). Obviously, this evidence represents the metabolic consequences of the binding of respective hormones to their specific receptor; regional differences in the number and/or affinity of adipocyte steroid receptors could explain regional differences in adipocyte response.

6 Estrogens and Adipogenesis

While genetic susceptibility cannot be discounted in human variation of fat distribution, a recent investigation has found, after statistical control for age, gender and total amount of subcutaneous fat, an additive genetic effect of about 20-25% of remaining human variance in amount of lower trunk fat and in the relative proportion of lower trunk versus extremity fat (Bouchard 1988). Undoubtedly, characteristics of regional adipose tissue metabolism are involved in mediating these genetic effects, as well as the sex hormones, but other regulatory mechanisms are probably implicated. Indeed, ever since the finding that 17ß-estradiol stimulated replication of human omental adipocytes in culture (Roncari et al. 1978), investigations

30

have been undertaken into the mechanism mediating this effect and the significance of this observation *in vivo*.

Various studies *in vitro* have established the fact that mammals, including adult humans, possess adipocyte precursors capable of replication and complete differentiation into mature fat cells (Roncari et al. 1978; Van et al. 1976; Van et al. 1977; Van et al. 1978). That these progenitor cells also multiply and mature *in vivo* has been confirmed (Klyde et al. 1979), indicating that cultured adipocyte precursors may reflect, at least to a certain extent, events that occur in intact organisms endowed with adipose tissue. This is important in view of the fact that the regional distribution of depot fat is regulated not only by the amount of triglyceride in each adipocyte (governed by metabolism) but also by the number of adipocytes with the capacity to store triglyceride. Thus, the effect of sex hormones on the regulatory steps of formation of new, differentiated adipocytes (adipogenesis) is of considerable interest.

Because it was believed that mature adipocytes do not multiply, most studies of the effect of sex hormones on adipocyte differentiation have been performed on adipose precursor cells which are known to divide, differentiate, and fill with lipid to become mature adipocytes. An investigation of adipose precursor cells in primary culture obtained from ovariectomized female rats and immature male rats suggested that new fat cells were formed by stimulation of differentiation of the adipose precursor cells by administration of both 17ß-estradiol and progesterone (Xu et al. 1987). It was therefore concluded that the sex steroid hormones might be partially responsible for the regulation of adipose tissue storage capacity by increasing the number of adipocytes by inducing differentiation of adipose precursor cells (Xu et al. 1987).

In order to account for some of the changes which occur in certain adipose tissue regions at puberty, the effects of 17ß-estradiol and androgens (testosterone and dihydrotestosterone) were studied on adipocyte precursors in culture, isolated from human omental fat tissue from non-obese male and female adults aged 20-60 years (Roncari et al., 1981). Addition of 17ß-estradiol significantly enhanced replication of the adipocyte precursors while, in contrast, androgens were found not to influence the precursors; it was concluded that these events support the hypothesis that the pubertal increment in the number of fat cells in certain adipose depots of women may be consequent to the stimulation of precursor replication by estrogens (rather than by androgen inhibition in men) (Roncari et al. 1981).

In genetically susceptible humans, a higher prevalence of obesity may be partially due to higher circulating levels of estrogens, promoting the production of mitogenic proteins; obesity and pregnancy are both associated with high levels of circulating estrogens, and therefore may represent particularly vulnerable periods (Cooper et al. 1989). It would appear that once begun, regional adipocyte hyperplasia or obesity in general may not be retractable due to increased numbers of adipocytes, as well as increased levels of local sex steroids produced by these additional adipocytes via peripheral aromatization.

7 Implications and Speculations

The central role of androgen/estrogen balance in both adiposity and adipose tissue distribution still requires further clarification, in particular the relationship between fatness and both timing and level of sex hormones throughout the full pubertal phase. Nonetheless, an understanding of the hormonal basis of body composition should prove invaluable in any attempts to change the amounts of fat, muscle or bone in the body. The degree of androgen/estrogen balance can be seen in many physiques, as a review of some of Sheldon's adult male somatotype subjects readily reveals (Sheldon 1954). Beginning first with the extreme endomorphs, we can separate two groups: those with little muscle and those with a moderate amount of muscle (there are no extreme endomorphs who are also highly mesomorphic). It is immediately clear that the fat distribution of the mesopenes is more gynoid. Of the 7-1-2 somatotype (Fig. 4, top), Sheldon notes that: "This is a female somatotype in the sense that it occurs more often, certainly five times as often, in women as in men." In addition many of these men show noticeable breast development, as in the 7-2-2 somatotype (Figure 4, bottom) of which Sheldon notes : "These are men who have invaded female territory." He also points out that they are often hypogenital. This spectrum of characteristics suggests estrogen dominance. The physique is reminiscent of some boys in early puberty, before the growth spurt, who pass through a brief phase of increased fatness and also display gynecomastia, shown to be related to transient increases in estrogen production. The gynoid men are generally low in another android index, the bi-acromial to bi-iliac breadth ratio (AIR). In the subjects with greater mesomorphy, the hips are narrower, the shoulders broader and the fat is seen more in the abdominal region. When high mesomorphy is accompanied by low endomorphy (Fig. 5), the bi-acromial to bi-iliac breadth ratio is at a maximum.

Since these bony dimensions are fixed by the end of the growth period, it may be possible to explain a significant part of some adult physiques on the basis of pubertal androgen/estrogen balance and timing. Thus the gynoid pattern in a young adult, either male or female, may reflect estrogenic predominance throughout adolescence, or perhaps only for some critical period during adolescence. Similarly, high levels of mesomorphy in young men may be associated with androgen dominance in puberty. Perhaps the genetic component of physique and body

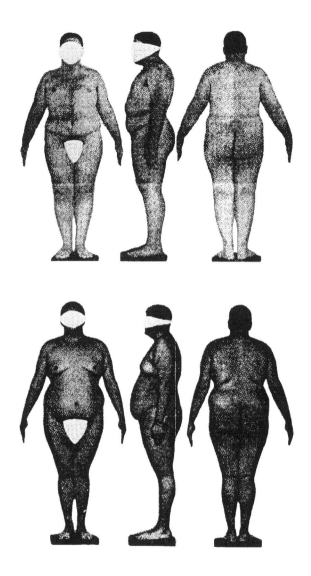

Fig. 4. Extreme endomorphy: the 7-1-2 somatotype (top) and the 7-2-2 somatotype (bottom), (Sheldon 1954).

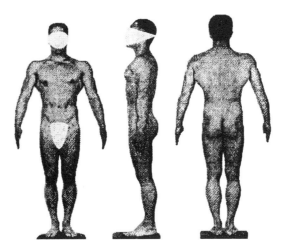

Fig. 5. Extreme mesomorphy; the 1-7-1 somatotype, (Sheldon 1954).

composition is expressed through androgen/estrogen balance in adolescence.

While it is generally believed that physical activity and caloric intake are the fundamental factors affecting fatness and muscularity, a variety of environmental factors affect the androgen/estrogen balance and therefore have the potential to alter body composition indirectly. In no particular order these are physical activity, parity, obesity, oral contraceptive use, alcohol consumption, diet (especially fat intake) and smoking. For example, evidence shows that smoking has an anti-estrogenic effect in women (Baron 1984; Hartz et al. 1987; Michnovicz et al. 1988) and smoking is associated with high WHR in men and women (Cox 1989; Haffner et al. 1986; Shimokata et al. 1989; Tonkelaar et al. 1989). As yet, no one has investigated whether serum estradiol is lower in smokers, which might be expected.

Looking at body composition from an endocrine perspective gives rise to other interesting questions. If gluteo-femoral fat is more labile in the hormonal milieu of lactation, what happens to fat patterning in women who do not nurse their infants? Do they become more gynoid? While exercise programs do not appear to induce changes in fat *patterning* in women (Després et al. 1988), what is the effect of exercise during lactation? Intense training in women is known to induce a hypothalamic amenorrhea that is associated with reduced levels of estradiol (Baker et al. 1988; Highet 1989). Such women are almost invariably very lean, but do they also undergo a shift in fat patterning away from the gynoid shape? One effect of beginning intense training before puberty is to delay menarche, perhaps by delaying the early pubertal rise of estrogen. Does this have an effect on fat patterning, and therefore health risk, over the short or long term? To resolve questions such as these and to reach a more complete understanding of why people have particular proportions of adipose tissue, muscle and bone, body composition researchers are encouraged to include hormonal assays in their measurement protocol where feasible and to make careful note of relevant environmental factors.

8 References

Arner, P. Engfedt, P. and Lithel, H. (1981) Site differences in the basal metabolism of subcutaneous fat in obese women. **J. Clin. Endocrinol. Metab.**, 53, 948-952.

Ashwell, M. Chinn, S. Stalley, S. and Garrow, J.S. (1978) Female fat distribution - a photographic and cellularity study. **Int. J. Obes.**, 2, 289-302.

Ashwell, M. Cole, T.J. and Dixon A.K. (1985) Obesity: new insight into the anthropometric classification of fat distribution shown by computed tomography. **Br. Med. J.**, 290, 1692-1694.

Baker, E. and Demers, L. (1988) Menstrual status in female athletes: correlation with reproductive hormones and bone density. **Obstet. Gynecol.**, 72 (5), 683-687.

Bani-Sacchi, T. Bianchi, S. Bani, G. and Bigazzi, M. (1987) Ultrastructural studies on white adipocyte differentiation in the mouse mammary gland following estrogen and relaxin. **Acta Anat.**, 129, 1-9.

Baron, J. A. (1984) Smoking and estrogen-related disease. **Am. J. Epidemiol.** 119 (1), 9-22.

Baumgartner, R.N. Roche, A.F. Chumlea, W.C. Siervogel, R.M. and Gluek, C.J. (1987) Fatness and fat patterns: associations with plasma lipids and blood pressures in adults, 18 to 57 years of age. **Am. J. Epidemiol.** 126, 614-629.

Baumgartner, R. N. Roche, A.F. Guo, S. Lohman, T. Boileau, R.A. and Slaughter, M. H. (1986) Adipose tissue distribution: the stability of principal components by sex, ethnicity and maturation stage. **Hum. Biol.**, 58(5), 719-735.

Björntorp, P. Enzi, G. Ohlson, R. Persson, B. Spongberg, P. and Smith, U. (1975) Lipoprotein lipase activity and uptake of exogenous triglycerides in fat cells of different size. **Horm. Metab. Res.**, 7, 230-237.

Bolinder, J. Kager, L. and Oestman, J. (1983) Differences at the receptor and postreceptor levels between human omental and subcutaneous adipose tissue in the action of insulin on lipolysis. **Diabetes**, 32, 117-123.

Bosello, O. Cigolini, M. Battaggia, A. Ferrari, F. Micciolo, R. Olivetti, R. and Corsato, M. (1984) Adipose tissue lipoprotein lipase in obesity. **Int. J. Obes.**, 8, 213.

Bouchard, C. (1988) Genetic factors in the regulation of adipose tissue distribution. **Acta Med. Scand.,** 723, 135-141.

Cooper, S.C. and Roncari, D.A.K. (1989) 17-beta-estradiol increases mitogenic activity of medium from cultured preadipocytes of massively obese persons. **J. Clin. Invest.,** 83, 1925-1929.

Cox, B. D. (1989) The relationship of smoking habits to waist/hip ratio in the Health and Lifestyle Survey (abstract) **Int. J. Obes.,** 13 (Suppl 1), 80.

Dark, J. Wade, G. N. and Zucker, I. (1984) Ovarian modulation of lipoprotein lipase activity in white adipose tissue of ground squirrels. **Physiol. Behav.,** 32, 75-78.

Després, J.-P. Tremblay, A. Nadeau, A. and Bouchard, C. (1988) Physical training and changes in regional adipose tissue distribution. **Acta Med. Scand.,** 723 (Suppl), 205-212.

Enriori, C. L. and Reforzo-Membrives, J. (1984) Peripheral aromatization as a risk factor for breast and endometrial cancer in post-menopausal women: a review. **Gynecol. Oncol.,** 17, 1-21.

Evans, D.J. Barth, J.H. and Burke, C.W. (1988) Body fat topography in women with androgen excess. **Int. J. Obes.,** 12, 157-162.

Evans, D.J. Hoffman, R.G. Kalkhoff, R.K. and Kissebah, A.H. (1983) Relationship of androgenic activity to body fat topography, fat cell morphology, and metabolic aberrations in premenopausal women. **J. Clin. Endocrinol. Metab.,** 57(2), 304-310.

Fried, S.K. and Kral, J.G. (1987) Sex differences in regional distribution of fat cell size and lipoprotein lipase activity in morbidly obese patients. **Int. J. Obes.,** 11, 129-140.

Frisancho, A.R. and Flegel, P.N. (1982) Advanced maturation associated with centripetal fat pattern. **Hum. Biol.,** 54(4), 717-727.

Frisch, R.E. (1976) Fatness of girls from menarche to age 18 years with a nomogram. **Hum. Biol.,** 48, 353-359.

Frisch, R.E. and McArthur, J.W. (1974) Menstrual cycles: fatness as a determinant of weight for height necessary for their maintenance and onset. **Science,** 185, 949-956.

Garn, S.M. (1986) Family-line and socioeconomic factors in fatness and obesity. **Nutr. Rev.,** 44(12), 381-386.

Garn, S.M. and Haskell, J.A. (1959) Fat and growth during childhood. **Science,** 130, 1710-1711.

Garn, S.M. LaVelle M. and Pilkington, J.J. (1983) Comparisons of fatness in premenarcheal and postmenarcheal girls of the same age. **J. Pediatrics,** 103, 328-331.

Garn, S.M. LaVelle, M. Rosenberg, K.R. and Hawthorne, V.M. (1986) Maturational timing as a factor in female fatness and obesity. **Am J. Clin. Nutr.,** 43, 879-883.

Grauer, W.O. Moss, A.A. Cann, C.E. and Goldberg, H.I. (1984) Quantification of body fat distribution in the abdomen using computed tomography. **Am. J. Clin. Nutr.,** 39, 631-637.

Gray, J.M. Nunez, A.A. Siegel, I. and Wade, G.N. (1979) Effects of testosterone on body weight and adipose tissue: role of aromatization. **Physiol. Behav.,** 23, 465-469.

Gray, J. M. and Wade, G. N. (1980) Cytoplasmic estrogen but not progestin binding sites in male rat adipose tissue. **Am. J. Physiol.,** 239, E237-E241.

Gray, J. M. and Wade, G. N. (1981) Food intake, body weight, and adiposity in female rats: actions and interactions of progestins and antiestrogens. **Am. J. Physiol.,** 240, E474-E481.

Greenblatt, R.B. Colle, M.L. and Mahesh, V.B. (1976) Ovarian and adrenal steroid production in the postmenopausal woman. **Obstet. Gynecol.,** 47(4), 383-387.

Haffner, S.M. Stern, M.P. Hazuda, H.P. Pugh, J., Patterson, J.K. and Malina, R. (1986) Upper body and centralized adiposity in Mexican Americans and non-Hispanic whites: relationship to body mass index and other behavioral and demographic variables. **Int. J. Obes.,** 10(6), 493-502.

Hamosh, M. and Hamosh, P. (1975) The effect of estrogen on the lipoprotein lipase activity in rat adipose tissue. **J. Clin. Invest.,** 55, 1132-1135.

Harsha, D.W. Voors, A.W. and Berenson, G.S. (1980) Racial differences in subcutaneous fat patterns in children aged 7-15 years. **Am. J. Phys. Anthrop.,** 53: 333-337.

Hartz, A.J. Kelber, S. Borkowf, H. Wild, R., Gillis, B.L. and Rimm, A.A. (1987) The association of smoking with clinical indicators of altered sex steroids - a study of 50,145 women. **Pub. Health Rep.,** 102(3), 254-259.

Highet, R. (1989) Athletic amenorrhea. An update on aetiology, complications and management. **Sport Med.,** 7(2), 82-108.

Jensen, J. Christiansen, C. and Rodbro, P. (1986) Oestrogen-progestogen replacement therapy changes body composition in early post-menopausal women. **Maturitas** , 8, 209-216.

Jensen, J. Riis, B.J. Hummer, L. and Christiansen, C. (1985) The effects of age and body composition on circulating serum oestrogens and androstenedione after the menopause. **Br. J. Obstet. Gynaecol.,** 92(3), 260-265.

Judd, H.L. Judd, G.E. Lucas, W.E. and Yen, S.S.C. (1974) Endocrine function of the post-menopausal ovary: Concentrations of androgens and estrogens in ovarian and peripheral vein blood. **J. Clin. Endocrinol. Metab.,** 39, 1020-1024.

Kather, H. Zöllig, K. Simon, B. and Schlierf, G. (1977) Human fat cell adenylate cyclase: regional differences in adrenaline responsiveness. **Eur. J. Clin. Invest.,** 7, 595-597.

Kirschner, M.A. Ertel, N. and Schneider, G. (1981) Obesity, hormones, and cancer. **Cancer Res.,** 41, 3711-3717.

Kissebah, A.H. Vydelingum, N. Murray, R.W. Evans, D.J. Hartz, A.J. Kalkhoff, R.K. and Adams, P.W. (1982) Relation of body fat distribution to metabolic complications of obesity. **J. Clin. Endocrinol. Metab.,** 54, 254-260.

Klyde, B.J. and Hirsch, J. (1979) Isotopic labelling of DNA in rat adipose tissue: evidence for proliferating cells associated with mature adipocytes. **J. Lipid. Res.,** 20, 691-704.

Krakower, G.R. James, R.G. Arnaud, C. Etienne, J. Keller, R. H. and Kissebah, A. H. (1988) Regional adipocyte precursors in the female rat: influence of ovarian factors. **J. Clin. Invest.,** 81, 641-648.

Krotkiewski, M. and Björntorp, P. (1978) The effects of estrogen treatment of carcinoma of the prostate on regional adipocyte size. **J. Endocrinol. Invest.,** 1(4), 365-366.

Krotkiewski, M. Björntorp, P. Sjöstrom, L. and Smith, U. (1983) Impact of obesity on metabolism in men and women: importance of regional adipose tissue distribution. **J. Clin. Invest.,** 72, 1150-1162.

Lafontan, M. Dang-Tran, L. and Berlan, M. (1979) Alpha-adrenergic antilipolytic effect of adrenaline in human fat cells of the thigh: comparison with adrenaline responsivenes of different fat deposits. **Eur. J. Clin. Invest.,** 9, 261-266.

Lafontan, M. Mauriege, P. Galitzky, J. and Berlan, M. (1985) Adrenergic regulation of regional adipocyte metabolism, in **Metabolic Complications of Human Obesities** (eds J. Vague, P. Björntorp, B. Guy-Grand, M. Rebuffé-Scrive and P. Vague), Excerpta Medica, Amsterdam, pp. 161-172.

Lanska, D.J. Lanska, M.J. Hartz, A.J. Kalkhoff, R.K. Rupley, D. and Rimm, A.A. (1985) A prospective study of body fat distribution and weight loss. **Int. J. Obes.,** 9, 241-246.

Lithell, H. and Boberg, L. (1978) Lipoprotein lipase activity of adipose tissue from different sites in obese women and relationship to cell size. **Int. J. Obes.,** 2, 47-52.

MacDonald, P.C. Edman, C.D. Hemsell, D.L. Porter, J.C. and Siiteri, P.K. (1978) The effect of obesity on conversion of androstenedione to estrone in postmenopausal women with and without endometrial cancer. **Am. J. Obstet. Gynecol.,** 130(107), 448-455.

MacMahon, B. Trichopoulos, D. Brown, J. Anderson, A.P. Cole, P. DeWard, F. Kauraniemi, T. Polychronopoulou, A. Ravnihar, B. Stormby, N. and Westlund, K. (1982) Age at menarche, urine estrogens and breast cancer risk. **Int. J. Cancer.,** 30, 427-431.

Michnovicz, J.J. Naganuma, H. Herschcopf, R.J. Bradlow, H.L. and Fishman, J. (1988) Increased urinary catechol estrogen excretion in female smokers. **Steroids,** 52(1-2), 69-83.

Mueller, W. H. (1982) The changes with age of the anatomical distribution of fat. **Soc. Sci. Med.,** 16, 191-196.

Pasquier, Y.N. Pecquery, R. and Giudicelli, Y. (1988) Increased adenylate cyclase activity explains how estrogens 'in vivo' promote lipolytic activity in rat white fat cells. **Biochem. Biophys. Res. Commun.,** 154(3), 1151-1159.

Per-Henrick, I. and Brunzell, J.D. (1988) Relationship between lipoprotein lipase activity and plasma sex steroid levels in obese women. **J. Clin. Invest.**, 82, 1106-1112.

Poissonnet, C.M. Burdi, A.R. and Garn, S.M. (1984) The chronology of adipose tissue appearance and distribution in the human fetus. **Early Hum. Dev.**, 10, 1-11.

Prior, J.C. Vigna, Y.M. and Watson, D. (1989) Spironolactone with physiological female steroids for presurgical therapy of male-to-female transsexualism. **Arch. Sex Behav.**, 18(1), 49-57.

Rebuffé-Scrive, M. and Björntorp, P. (1985) Regional adipose tissue metabolism in man, in **Metabolic Complications of Human Obesities**. (eds J. Vague, P. Björntorp, B. Guy-Grand, M. Rebuffé-Scrive and P. Vague), Excerpta Medica, Amsterdam, pp. 149-159.

Rebuffé-Scrive, M. Eldh, J. Hafström, L.-O. and Björntorp, P. (1986) Metabolism of mammary, abdominal, and femoral adipocytes in women before and after menopause. **Metabolism** , 35(9), 792-797.

Rebuffé-Scrive, M. Enk, L. Crona, N. Lönnroth, P. Abrahamsson, L. Smith, U. and Björntorp, P. (1985) Fat cell metabolism in different regions in women. **J. Clin. Invest.**, 75, 1973-1976.

Rebuffé-Scrive, M. Lönnroth, P. Mårin, P. Wesslau, C. Björntorp, P. and Smith, U. (1987) Regional adipose tissue metabolism in men and postmenopausal women. **Int. J. Obes.**, 11, 347-355.

Rice, P. L. (1988) Relationship of estrogen to strength, percent body fat and oxygen uptake in women. **J Sports Med. Phys. Fit.**, 28, 145-150.

Rolland-Cachera, M. F. Bellisle, F. and Sempé, M. (1989) Development and prediction of body fat distribution (abstract). **Int. J. Obes.**, 13 (Suppl.1), 76.

Roncari, D.A.K. Lau, D.C.W. and Kindler, S. (1981) Exaggerated replication in culture of adipocyte precursors from massively obese persons. **Metabolism**, 30, 425-427.

Roncari, D.A.K. and Van, R.L.R. (1978) Adipose tissue cellularity and obesity: new perspectives. **Clin. Invest. Med.**, 1, 71-79.

Roncari, D.A.K. and Van, R.L.R. (1978) Promotion of human adipocyte precursor replication by 17-beta-estradiol in culture. **J. Clin. Invest.**, 62, 503-508.

Ross, W.D. and Marfell-Jones, M.J. (1982) Kinanthropometry, in **Physiological Testing of the Elite Athlete** (eds S. D. McDougall, M. A. Wenger and H. A. Green), Mutual., Ottawa, pp. 75-115.

Samoljik, E. Santen, R.J. and Wells, S.A. (1977) Adrenal suppression with aminoglutethimide. II. Differential effects of aminoglutethimide on plasma androstenedione and estrogen levels. **J. Clin. Endocrinol. Metab.**, 45, 480-487.

Santen, R.J. Friend, J.N. Trojanowski, D. Davis, B. Samoljik, E. and Wayne, B. C. (1978) Prolonged negative feedback suppression after estradiol administration: Proposed mechanism of eugonadal secondary amenorrhea. **J. Clin. Endocrinol. Metab.**, 47, 1220-1229.

Seidell, J.C. Tonkelaar, D.I. van Noord, P.A.H. and Baanders-van Halewijn, E.A. (1989) Obesity and fat distribution in 11,653 Dutch women - effects of smoking, oestrogen use, parity and age of menarche (abstract). **Int. J. Obes.,** 13 (Suppl 1), 69.

Sheldon, W.S. (1954) **Atlas of Men.** Gramercy Publishing, New York, pp. 357.

Shimokata, H. Muller, D.C. and Andres, R. (1989) Studies in the distribution of body fat. III. Effects of cigarette smoking. **J. Am. Med. Assoc.,** 261(8), 1169-1173.

Sjöström, L. Smith, U. Krotkiewski, M. and Björntorp, P. (1972) Cellularity in different regions of adipose tissue in young men and women. **Metab. Clin. Exp.,** 21, 1143-1153.

Smith, U. (1985) Regional differences in adipocyte metabolism and possible consequences in vivo, in **Recent Advances in Obesity Research IV.** (eds J. Hirsch and T.B. Van Itallie), Libbey, London, pp. 33-36.

Smith, U. Hammersten, J. Björntorp, P. and Kral, J.G. (1979) Regional differences and effect of weight reduction on human fat cell metabolism. **Eur. J. Clin. Invest.,** 9, 327-332.

Sparrow, D. Bosse, R. and Rowe, J. W. (1980) The influence of age, alcohol consumption and body build on gonadal function in men. **J. Clin. Endocrinol. Metab.,** 51, 508-517.

Steingrimsdottir, L. Brasel, J. and Greenwood, M.R.C. (1980) Hormonal modulation of adipose tissue lipoprotein lipase may alter food intake in rats. **Am. J. Physiol.,** 239, E162-E167.

Tanner, J.M. (1978) **Foetus into Man: Physical Growth from Conception to Maturity.,** Harvard University Press, Cambridge.

Taskinen, M.R. and Nikkilä, E. (1981) Lipoprotein lipase of adipose tissue and skeletal muscle in human obesity: response to glucose and semi-starvation. **Metabolism,** 30, 801-817.

Taskinen, M.R. Nikkilä, E.A. Huttunen, J. K. and Hilden, H. (1980) A micromethod for assay of lipoprotein lipase in needle biopsy samples of human adipose tissue and skeletal muscle. **Clin. Chim. Acta** , 104, 107-117.

Tomita, T. Yonekura, I. Okada, T. and Hayashi, E. (1984) Enhancement of cholesterol-esterase activity and lipolysis due to 17ß-estradiol treatment in rat adipose tissue. **Horm. Metab. Res.,** 16, 525-528.

Tonkelaar, I.D. Seidell, J.C. van Noord, P.A.H. Baanders-van Halewijn, E. A. Jacobus, J. H. and Bruning, P. F. (1989) Factors influencing waist/hip ratio in randomly selected pre- and post-menopausal women in the Dom - Project (Preliminary Results). **Int. J. Obes.,** 13(6), 817-824.

Vague, J. (1956) The degree of masculine differentiation of obesities. **Am. J. Clin. Nutr.,** 4(1), 20-34.

Vague, J. Meignen, J.M. and Negrin, J.F. (1984) Effects of testosterone and estrogens on detoid and trochanter adipocytes in two cases of transsexualism. **Horm. Metabol. Res.,** 16, 380-381.

Vague, J. Rubin, P. Jubelin, J. Lam-Van, G. Aubert, F. Wasserman, A. M. and Fondari, J. (1974) Regulation of the adipose tissue mass: histometric and anthropometric aspects, in **The Regulation of the Adipose Tissue Mass** (eds J. Vague and J. Bayer), Excerpta Medica, Amsterdam, pp. 296.

Van, R.L.R. Bayliss, C.E. and Roncari, D.A.K. (1976) Cytological and enzymological characterization of adult human adipocyte precursors in culture. **J. Clin. Invest.,** 58, 699-704.

Van, R.L.R. and Roncari, D.A.K. (1977) Isolation of fat cell precursors from adult rat adipose tissue. **Cell. Tiss. Res.,** 181, 197-203.

Van, R.L.R. and Roncari, D.A.K. (1978) Complete differentiation of adipocyte precursors. A culture system for studying the cellular nature of adipose tissue. **Cell. Tiss. Res.,** 195, 318-329.

Vansant, G. Den Besten, D. Weststrate, J. and Deurenberg, P. (1988) Body fat distribution and the prognosis for weight reduction: preliminary observations. **Int. J. Obes.,** 12, 133-140.

Vermeulen, A. and Verdonck, L. (1978) Sex hormone concentrations in post-menopausal women. **Clin. Endocrinol.,** 9, 59-66.

Vermeulen, A. and Verdonck, L. (1979) Factors affecting sex hormone levels in postmenopausal women. **J. Steroid. Bioch.,** 11, 899-904.

Wade, G.N. and Gray, J.M. (1978) Cytoplasmic 17ß-[^{3}H]Estradiol binding in rat adipose tissues. **Endocrinology,** 103(5), 1695-1701.

Wade, G.N. Gray, J.M. and Bartness, T.J. (1985) Gonadal influences on adiposity. **Int. J. Obes.,** 9 (Suppl.1), 83-92.

Wilson, D.E. Flowers, C.M. Carlile, S.I. and Udal, K.S. (1976) Estrogenic treatment and gonadal function in the regulation of lipoprotein lipase. **Atherosclerosis,** 24, 491-499.

Xu, X. and Björntorp, P. (1987) Effects of sex steroid hormones on differentiation of adipose tissue precursor cells in primary culture. **Exp. Cell. Res.,** 173, 311-321.

2

MINERAL AND WATER CONTENTS OF THE FAT FREE BODY : EFFECT OF THE GENDER, ACTIVITY LEVEL, AGE AND MATURATION

M.H. SLAUGHTER, C.B. CHRIST, R.A. BOILEAU, R.J. STILLMAN and
T.G. LOHMAN
Dept. of Kinesiology, University of Illinois at Urbana-Champaign, USA

Keywords : Body composition, Bone mineral content, Fat-free body.

1 Introduction

The effect of exercise conditioning and physical training on body composition in the pediatric population has been studied in recent years by Malina (1978, 1983, 1984) Bailey (1985), Borms (1986), Hebbelinck, Bouchard and Malina (1983) and Parizkova (1973). Their findings suggest that exercise does play a role in body weight control and body composition modification. Furthermore, children who engage in sports programs and have a chronic history of such activity appear to be leaner and develop fat-free body at a greater rate than expected from normal growth patterns.

Research has been hindered by the lack of control groups, insensitive body composition techniques and a disregard for changes in body composition which take place during growth and development.

Our recent work on the development of a multicomponent equation for the estimation of body composition is more applicable to the pediatric population than the equation based on density or one component alone (Boileau et al. 1985). Using this equation, we are now able to have a better estimation of fat-free body and by actually measuring body water and bone mineral content, we are able to examine the effects of gender, activity level (AL), maturation level (ML), and age on the mineral (M/FFB) and water (W/FFB)contents of the FFB.

The hypotheses for the study were that W/FFB would decrease and M/FFB would increase across maturational levels for both males and females. Additional hypotheses were that the M/FFB would be greater in swimmers than non-swimmers and the W/FFB would be less in swimmers than their non-swimmers counterparts.

2 Methods

The 176 subjects in this study included three maturational groups of male and female swimmers and non-swimmers arranged in a 3 x 2 x 2 factorial

42

plan. There were 23 male swimmers, including 10 prepubescents, 9 pubescents, and 4 postpubescents; 73 male non-swimmers including 36 prepubescents, 25 pubescents, 12 postpubescents; 24 female swimmers including 4 prepubescents, 12 pubescents and 8 postpubescents; and 56 female non-swimmers including 10 prepubescents, 32 pubescents and 14 postpubescents.

The maturational level of the subjects was assessed by the Tanner Scale (1962) of pubertal stage developed to classify each subject as prepubescent (stages 1 and 2), pubescent (stage 3), postpubescent (stages 4 and 5) or adult (stage 6 and higher). The project was approved by both the University of Illinois and University of Arizona Institutional Review Boards, and a written informed consent was obtained for each subject and from the guardian of each minor child prior to participation. The study has been previously described (Slaughter et al. 1984; Boileau et al. 1984 and Lohman et al. 1984a).

Body density was measured by underwater weighing with the body volume estimate from underwater weight corrected for pulmonary residual volume (Boileau et al. 1981).

Body water was measured by deuterium oxide dilution using a modification of the method of Byers (1979) as described by Boileau et al. (1984). Bone mineral measurements were made on both the right and left radius and ulna using photon absorptiometry (Cameron and Sorenson 1963) with a Norland Cameron Bone Mineral Analyser as described by Lohman et al. (1984a). The mean of the two measurements was used as the representative value.

The equation used for prediction of percent body fat from density, water and bone was:

PFDWB = [(2.747/BD) - .727 (PWBWT) + 1.146 x MW- 2.053] x 100

where MW = Total body mineral (kg)/Body Weight (kg)

Total body Mineral = Mineral Content of FFB x Fat-Free Body Weight

Mineral Content of FFB = 2.1 x Radius Bone Mineral + 4.05

FFBDWB = Body Weight - (PFDWB x Body Weight)

PWBWT = Total Body Water (l)/ Body Weight (kg)

The derivation of the equation for estimating the mineral content of the fat-free body is discussed in Lohman et al. (1984), Boileau et al. (1985) and Lohman (1986). There is evidence that the estimates of bone mineral content in small cross-section of the radius and ulna by single photon absorptiometry give reliable estimates of total bone mineral content. The significant partial correlations between bone mineral content and body density, holding constant skinfolds, enabled Lohman and co-workers (1984) to develop a partial regression for the change in density as a function of the change in radius bone mineral content. For each 1 g/cm increase in radius bone mineral, body density increased by 0.0013 g/cc. To account for the increase in body density, the bone mineral content would increase 0.2 percent for each 0.1 g/cm increase in radius bone mineral. Bone mineral content was then estimated for prepubecent, pubescent, postpubescent and adult males and females.

3 Results

The age and physical characteristics in this sample are similar to those found in the literature of equivalent ages (Parizkova 1961a, 1961b, Boileau et al. 1981; Young et al. 1968) and for youth (Parizkova 1961a; Young et al. 1968; Katz and Michael 1969) (see Table 1).

The mean values for the radius measured at the distal third of the bone and total body water in liters are presented for each pubertal stage within sex and activity level group (see Table 2). The representative values for these two measures were similar to our previous work for the prepubescent and pubescent groups, but in the postpubescent groups, the bone mineral means were less while the water values were higher. The reason for this difference can be explained by the fact that the children in the postpubescent groups in this study were younger than those children who made up the postpubescent groups in our previous work.

The effect of gender, ML, AL and age on M/FFB and W/FFB were statistically determined utilizing least squares multiple regression analysis coding for gender, ML and AL with weighted orthogonal contrasts to account for sample size differences.

For the total sample, the analysis revealed a significant maturation effect (linear) on M/FFB indicating that the M/FFB of the pubescents was significantly less than that of the postpubescents. Although there were no significant differences in M/FFB between males and females, the gender x AL interaction approached significance, suggesting that there may be a differences between swimmers and non-swimmers, but the difference depends on whether the male or female is considered. Hence, a within gender analysis was employed to determine the effects of ML, age, and AL within the males and females separately (see Table 3 and Figures 1 & 2).

The maturation effect (linear) on the M/FFB observed in the analysis of the total sample was upheld in the within gender analysis separately, as it was significant ($p < .001$) in both male and female samples. However, there were no significant differences in M/FFB between male swimmers and non-swimmers. In fact, within the male sample the independent variable of AL was the least significant of all the effects examined. The increase in M/FFB across maturation for the male swimmers was: .14 (2.7%) between prepubescent and pubescent groups, .28 (5.3%) between the pubescent and postpubescent groups, and .42 (8.1%) overall between the prepubescent and postpubescent groups. Similarly, the increase in M/FFB

Table 1. Age and Physical Characteristics of Swimmers and Non-Swimmers

		Age (yr)	Height (cm)	Weight (kg)	Fat-Free Body (kg)
Male Prepubescent	X	10.6	142.6	36.0	30.6
Swimmers (10)	SD	1.0	7.2	5.0	4.5
Male Pubescent	X	11.4	148.3	39.3	33.8
Swimmers (9)	SD	1.1	11.3	9.0	6.4
Male Postpubescent	X	13.5	164.0	51.4	44.6
Swimmers (4)	SD	0.3	6.2	4.6	5.7
Male Prepubescent	X	10.0	139.6	32.3	27.4
Non-Swimm. (36)	SD	1.1	6.9	4.2	3.5
Male Pubescent	X	12.0	151.8	40.9	34.3
Non-Swimm. (25)	SD	1.2	10.2	6.9	5.3
Male Postpubescent	X	13.5	164.5	53.4	43.9
Non-Swimm. (12)	SD	0.7	4.5	6.5	3.9
Female Prepubescent	X	11.6	144.4	36.2	30.8
Swimmers (4)	SD	1.4	6.0	2.0	1.0
Female Pubescent	X	12.3	152.4	44.1	35.2
Swimmers (12)	SD	0.9	7.1	6.3	5.3
Female Postpubesc.	X	13.2	161.9	51.2	43.2
Swimmers (8)	SD	1.6	6.0	6.2	6.2
Female Prepubescent	X	9.6	139.9	34.3	28.2
Non-Swimm. (10)	SD	1.1	7.8	4.7	3.3
Female Pubescent	X	11.5	149.5	40.2	32.2
Non-Swimm. (32)	SD	1.1	9.2	6.1	4.8
Female Postpubesc.	X	13.2	161.8	51.2	41.4
Non-Swimm. (14)	SD	0.9	7.2	7.5	5.1

Table 2. Mean and Standard Deviations of Bone Mineral Content and Total Body Water

	Bone Mineral Content (gm/cm)		Total Body Water (l)	
	X	SD	X	SD
Male Prepubescent Swimmers (10)	.538	.06	22.7	3.6
Male Pubescent Swimmers (9)	.605	.08	25.4	4.9
Male Postpubescent Swimmers (4)	.739	.11	33.3	5.2
Male Prepubescent Non-Swimm. (36)	.529	.07	20.6	3.1
Male Pubescent Non-Swimm. (25)	.615	.09	25.6	3.4
Male Postpubescent Non-Swimm. (12)	.752	.11	33.4	3.5
Female Prepubesc. Swimmers (4)	.595	.06	23.5	1.24
Female Pubescent Swimmers (12)	.637	.09	26.3	3.72
Female Postpubesc. Swimmers (8)	.716	.13	35.5	4.97
Female Pubescent Non-Swimm. (10)	.519	.06	21.2	2.55
Female Pubescent Non-Swimm. (32)	.585	.08	24.0	3.68
Female Postpubesc. Non-Swimm. (14)	.742	.08	30.8	4.12

Table 3. Adjusted Means of Bone Mineral Content in Grams Per Kilogram of Fat-Free Body of Swimmers and Non-Swimmers.

	N	Males	N	Females
Prepubescent Swimmers	10	5.18	4	5.14
Prepubescent Non-Swimmers	36	5.17	10	5.16
Pubescent Swimmers	9	5.32	12	5.41
Pubescent Non-Swimmers	25	5.35	32	5.30
Postpubescent Swimmers	4	5.60	8	5.58
Postpubescent Non-Swimmers	12	5.63	14	5.63

across maturation for the male non-swimmers was .18 (3.5%), .28 (5.4%) and .46 (8.9%), between the prepubescent and pubescent, pubescent and postpubescent, and prepubescent and postpubescent groups, respectively. Within the female sample, in addition to the linear effect of maturation, the effect of maturation (quadratic) was significant (p = . 002), indicating that the female pubescent group was not equally spaced between the prepubescent and postpubescent groups. Modified Newman-Keul's multiple-range tests accounting for disparate sample sizes revealed that for the non-swimmers the M/FFB of the postpubescent group was significantly greater than the pubescent but the pubescent was not greater

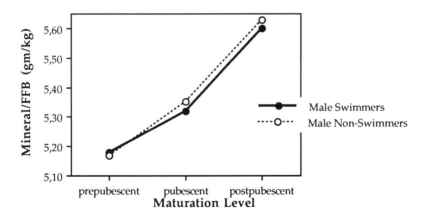

Fig. 1. Mineral Content of the Fat-Free body across Maturation Levels in Male Swimmers and Non-Swimmers.

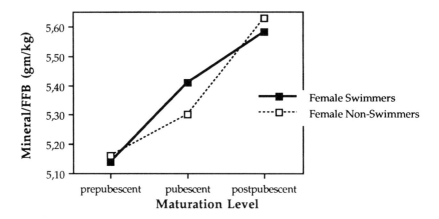

Fig. 2. Mineral Content of the Fat-Free body across Maturation Levels in Female Swimmers and Non-Swimmers.

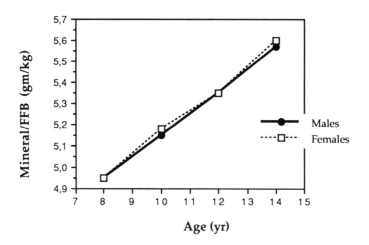

Fig. 3. Mineral Content of the Fat-Free body across Age in Swimmers and Non-Swimmers.
Regression equations:
Males: Y = .105419 (age) + 4.11; SEE = .16
Females   Y = .108521 (age) + 4.08; SEE = .16

than the prepubescent group. In the swimmers, the M/FFB of the postpubescent group was greater than that of the pubescent and the M/FFB of the pubescent group was greater than that of the prepubescent group. Furthermore, the post-hoc analysis revealed that within each ML there were no significant differences ($p < .05$) in M/FFB between the swimmers and non-swimmers; however, the mean difference between the pubescent groups approached significance ($p = .06$).

In the female swimmers, the increase in the M/FFB across maturation was: .27 (5.3%) between the prepubescents and pubescents, .17 (3.1%) between the pubescents and postpubescents, and .44 (8.6%) overall between the prepubescent and postpubescent groups. In the female non-swimmers, the increase in the M/FFB between the prepubescent and pubescent groups was only 1.4 (2.7%), half as great as their swimmers counterparts. However, the increase in M/FFB between the pubescent and postpubescent groups was twice as great for the non-swimmers .33 (6.2%) than the swimmers; hence, the overall increase across ML, between the prepubescent and postpubescent groups .47 (9.1%) was similar to that observed in the female swimmers sample.

When age, rather than maturation was used as an independent variable, it too was significant ($p < .001$) for both genders, indicating that the M/FFB increases with age as well as with maturation (see Fig. 3). Similar increases in M/FFB across age (from 8 to 15 years) were observed for both genders. The M/FFB of the males increased .74 (14.9%) from 4.95 to 5.69, while that of the females increased .76 (15.3%) from 4.95 to 5.71. Hence, the increase in M/FFB per year in males and females aged 8 to 15 years was 2.1% and 2.2%, respectively.

None of the effects of W/FFB examined in this study were significant for either males or females, suggesting that the within group variability of the W/FFB exceeded that between groups (see Table 4 and Figures 5 & 6 This result was surprising since in our previous work on a larger sample, W/FFB decreased 2.8% in children 8-18 years. In this sample there were no significant W/FFB differences observed across age.

In conclusion, the consideration of ML or age, and not gender or AL are important in body composition estimates that are affected by M/FFB. Limitations in studies that have compared athletes and non-athletes during childhood and adolescence have been documented (Malina 1984). Tenuous assumptions about the training regimes of the athletes (i.e., that they train regularly) may lead to false inferences and conclusions, namely, that the differences observed in the growth and development of athletes and non-athletes can be attributed to the training programs required for the specific sports. It may be that potential genetic, nutritional and lifestyle influences outweigh those typically attributed to training.

Table 4. Adjusted Means of the Total Water Content in Liters per Kilogram of Fat-Free body in Swimmers and Non-Swimmers.

	N	Males	N	Females
Prepubescent Swimmers	10	75.9	4	76.3
Prepubescent Non-Swimmers	36	75.5	10	75.3
Pubescent Swimmers	9	75.2	12	74.7
Pubescent Non-Swimmers	25	74.7	32	74.9
Postpubescent Swimmers	4	74.2	8	75.3
Postpubescent Non-Swimmers	12	75.8	14	74.1

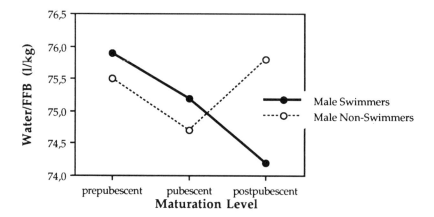

Fig. 4. Water Content of the Fat-Free body across Maturation Levels in Male Swimmers and Non-Swimmers.

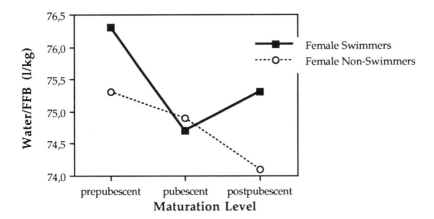

Fig. 5. Water Content of the Fat-Free body across Maturation Levels in Female Swimmers and Non-Swimmers.

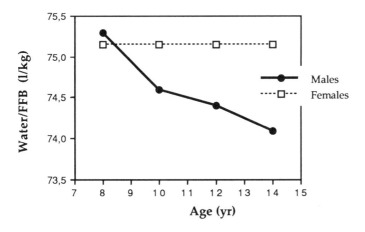

Fig. 6. Water Content of the Fat-Free body across Age in Swimmers and Non-Swimmers.
Regression equations:
Males: Y = (-.002157 (age) + .77) x 100; SEE = .03
Females   Y = (.000082 (age) + .751)x 100; SEE = .03

4 References

Bailey, D.A. Malina, R.M. and Mirwald, R.L. (1985) The child, physical activity and growth, in **Human Growth**, Vol. 2. (2nd ed), (ed F. Falkner and J.M. Tanner), Plenum Publ. Comp., New York, pp. 147-70.

Boileau, R.A. Lohman, T.G. Slaughter, M.H. Ball, T.E. Going, S.B. and Hendrix M.K. (1984) Hydration of the fat-free body in children during maturation. **Hum. Biol.** 56, 651-666.

Boileau, R.A. Wilmore, J.H. Lohman, T.G. Slaughter M.H. and Riner W.F. (1981) Estimation of body density from skinfold thicknesses, body circumferences and skeletal widths in boys aged 8 to 11 years: Comparison of two samples. **Hum. Biol.**, 58, 575-592.

Borms, J. (1986). The child and exercise: an overview. **J. Sport Sci.**, 4, 3-20.

Byers, F.M. (1979) Extraction and measurement of deuterium oxide at tracer levels in biological fluids. **Analytical Biochem.**, 98, 208-213.

Cameron, J.R. and Sorenson, J.A. (1963) Measurement of bone mineral in vivo: An improved method. **Sci.**, 140, 230-232.

Katch, F.I. and Michael, E.D. (1969) Prediction of body density form skinfold and girth measurements of college females. **J. Appl. Physiol.**, 26, 92-94.

Lohman, T.G. Slaughter, M.H. Boileau, R.A. Bunt, J.C. and Lussier, L. (1984) Bone mineral measurements and their relation to body density in children, youth and adults. **Hum. Biol.**, 56, 667-679.

Malina, R.M. (1978) Physical growth and maturity characteristics of young athletes, in **Children in Sports** (eds R.A. Magill, M.J. Ash and F.L. Smoll), Human Kinetics, Champaign, Illinois, pp. 79-101.

Malina, R.M. (1983) Menarche in athletes: a synthesis and hypothesis. **Ann. Hum. Biol.**, 10, 1-24.

Malina, R.M. (1984) Human growth, maturation, and regular physical activity, in **Advances in Paediatric Sport Sciences** (ed R.A. Boileau), Human Kinetics, Champaign, Ill., pp. 59-83.

Malina, R.M. Spirduso, W.W. Tate, C. and Baylor, A.M. (1978) Age at menarche and selected menstrual characteristics in athletes at different competitive levels and different sports. **Med. Sci. Sports**, 10, 218-222.

Parizkova, J. (1961a) Total body fat and skinfold thickness in children. **Metab.**, 10, 794-807.

Parizkova, J. (1961b) Age trends in fat in normal and obese children. **J. Appl. Physiol.**, 16 : 173-174.

Parizkova, J. (1973) Body composition and exercise during and development, in **Physical Activity: Human Growth and Development** (ed G.L. Rarick), Academic Press, New York, pp. 97-124.

Tanner, J.M. (1962) **Growth and Adolescence** (2nd ed.) Blackwell Scientific Publication, Oxford.

Young, G.M., Sipin, S.S. and Roe, D.A. (1968) Body composition of pre-adolescent and adolescent girls. I. Density and skinfolds measurements. **J. Amer. Diet. Assoc.,** 53, 25-31.

3

LONGITUDINAL STUDY OF THE STABILITY OF THE SOMATOTYPE IN BOYS AND GIRLS

W. DUQUET [1] J. BORMS [1], M. HEBBELINCK [1], J.A.P. DAY [2] and P. CORDEMANS [1]

[1] Human Biometry Laboratory, Vrije Universiteit Brussel, Belgium
[2] University of Lethbridge, Canada

Keywords : Growth, Somatotype, Longitudinal study, Children

1 Introduction

A person's phenotypical appearance is by definition the physical reflection of the many influences of all possible environmental factors on the human body build. The structural changes that evolve from this have been described extensively as far as longitudinal evolution of the principal anthropometric characteristics is concerned. Long term longitudinal descriptions of human physique as a whole are, however, less numerous.

In the specific field of growth studies, most reports deal with either mixed-longitudinal designs or short term projects, or with a very limited number of measuring occasions within the same individual. Descriptions of body type changes from early childhood through puberty to adulthood are rare (Carter and Heath 1990, p. 146), and studies of the interactions of these changes with other factors are as yet unavailable.

The Belgian Longitudinal and Experimental Growth Study (LEGS) (Hebbelinck et al. 1980) has the potential to fill this gap. In the present study, as a first step in the approach to this objective, the consecutive somatotypes of a series of children, followed from 6 to 17 years of age, will be described and discussed.

2 Methods

The LEGS study encompasses a group of over 500 children, belonging to 5 consecutive generations or cohorts, who participated in the measurements from the last year of Kindergarten (ages 5-6) until, if feasible, the last year of secondary school (age 18 or more). The data collection took place from 1969 until 1986. Next to anthropometric and physical performance capacity measurements, data were also assembled on traits, behaviour and influences in the psychological, social, environmental, educational, medical, and psychomotor domain. The anthropometric and motor performance variables were collected annually, and the principal anthropometric variables semi-annually from the onset of puberty on. All measures were taken by the same examiners throughout the whole project.

For this analysis, only those children were selected who had been present at each measurement occasion in a period starting before their sixth birthday and ending after their seventeenth birthday, and for whom a complete data set for calculating the Heath-Carter somatotype was available at each of these measurement occasions. This rather severe screening resulted in a sample of 30 girls and 52 boys. Their anthropometric somatotypes were calculated according to the Heath-Carter method (Heath and Carter 1967; Carter 1980). Each endomorphy value was corrected for body height as suggested by Hebbelinck et al. (1973) and validated by Duquet (1980). The obtained component values were then converted to point age values by means of linear interpolation.

This resulted in a complete set of 82 pure longitudinal individual somatotype evolutions with values at age points 6 to 17.

Between-age differences and associations in component values were tested for significance using repeated-measures ANOVA and product-moment correlations. For the between-age comparisons of global somatotypes, the Somatotype Attitudinal Distance (SAD) techniques were used as outlined by Duquet and Hebbelinck (1977) and Carter et al. (1983).

3 Results and discussion

3.1 Evolution of the mean component values

Judging from the mean values of the separate components at the different ages (Table 1), one would be inclined to conclude that each component changes slowly with time.

Endomorphy or relative fatness seems to be the least important factor of body build at all ages, undulating slightly around a value of 2 in boys, and increasing slowly around a value of 3 in girls.

Mesomorphy or relative musculo-skeletal development is at all ages dominant over endomorphy for both sexes. This component decreases around a value of 4 with increasing age.

Ectomorphy or relative height for weight has a different evolution. In boys, this component is almost as low as endomorphy at age 6, but then increases and becomes the dominant factor of body build at age 13, then decreases again towards a general balanced ectomorph-mesomorph physique in 17 year old boys. In girls, the ectomorphy value is the least dominant at age 6. It increases to a 3.5 value at ages 11 and 12, but then decreases again at older ages, ending slightly under the mean values for endo- and mesomorphy at age 17.

The between-age differences per component, tested for significance by means of a repeated-measures ANOVA, are also indicated in Table 1. Common underlining of age values means that there were no significant

55

Table 1. Mean values of the somatotype components in 52 boys and 30 girls followed longitudinally from age 6 to 17. Common underlined means are not significantly different (p< .05).

						Ages						
	6	7	8	9	10	11	12	13	14	15	16	17
Boys												
Endo	2.1	2.0	2.0	2.1	2.2	2.3	2.4	2.3	2.0	1.8	1.8	1.8
Meso	4.2	4.1	4.1	4.0	4.0	3.9	3.9	3.9	3.9	3.8	3.8	3.8
Ecto	2.6	3.0	3.3	3.5	3.6	3.7	3.8	3.9	4.1	4.1	4.0	3.9
Girls												
Endo	2.8	2.7	2.8	2.9	3.1	3.1	3.0	3.1	3.2	3.1	3.2	3.4
Meso	4.4	4.2	4.1	4.0	3.9	3.9	3.8	3.5	3.5	3.5	3.5	3.6
Ecto	2.3	2.8	2.9	3.2	3.3	3.5	3.5	3.4	3.4	3.3	3.1	2.9

differences (p≤0.05). This is the case for all age values of endomorphy in both sexes, and also for mesomorphy in boys. In girls, the decreasing mesomorphy becomes at the age of 12 years significantly different from the dominant starting value at 6, but not from the value at 7, and this continues until 17 years. Ectomorphy in girls is at no age significantly different from other ages. In boys, the increase in ectomorphy is significant between 6 years and older ages, between 7 and ages older than 8, and between 8 and ages older than 12.

The foregoing approach, showing few significant differences, may be misleading. The lack of significance is caused by the small means of yearly increases and decreases of component values with regard to the much higher standard deviations of these changes in individual component values. But, in our opinion, this kind of analysis, in which each indicator of body build is checked separately for its eventual change, masks the overall plasticity of body build that can be observed when several of these indicators are checked simultaneously. This is one of the advantages of the somatotype analysis technique. It is therefore indispensable to inspect more closely the changes in within-individual component combinations and somatotype growth values.

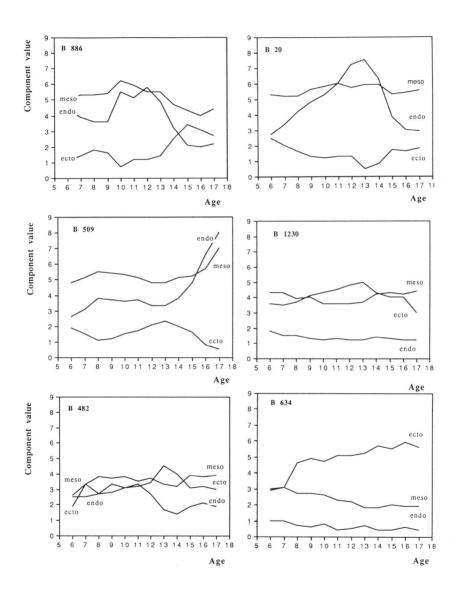

Fig. 1. Individual longigtudinal evolution of the somatotype components in 6 boys.

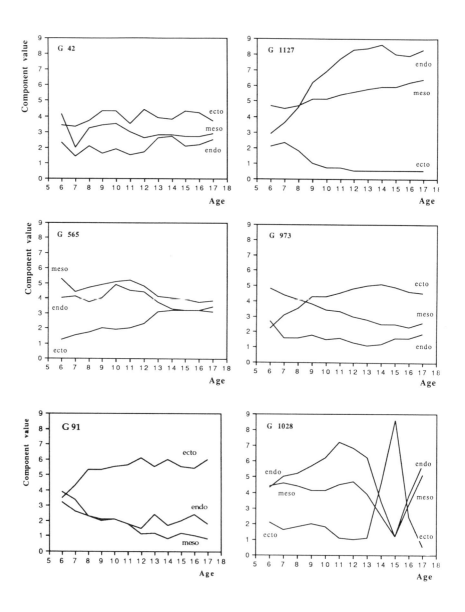

Fig. 2. Individual longigtudinal evolution of the somatotype components in 6 girls.

3.2 Evolution of the individual component values

Fig. 1 and 2 demonstrate 6 examples of boys' and girls' individual component evolutions. They were chosen from the total of 82 subjects, to show the great diversity of possible individual body type developments.

Some of these patterns can be considered as examples of common evolutions in type. Boy 1230, e.g., is the typical 'healthy boy', showing from the age of 6 on a constant mesomorph-ectomorph physique with moderate to low adiposity. Boy 634 is the typical consistent ectomorph from the age of 8 years on. Boy 509 is the endomorphic mesomorph who gets fatter and stockier, and becomes a rather extreme mesomorphic endomorph at 17 years. Boy 20 is the example of a child that tended to go in the same direction. His increase in relative fatness turned the balanced mesomorph at age 6 into an endomorph with mesomorphic traits at the age of 13, without any remarkable change in mesomorphy during this period. His drop in ectomorphy at age 13 reflects clearly the gain in fat mass. Starting a sports training program and changing his nutritional habits around age 13 brought him back to more or less his original somatotype. He is now an athletic physical education teacher with a moderate, well controlled tendency to endomorphy. This pattern of somatotype evolution appeared in several children, although mostly to a less extreme extent. Boy 886 is an example of this. Boy 482 is the central type, with almost equal dominance of the 3 components until the age of 12, and so is girl 42. Girl 1127 shows the same pattern as boy 509, but with an earlier dominance switch from endomorphic mesomorphy to mesomorphic endomorphy. Girl 565 is an example of a child with a clear dominance situation at 6, who changes into a central type with no dominant component at 17. Girl 973 is a perfect example of the overall pattern of somatotype means in girls that we found in an earlier cross-sectional sample of 4743 six to thirteen year old Flemish girls (Duquet et al. 1975). Girl 91 follows a similar pattern. The last example, girl 1028, is the most spectacular. It is a unique longitudinal recording of the dramatic but true changes in body build of an anorexic girl, who was, fortunately, treated successfully, and regained her former profile.

3.3 Predictability of the somatotype components

Between age correlations were calculated per component in each group (Tables 2 to 4). Each table displays the correlation coefficients for boys in the upper right triangle, and for girls in the lower left triangle. The results indicate for each age a high level of predictability from the value one year earlier. The correlations run up to .98 in adjacent years (on the diagonal). Only 5 out of 66 of these were less than .80, 8 were higher than .80 but less than .90, and all remaining 53 were above .90. As could be expected, the correlation coefficient decreases with an increasing distance in years between predicting and predicted age. This is especially true in endomorphy.

How well is a somatotype component at 17 years predictable from earlier component assessments ? If we use an r of .90 as the standard, then

Table 2. Between-age correlations for endomorphy in boys (upper right triangle) and in girls (lower left triangle) (underlined values are not significant at p < .05).

AGE	6	7	8	9	10	11	12	13	14	15	16	17
6	-	.77	.74	.66	.67	.60	.53	.46	.48	.50	.44	<u>.38</u>
7	.89	-	.93	.90	.87	.81	.73	.65	.68	.68	.64	.58
8	.70	.83	-	.95	.91	.85	.78	.71	.73	.73	.71	.63
9	.73	.87	.89	-	.96	.91	.83	.76	.76	.72	.72	.65
10	.75	.87	.83	.97	-	.96	.91	.85	.80	.73	.73	.67
11	.72	.83	.79	.93	.96	-	.96	.91	.86	.78	.77	.70
12	.71	.81	.80	.92	.93	.95	-	.97	.89	.77	.73	.67
13	.68	.78	.78	.89	.90	.92	.96	-	.93	.78	.75	.68
14	.55	.58	.60	.70	.71	.70	.74	.83	-	.90	.81	.70
15	<u>.45</u>	<u>.49</u>	.55	.65	.67	.68	.70	.77	.82	-	.92	.78
16	.54	.65	.65	.77	.79	.82	.83	.89	.84	.92	-	.94
17	.55	.70	.69	.83	.82	.84	.87	.89	.75	.78	.92	-

Table 3. Between-age correlations for mesomorphy in boys (upper right triangle) and in girls (lower left triangle) (all values are significant at p < .05).

AGE	6	7	8	9	10	11	12	13	14	15	16	17
6	-	.60	.52	.54	.51	.52	.46	.48	.59	.47	.47	.44
7	.66	-	.80	.77	.72	.72	.69	.65	.70	.66	.63	.63
8	.64	.88	-	.95	.92	.90	.88	.86	.88	.86	.86	.84
9	.60	.75	.94	-	.96	.94	.91	.88	.90	.87	.87	.83
10	.61	.74	.92	.97	-	.98	.95	.92	.90	.86	.85	.81
11	.58	.76	.90	.95	.97	-	.98	.95	.92	.88	.86	.82
12	.52	.74	.88	.94	.93	.97	-	.96	.94	.90	.87	.82
13	.56	.72	.87	.92	.92	.94	.96	-	.96	.90	.89	.84
14	54	.65	.81	.86	.87	.87	.87	.94	-	.96	.94	.90
15	.53	.60	.74	.79	.80	.77	.76	.86	.96	-	.97	.92
16	.52	.65	.80	.84	.85	.85	.86	.93	.97	.94	-	.96
17	.52	.66	.81	.84	.86	.87	.90	.92	.98	.81	.94	-

endomorphy at 17 can only be predicted from age 16 on. Mesomorphy at 17 years can be predicted from age 14 on in boys, and from age 12 in girls. In ectomorphy, these ages are 14 years in boys and 11 years in girls. Endomorphy is the least predictable of the 3, and girls' values are less predictable than boys'.

Table 4. Between-age correlations for ectomorphy in boys (upper right triangle) and in girls (lower left triangle) (all values are significant at $p < .05$).

AGE	6	7	8	9	10	11	12	13	14	15	16	17
6	-	.79	.72	.69	.68	.64	.63	.58	.60	.62	.64	.58
7	.85	-	.91	.87	.86	.84	.84	.81	.84	.83	83	.80
8	.81	.89	-	.95	.91	.87	.87	.84	.87	.86	.88	.86
9	.76	.88	.92	-	.95	.91	.90	.87	.90	.86	.86	.85
10	.76	.89	.90	.98	-	.96	.95	.91	.88	.83	.85	.84
11	.74	.88	.84	.95	.98	-	.98	.93	.90	.85	.86	.85
12	.70	.84	.82	.94	.96	.97	-	.96	.92	.88	.88	.86
13	.69	.80	.79	.91	.93	.93	.96	-	.95	.88	.88	.85
14	.68	.72	.73	.83	.84	.82	.85	.91	-	.96	.94	.91
15	.61	.57	.60	.70	.70	.67	.68	.77	.95	-	.97	.94
16	.68	.74	.75	.84	.87	.87	.89	.94	.94	.86	-	.97
17	.66	.78	.77	.84	.87	.90	.92	.92	.86	.72	.95	-

To predict a somatotype component in young adults one obviously needs more than the same component's value at a younger age. The question arises if the same applies to the prediction of the young adult somatotype as a whole, and if so, which other indicators can add enough predictive power.

3.4 Longitudinal evolution of global somatotypes

Fig. 3 and 4 illustrate the changes with age of the mean somatotype at each age level in the boys' and the girls' group. Here too, the changes in means over the years seem not to be spectacular. Girls change on the average from a low but balanced mesomorphy with slight tendency to endomorphy at 6 years to a central type with equal importance of all components at later ages. Boys are, on the average, low balanced mesomorphs with slight ectomorphic traits at 6, then move towards a mesomorph-ectomorph physique.

Inspection of individual somatotype changes reveals again the existence of inter-individual differences in patterns of somatotype changes. These are exemplified in fig. 5 and 6 for the same 12 children as in fig. 1 and 2.

It should be clear from the examples in fig. 1, 2, 5 and 6 that the unique combination of three component values within one individual adds considerably more information to the analysis of changes in separate component values. The year to year change in body type as a whole was also calculated (Table 5). The values indicate the means of the individual somatotype changes, and not the change in group mean. The latter may, again, hide the magnitude of the individual changes. These show important, significant differences at most ages. The change in somatotype is not significant between ages 10 to 12 and between 14 to 17 in boys, and between ages 10 to 16 in girls.

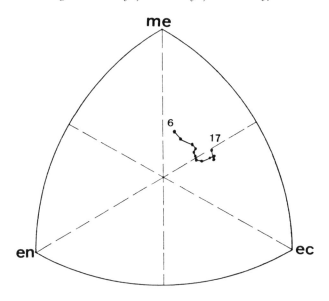

Fig. 3. Longitudinal evolution in means of somatotypes of 52 boys from age 6 to 17.

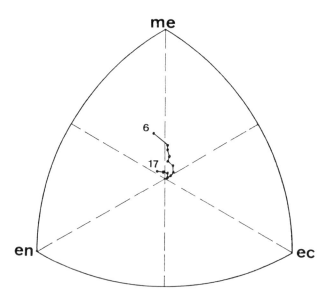

Fig. 4. Longitudinal evolution in means of somatotypes of 30 girls from age 6 to 17.

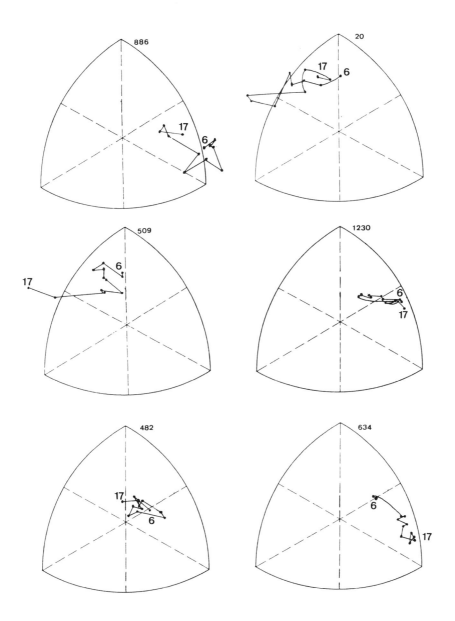

Fig. 5. Individual longitudinal evolution of somatotype in 6 boys from age 6 to 17.

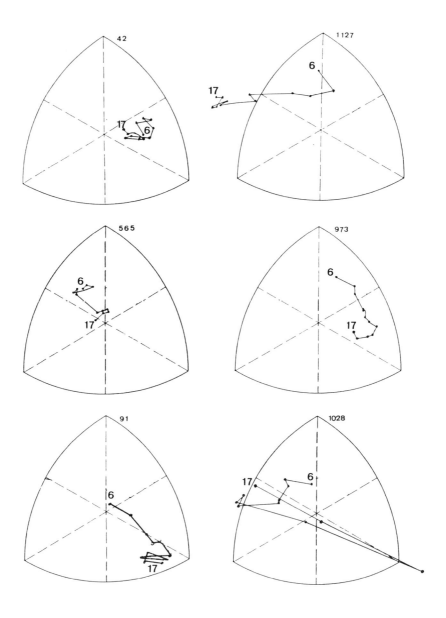

Fig. 6. Individual longitudinal evolution of somatotype in 6 girls from age 6 to 17.

Table 5. Means of individual year-to-year changes in somatotype, expressed in component units, in 52 boys (upper right triangle) and 30 girls (lower left triangle). Non-significant changes are underlined (p < .05).

AGE	6	7	8	9	10	11	12	13	14	15	16	17
6	-	1.04	1.37	1.66	1.87	2.02	2.18	2.29	2.26	2.22	2.16	2.16
7	1.02	-	.67	.98	1.31	1.48	1.64	1.77	1.70	1.67	1.62	1.61
8	1.37	.79	-	.56	.89	1.11	1.25	1.39	1.33	1.29	1.24	1.29
9	1.70	1.11	.77	-	.53	.82	1.01	1.14	1.13	1.17	1.13	1.19
10	1.92	1.34	1.10	.51	-	.47	.72	.91	1.04	1.22	2.15	1.22
11	2.30	1.69	1.52	.92	.63	-	.43	.68	.92	1.18	1.16	1.25
12	2.39	1.76	1.58	1.05	.88	.57	-	.50	.89	1.16	1.19	1.29
13	2.27	1.73	1.55	1.14	1.00	.95	.69	-	.69	1.04	1.07	1.18
14	2.27	1.89	1.76	1.49	1.41	1.47	1.29	.82	-	.54	.75	.94
15	2.28	1.95	1.83	1.60	1.51	1.55	1.51	1.10	.72	-	.47	.75
16	2.05	1.68	1.59	1.43	2.01	1.43	1.37	.98	.79	.59	-	.47
17	2.16	1.76	1.64	1.42	1.40	1.42	1.26	1.06	1.05	1.02	.65	-

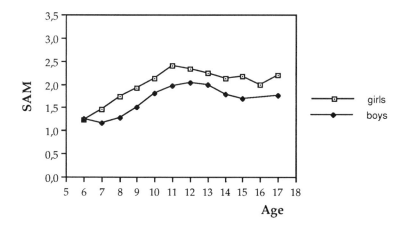

Fig. 7. Heterogeneity of somatotypes (SAM) in boys (n=52) and girls (n=30) followed longitudinally from age 6 to 17.

Fig. 7 demonstrates the changes with age of the somatotype heterogeneity within both groups, expressed as somatotype attitudinal mean (SAM). The mean scatter of the individual somatotypes around their age group mean is about 1 component unit at age 6, and then increases to values of 2 in girls and 2.5 in boys towards puberty. This change in somatotype heterogeneity was also tested for its significance. The increasing variances from ages 6 to 9 are not different within these age groups, and neither are the stabilized variances between age groups 9 to 17. The variances are significantly different between these two age blocs.

Migratory distances (MD), or sums of consecutive within-subject changes, reflect total absolute change in somatotype with time. They are expressed in component units, as are all SAD-based parameters. The mean MD in boys was 6.4 in 11 years, or .58 as average component change per boy per year. The most stable boy in terms of physique had a MD of 3.6 over 11 years, the most unstable boy a MD of 12.9, or more than one component unit change per year during 11 years. In girls, the mean MD was 7.8. The lowest MD in girls was 3.9. If one does not consider the special case of the anorexic girl 1028, who had an extremely high MD of 21.7 over 11 years, the mean MD for girls is 7.3 in 11 years. This means an average somatotype change of .66 component units per girl per year. The girls in our study seem to have a more unstable somatotype than the boys.

4 Conclusions

This first attempt to study a complete set of individual somatotype changes from childhood to adulthood gives an impression of the diversity and possible plasticity of the physique of the growing child. The Heath-Carter somatotype method, with its phenotypical approach, is able to describe a number of aspects of these changes. Using the Somatotype Attitudinal Distance and its derived parameters helps to express these global changes in the same units as the initial components.

The screening that was used for this study may have been too severe, possibly resulting in a not representative, because too small, sample of subjects. The observed longitudinal changes of the component values should be our basis for a forthcoming better fitting procedure, that will result in larger samples. This will later permit us to explore on a longitudinal basis the interactions of the changing physique with other maturational processes and the other mentioned characteristics of the child, not in the least its motor functions.

As for now, the present results at the same time stress the possible intra-individual changes and the subsequent low predictability within the somatotype components. The patterns of individual somatotype change that we suppose to have recognized can, if confirmed in larger samples, offer a new perspective to dealing with this problem.

5 Acknowledgements

This investigation was supported in part by the National Research Fund (NFWO) of Belgium, by the Fund for Medical Research (FGWO), contract number 935.

6 References

Carter, J.E.L. (1980) **The Heath-Carter somatotype method.** San Diego State University Syllabus Service, San Diego.

Carter, J.E.L. Ross, W.D. Duquet, W. and Aubry, S. (1983) Advances in somatotype methodology and analysis. **Y. Phys. Anthropol.,** 26, 193-213.

Duquet, W. (1980) **Studie van de toepasbaarheid van de Heath & Carter-somatotypemethode op kinderen van 6 tot 13 jaar. (Applicability of the Heath & Carter somatotype method to 6 to 13 year old children).** PhD Dissertation, Vrije Universiteit Brussel, Belgium.

Duquet, W. Borms, J. and De Meulenaere, F. (1979) A method for detecting errors in data of growth studies. **Ann. Hum. Biol.,** 6(5), 431-441.

Duquet, W. and Hebbelinck, M. (1977) Application of the somatotype attitudinal distance to the study of group and individual somatotype status and relations, in **Growth and Development : Physique** (ed O. Eiben), Akadémiai Kiado (Hungarian Academy of Sciences), Budapest, pp. 377-384.

Duquet, W. Hebbelinck, M. Borms, J. (1975) Somatotype distributions of primary school boys and girls, in **Proceedings of the 18th International Congress of ICHPER** (ed D. Schmull), The Jan Luiting Foundation, Zeist, The Netherlands, pp. 326-334.

Heath, B. H. and Carter, J.E.L. (1967) A modified somatotype method. **Am. J. Phys. Anthropol.,** 27, 57-74.

Hebbelinck, M. Blommaert, M. Borms, J. Duquet, W. Vajda A. and Van Der Meer J. (1980) Een multidisciplinaire longitudinale groeistudie, een inleiding tot het project "LEGS", **Geneeskunde en Sport,** 13(2), 48-52.

Hebbelinck, M. and Ross, W.D. (1974) Body type and performance, in **Fitness, Health, and Work Capacity** (ed L.A. Larson), Macmillan, New York, pp. 266-283.

4

THE ANALYSIS OF INDIVIDUAL AND AVERAGE GROWTH CURVES: SOME METHODOLOGICAL ASPECTS

R.C. HAUSPIE [1] and H. CHRZASTEK-SPRUCH [2]
[1] NFWO, Vrije Universiteit Brussel, Belgium
[2] Institute of Pediatrics of the Medical Academy, Lublin, Poland

Keywords: Growth, Growth models, Curve fitting, Logistic, Gompertz, Triple logistic, Centiles, Growth standards.

1 Introduction

The outcome of any growth study, whether it is longitudinal or cross-sectional, is a set of discrete measures of size, individual or average, in function of age. Consequently, growth data consist of a discontinuous series of images of a process which is naturally continuous. However, quite often interest lies in estimating this continuous process, i.e. to establish a smooth curve describing the pattern observed in the growth data. It is at this level that growth modelling can be of great help. Besides the fact that curve fitting is an elegant smoothing technique, it also summarizes the growth data in a limited number of constants, the values of the fitted function parameters. These constants or parameters have the same meaning for each curve and thus allow easy comparison between individuals or between groups of individuals. Moreover, it is possible to derive various 'biological parameters' from a fitted curve, such as age, size and velocity at take-off or at maximal velocity of the adolescent growth spurt, for example. These biological parameters may then form a basis for further analysis of the growth data.

In this contribution, we will not attempt to review the great number of mathematical equations proposed for describing human growth data, but we will focus on some aspects, possibilities and limitations of a few commonly used equations. For a more extensive review of growth models we refer to Hauspie (1989). We will also briefly discuss Healy's method for distribution-free estimation of age-related centiles (Healy et al. 1988), illustrating the technique by an application to growth data for height.

2 Logistic and Gompertz function

Various growth models have been derived from the generalized logistic model (Von Bertalanffy 1941, 1957, 1960; Richards 1959):

$$y = K[1 + c\,e^{-bt}]^{1/(1-m)}$$

For $m > 1$, this curve is S-shaped, having a lower and upper asymptote, respectively equal to zero and K, and a single point of inflection. Parameter b is a rate constant and parameter c is an integration constant. Of particular interest are the special cases whereby $m = 2$ and $m \to 1$. For $m = 2$ the generalized logistic leads to the autocatalytic or logistic function which, after re-parameterization, takes the form:

$$y = \frac{K}{1 + e^{a-bt}}$$

For $m = 1$ the generalized logistic breaks down, but Richards (1959) demonstrated that for $m \to 1$, the model leads to the Gompertz curve:

$$y = P + Ke^{-e^{a-bt}}$$

In both the logistic and Gompertz curve, y = size, t = age, P, K, a and b are the function parameters. These models have been frequently used to describe the adolescent growth cycle (Deming 1957; Marubini et al. 1971, 1972; Hauspie 1981; Hauspie et al. 1980; Tanner et al. 1976). The following biological parameters can be easily obtained:

	LOGISTIC	GOMPERTZ
age at peak velocity	a/b	a/b
size at peak velocity	$P + K/2$	$P + K/e$
peak velocity	$bK/4$	bK/e

Fig. 1 shows an example of the fit of the logistic and the Gompertz function to part of the growth data of Girl N° 7 from the Lublin Longitudinal Growth Study (Chrzastek-Spruch et al. 1989). The residual mean square was 0.169 cm^2 for the logistic and 0.341 cm^2 for the Gompertz function (d.f. = 5). Graphical inspection of the data shows that the yearly increments reach a maximum of 8.0 cm/year at 12.5 years. The values for these features obtained by the logistic and Gompertz function are respectively 12.4 years - 8.1 cm/year and 12.1 years - 8.5 cm/year. It seems

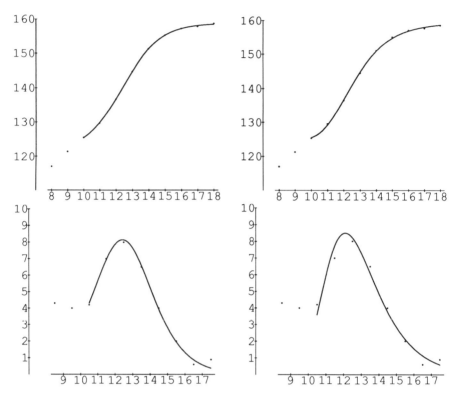

Fig. 1. Fit of logistic and Gompertz function to the adolescent growth data of Girl N° 7 from the Lublin Longitudinal Growth Study (Chrzastek-Spruch et al. 1989).

that, in this particular individual, the logistic function fits the growth data slightly better than the Gompertz function. Hauspie (1981) found that this was also true when analyzing the logistic and Gompertz fits to the height data of 68 boys. In this study, it was shown that the pooled residual variance was 0.353 cm^2 for the logistic and 0.450 cm^2 for the Gompertz function. The difference was statistically significant: probability of Wilcoxon's matched-pairs ranked-sign test was 0.021. Both the logistic and the Gompertz function also have the drawback that the lower age boundary of the data to be fitted (i.e. the cut-off point between the pre-pubertal and adolescent growth cycle) has to be determined arbitrarily for each individual. This is usually done by inspecting a plot of the yearly increments and taking the age at minimal velocity before the adolescent growth spurt as the cut -off point. However, this procedure is like having an extra parameter to estimate.

3 Triple logistic function

In an attempt to overcome the problem of estimating the point at take-off and, at the same time, to provide a model describing the growth process from early childhood to full maturity Thissen et al. (1976) have tested four two-component combinations of logistic and Gompertz functions. They found that the linear summation of two logistic functions, yielding a model with 6 parameters, was superior to the other three combinations (Bock et al. 1973). Later, Bock and Thissen (1980) developed the triple logistic function (with 9 parameters) which is based on the conception that mature size is a summation of three processes, each of which can be represented by a logistic component.

$$y = a_1 \left[\frac{1-p}{1 + e^{-b_1(t-c_1)}} + \frac{p}{1 + e^{-b_2(t-c_2)}} \right] + \frac{a_2}{1 + e^{-b_3(t-c_3)}}$$

The triple logistic function also allows for a small prepubertal growth spurt. Fig. 2 shows the decomposition of the triple logistic function.

Fig. 3 shows an example of the fit of the triple logistic function (TRL) to the growth data of Girl N° 56 of the Lublin Longitudinal Growth Study (ages 0 - 18 years). Age at peak velocity is estimated by the triple logistic function at 10.9 years with a peak velocity of 9.6 cm/year. The prepubertal spurt was estimated by TRL at 3.9 years with a peak velocity of 7.6 cm/year. However, graphical inspection of the pattern of the yearly increments shows that the pre-pubertal spurt is actually later (4.8 years) and sharper than what is shown by the TRL-fit (graphically estimated prepubertal peak velocity is 8.2 cm/year). It seems that the TRL model is apparently not flexible enough to adequately represent the short-lasting sharp rise in prepubertal growth velocity in this particular girl.

Moreover, there is also the fact that many individuals do not show just one single prepubertal growth spurt, but may have several such spurts (Butler et al. 1989). Figure 4 shows two examples, taken from the Lublin Longitudinal Growth Study: Girl N° 8 with 2 and Girl N° 21 with 3 prepubertal growth spurts. The triple logistic function which, by the nature of its mathematical equation, allows for only one prepubertal spurt, clearly smooths out the prepubertal growth pattern of subjects who actually show more than one prepubertal spurt in their growth data.

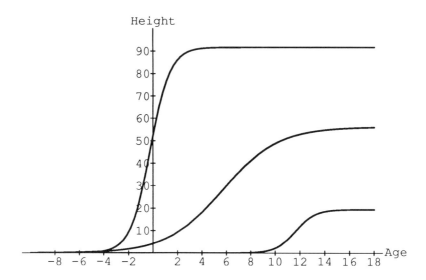

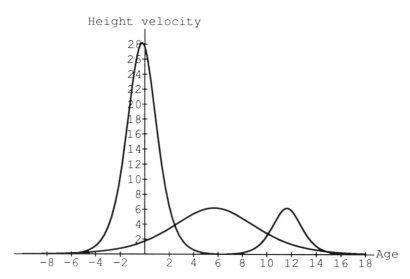

Fig. 2. Decomposition of the triple logistic function into three additive logistic components. Distance curves in upper part, velocity curves in lower part.

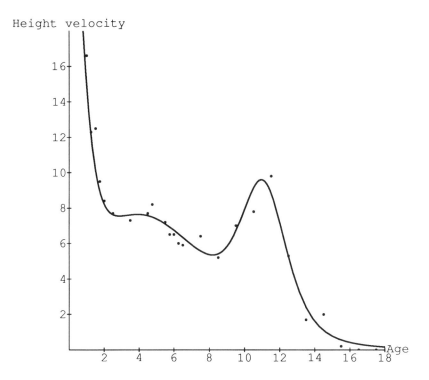

Fig. 3. Fit of the triple logistic function to the growth data of Girl N°56 of the Lublin Longitudinal Growth Study. Plot of the yearly increments in height, based on the raw data, together with the first derivative of the fitted curve.

Graphical analysis of the yearly increments of 56 girls from the Lublin Longitudinal Growth Study revealed that, actually, a few subjects had no prepubertal growth spurt at all, and that most showed at least two such spurts. Table 1 gives the frequency distribution of the number of prepubertal spurts observed in these 56 subjects. We have considered as 'prepubertal spurt' each peak in the pattern of the yearly increments which was confirmed by at least three values. Fluctuations in the yearly increments, giving rise to peaks, but composed of fewer than 3 data points have been considered as random fluctuations. Figure 5 shows a graphical representation of the mean ages at maximal velocity (± 1 SD) of these prepubertal spurts for curves with varying numbers of such peaks.

73

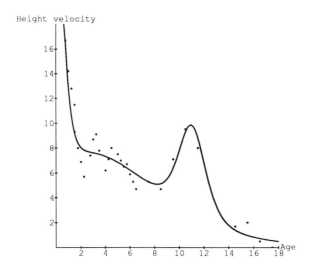

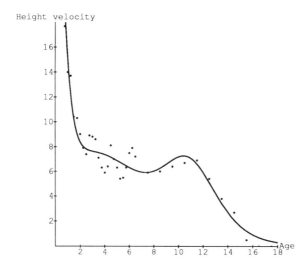

Fig. 4. Fit of the triple logistic function to the growth data of Girl N° 8 (with 2 prepubertal growth spurts) and Girl N° 21 (with 3 prepubertal growth spurts) from the Lublin Longitudinal Growth Study.

Table 1. Frequency distribution of the number of prepubertal growth spurts observed by graphical inspection of the yearly increments of 56 girls (Lublin Longitudinal Growth Study).

Number of peaks	Frequency (count)	Relative frequency (percentage)
0	4	7
1	17	30
2	22	39
3	11	20
4	2	4

Out of the 35 girls showing graphically more than 1 prepubertal growth spurt, the TRL fit came up with a prepubertal spurt in about 50% of the cases. Obviously, the outcome of these TRL-fits were misleading with respect to the prepubertal growth spurt.

On the other hand, in the 4 girls with graphically no prepubertal spurt (i.e. with a steadily decreasing trend in the yearly increments), one of the TRL velocity curves showed a small prepubertal growth spurt. This was obviously erroneous. In the other three cases, there was a small bump present in the prepubertal TRL velocity curve, reflecting the presence of the mid-childhood component in the mathematical model.

Finally, out of the 17 subjects showing graphically one single spurt, TRL detected the spurt in only 10 cases. Table 2 shows some statistics concerning age at peak velocity and peak velocity of the prepubertal spurt for these cases. It seems that the TRL estimates the age at prepubertal peak velocity significantly too early in these subjects. The mean value of prepubertal peak velocity itself is also lower in the TRL-fits than in the graphically obtained estimates. The difference is at the border of significance.

It can be concluded that the ability of the TRL model to describe the prepubertal growth spurt should not be over-emphasized. Indeed, it appears that the growth pattern in the mid-childhood period is in many cases far too complex (showing a variable number of small spurts) to be described adequately by a model allowing for only one single spurt in this age range. Otherwise, the present results show that the prepubertal spurt estimated by the TRL model in those cases with one single such spurt in the raw data may be misleading (underestimation of age at peak velocity and peak velocity). However, it should be noticed that the TRL model is

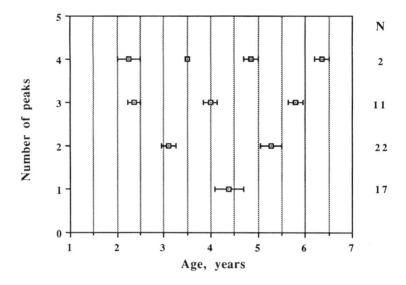

Fig. 5. Mean age at peak velocity (± 1 SD) of the prepubertal growth spurt in curves with varying number of such spurts. N: number of cases. Based on graphical analysis of the yearly increments of 52 girls taken from the Lublin Longitudinal Growth Study.

Table 2. Comparison of mean age at peak velocity and peak velocity of the prepubertal spurt in 10 girls showing one single prepubertal spurt in the pattern of the yearly increments (raw data) and coming up also with a prepubertal spurt in the fit of the TRL function.

	GRAPHICAL	TRL	Probability of paired t-test
Age at peak velocity (years)			
Mean	4.8	4.1	
SD	0.9	0.8	0.02
Peak velocity (cm/year)			
Mean	8.1	7.3	
SD	1.6	0.8	0.05

very suitable to provide a fit of the overall pattern of growth from birth to adulthood, usually providing a fairly unbiased description of the adolescent growth spurt.

4 Healy's method for estimating centile lines

In the analysis of growth data for a group of individuals (sample) we usually need to calculate some measure of central tendency and of dispersion of the data at particular target ages (centile distribution). Since in all cross-sectional growth surveys but also in many longitudinal growth studies, subjects are not measured at fixed target ages (let's say birthdays), it is common practice to group the information into age classes of a fixed length (usually of one year) and to calculate the centile distribution corresponding to the center of each age class. On the basis of the so obtained centile values, we often wish to estimate smooth centile lines, particularly if the purpose of the study is to produce growth standards, for example. Healy proposed a number of important methodological approaches to tackle these problems.

4.1 Estimating centile distribution within each age class
Assuming that, *within an age class,* 1) the growth variable is normally distributed, 2) growth is linear, and 3) the ages are distributed homogeneously, then the arithmetic mean is a correct estimate of the central tendency with respect to the center of that age class. However, this is not necessarily the case for the variance. Particularly, in age periods of rapid changes in growth rate (around adolescence, for example), the values of the growth variable will show an increase or decrease with age, even within an age class of one year. In such situations, the variance calculated on all raw data of a single age class will be greater than the variance corresponding to the center of that age class (instantaneous measure of the variance). Healy (1962, 1978) has proposed the following correction for the variance:

$$s^{2'} = s^2 - b^2/12$$

b, being the regression coefficient of the growth variable on age, calculated within the considered age class. Hauspie (1986) showed that this correction reduces the estimation of the standard deviation of height in girls, age 5-6 years, by 6.3 % . Using the mean and the corrected estimate of the variance, we can then calculate parametrically various centiles using a table of the standard normal distribution. More recently, Healy et al. (1988) also proposed a method for estimating age-related centile values for growth variables which depart from the Gaussian distribution.

4.2 Estimating smooth centile curves

Healy's method for estimating smooth centile curves basically assumes that each centile line can be represented by a polynomial of degree p:

$$y_i = a_{0i} + a_{1i}t + a_{2i}t^2 + \dots + a_{pi}t^p$$

with t = age and y_i the smoothed value of the ith centile. The coefficients a for fixed j can be represented by a polynomial in z_i, z_i being the value of the normal equivalent deviate (Gaussian position) of the ith centile:

$$a_{ji} = b_{j0} + b_{j1}z_i + \dots + b_{jq_j}z_i^{q_j}$$

Fig. 6 shows six theoretical examples. The equations of the centile lines are:

(A) $y_i = (b_{00} + b_{01}z_i) + (b_{10})t$

(B) $y_i = (b_{00} + b_{01}z_i) + (b_{10} + b_{11}z_i)t$

(C) $y_i = (b_{00} + b_{01}z_i + b_{02}z_i^2) + (b_{10})t$

(D) $y_i = (b_{00} + b_{01}z_i + b_{02}z_i^2) + (b_{10} + b_{11}z_i)t$

(E) $y_i = (b_{00} + b_{01}z_i) + (b_{10} + b_{11}z_i)t + (b_{20})t^2$

(F) $y_i = (b_{00} + b_{01}z_i + b_{02}z_i^2) + (b_{10} + b_{11}z_i)t + (b_{20})t^2$

The various examples can be interpreted as follows:

(A) *Gaussian-distributed straight centile lines showing constant spread over age*
  $p = 1$: the centiles curves are straight lines (1st degree polynomial in t).
  $q_0 = 1$: the distribution of the centile lines is Gaussian (1st degree polynomial relationship of the intercepts of the centile lines with respect to the respective Gaussian position z_i).

  $q_1 = 0$: the spread of the various centile lines (or the standard deviation) is constant over the ages (0 degree polynomial relationship of the slope of the centile lines with respect to the respective Gaussian position z_i).

(B) *Gaussian-distributed straight centile lines showing a gradually changing spread over age*
  $p = 1$: idem as in (A).
  $q_0 = 1$: idem as in (A).
  $q_1 = 1$: the spread of the various centile lines (or the standard deviation) changes linearly with age (1st degree polynomial relationship of the slope of the centile lines with respect to the respective Gaussian position z_i).

(C) *non-Gaussian-distributed straight centile lines showing constant spread over age*
  $p = 1$: idem as in (A).

$q_0 = 2$: the distribution of the centile lines is non-Gaussian (2nd degree polynomial relationship of the intercepts of the centile lines with respect to the respective Gaussian position z_i).

$q_1 = 0$: idem as in (A).

(D) *non-Gaussian-distributed straight centile lines showing a gradually changing spread over age*

$p = 1$: idem as in (A).

$q_0 = 2$: idem as in (C).

$q_1 = 1$: idem as in (B).

(E) *Gaussian-distributed curved centile lines showing a gradually changing spread over age*

$p = 2$: the centiles curves are curved lines (2nd degree polynomial in t).

$q_0 = 1$: idem as in (A).

$q_1 = 1$: idem as in (B).

(F) *non-Gaussian-distributed curved centile lines showing a gradually changing spread over age*

$p = 2$: idem as in (E).

$q_0 = 2$: idem as in (D).

$q_1 = 1$: idem as in (B).

In practical situations, where the growth data cover a wide age span and where the centile distribution changes in a rather complex manner with respect to age, higher powers of the basic polynomial (p) and of the polynomials of the various coefficients (q_i) are required. A polynomial function may also not be appropriate to describe the general pattern of the average growth pattern. Healy suggested that, in such situations, one could try to fit a typical growth model (like the TRL or Preece Baines function, for example) to the P50 values and then use the centile deviations from the fitted P50 curve to analyze with the above described method.

We have adopted this approach to construct centile charts for growth in height of Bengali boys (unpublished material from Hauspie et al. 1980). Figure 7a shows the values of P3, P5, P10, P25, P50, P75, P90, P95 and P97 at each half-year between age 1.5 and 18.0 years. The Preece Baines model 1 was fitted to the P50 values in order to define the basic pattern of the average growth curve (Preece and Baines 1978). The residual mean square was 0.30 cm^2 (d.f. = 20). Healy's model was then fitted to the centile deviations from the fitted curve. We used a 7th degree polynomial as the basic curve ($p = 7$); the powers of the polynomials for the various coefficients were taken as follows: $q_0 = 3, q_1 = 4, q_2 = 3, q_3 = 3, q_4 = 2, q_5 = 1,$ $q_6 = 1, q_7 = 1$. The resulting residual variance was 0.58 cm^2 (d.f. = 174). The results of this fit is shown in Figure 7b. Finally, by adding the smooth centile curves to the Preece Baines fitted P50 curve, we obtain the smooth centile lines shown in Figure 7c. There is no strict rule to make choices about the various values of p and q_j to be used in Healy's model. The author states that the values of q_j will usually be higher for the low-order

79

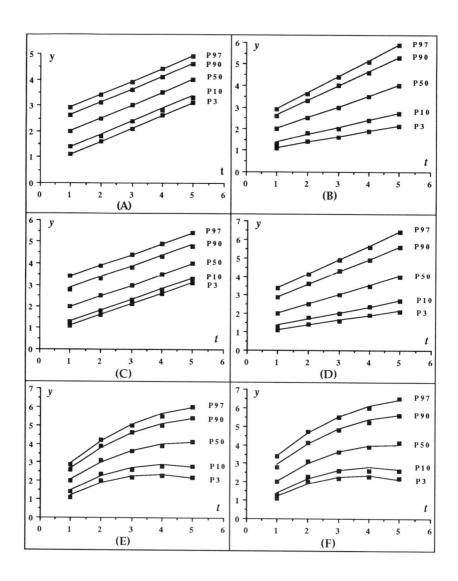

Fig. 6 Some theoretical examples of Healy's method for distribution-free estimation of age-related centiles. See text for explanations.

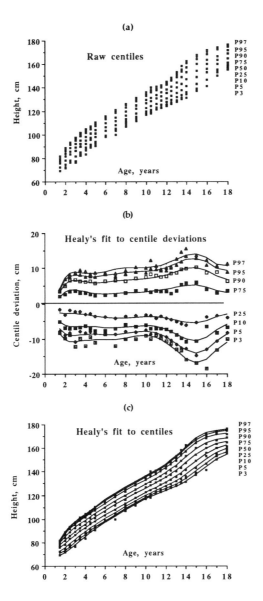

Fig. 7: Application of Healy's method of distribution-free estimates of age-related centiles for growth data in height of Bengali boys (Hauspie et al. 1980). (a): raw centiles; (b): Healy's fit to the centile deviations from the Preece Baines fitted P50; (c): centiles estimated according to Healy's method together with the raw centile values

81

coefficients of the basic polynomial and may be zero for the high-order ones but that in practice a good deal of experimentation may be needed to obtain good values for the parameters p and q_j.

6 References

Bock, R.D. and Thissen, D.M. (1980) Statistical problems of fitting individual growth curves, in **Human physical growth and maturation** (eds F.E. Johnston, A.F. Roche and C. Susanne), Plenum Press, New York and London, pp. 265-290.

Bock, R.D. Wainer, H. Petersen, A. Thissen, D. Murray, J. and Roche, A.F. (1973) A parameterization for individual human growth curves. **Hum. Biol.**, 45, 63-80.

Butler, G.E. McKie, M. and Ratcliffe, S.G. (1989) An analysis of the phases of mid-childhood growth by synchronization of growth spurts, in **AUXOLOGY 88, Perspectives in the Science of Growth and Development** (ed J.M. Tanner), Smith-Gordon and Comp. Ltd., London, pp. 77-84.

Chrzastek-Spruch, H. Susanne, C. Hauspie, R.C. and Kozlowska, M.A. (1989) Individual growth patterns and standards for height and height velocity based on the Lublin Longitudinal Growth Study, in **AUXOLOGY 88, Perspectives in the Science of Growth and Development** (ed J.M. Tanner), Smith-Gordon and Comp. Ltd., London, pp. 161-166.

Deming, J. (1957) Application of the Gompertz curve to the observed pattern of growth in length of 48 individual boys and girls during the adolescent cycle of growth. **Hum. Biol.**, 29, 83-122.

Hauspie, R.C. (1981) L'ajustement de modèles mathématiques aux données longitudinales. **Bull. Soc. r. belge Anthropol. Préhis.**, 92, 157-165.

Hauspie, R.C. (1986) Croissance, in **L'Homme, son Evolution, sa Diversité: manuel d'anthropologie physique** (eds D. Ferembach, C. Susanne, M.-C. Chamla), Doin, Paris, pp. 359-368.

Hauspie, R.C. (1989) Mathematical models for the study of individual growth patterns. **Rev. Epidém. et Santé Publ.**, 37, 461-476.

Hauspie, R.C. Das, S.R. Preece, M.A. and Tanner, J.M. (1980) A longitudinal study of the growth in height of boys and girls of West Bengal (India) age six months to 20 years. **Ann. Hum. Biol.**, 7, 429-441.

Hauspie, R.C. Wachholder, A. Baron, G. Cantraine, F. Susanne, C. and Graffar, M. (1980) A comparative study of the fit of four different functions to longitudinal data of growth in height of Belgian girls. **Ann. Hum. Biol.**, 7, 347-358.

Healy, M.J.R. (1962) The effect of age-grouping on the distribution of a measurement affected by growth. **Am. J. Phys. Anthrop.**, 20, 49-50.

Healy, M.J.R. (1978) Statistics of growth standards, in **Human Growth** (eds F. Falkner and J.M. Tanner), Ballière Tindall, London, pp. 169-181.

Healy, M.J.R. Rasbash, J. and Yang, M. (1988) Distribution-free estimation of age-related centiles. **Ann. Hum. Biol.**, 15, 17-22.

Marubini, E. Resele, L.F. and Barghini, G. (1971) A comparative fit of the Gompertz and logistic functions to longitudinal height data during adolescence in girls. **Hum. Biol.** , 43, 237-252.

Marubini, E. Resele, L.F. Tanner, J.M. and Whitehouse, R.H. (1972) The fit of the Gompertz and logistic curves to longitudinal data during adolescence on height, sitting height, and biacromial diameter in boys and girls of the Harpenden Growth Study. **Hum. Biol.** , 44, 511-524.

Preece, M.A. and Baines, M.K. (1978) A new family of mathematical models describing the human growth curve. **Ann. Hum. Biol.** , 5, 1-24.

Richards, F.J. (1959) A flexible growth function for empirical use. **J. Exp. Botany** , 10, 290-300.

Tanner, J.M. Whitehouse, R.H. Marubini, E. and Resele, L. (1976) The adolescent growth spurt of boys and girls of the Harpenden Growth Study. **Ann. Hum. Biol.** , 3, 109-126.

Thissen, D. Bock, R.D. Wainer, H. and Roche, A.F. (1976) Individual growth in stature. A comparison of four growth studies in the U.S.A. **Ann. Hum. Biol.**, 3, 529-542.

Von Bertalanffy, L. (1941) Stoffwechseltypen und wachstumstypen. **Biol. Zentralbl.** , 61, 510-532.

Von Bertalanffy, L. (1957) Quantitative laws in metabolism and growth. **Quart. Rev. Biol.** , 32, 217-231.

Von Bertalanffy, L. (1960) Principles and theory of growth, in **Fundamental aspects of normal and malignant growth** (ed W.W. Nowinski), Elsevier, London, pp. 137-259.

Part Two

Physical Activity, Health and Fitness

5

NUTRITION AND PHYSICAL ACTIVITY

J. PARIZKOVA
Charles University, Prague, Czechia.

Keywords : Dietary intake, Nutritional status, Exercise, Sport training, Preschool children, Youth, Adolescents.

1 Introduction

Some nutritionists maintain that the nutritional status of a population e.g. in a developing country can be recognized according to the level of spontaneous physical activity of children. A bad nutritional status is rapidly apparent when they move very little and are apathetic. Marginal malnutrition, however, may not necessarily interfere with an adequate development of cardiorespiratory efficiency, as shown in various developing countries.

Children of smaller body size may have quite a good level of aerobic power (VO_2 max kg^{-1} body mass). Work output and muscle strength which depend more on body size and muscle mass are in this case lower. Needless to say that in seriously malnourished children all parameters of functional capacity are deteriorated (Parizkova 1987).

In the industrially developed countries nutritional problems of an opposite character appear - too abundant and unbalanced dietary intake as related to the energy output result in apparent, and/or "hidden" obesity (i.e. high ratio of depot fat without much increased body mass), and low level of fitness as a consequence of hypokinesia.

2 Recommended dietary allowances (RDA)

When considering the adequacy of the recommended allowances for energy intake, energy output - the above-basal level of which depends mainly on the level of physical activity - must be considered. Such were the conclusions of Expert Consultation of FAO / WHO/ UNO (Rome 1981; WHO Geneva 1985). The amount of energy ingested ought to be individually calculated on the basis of the estimation of basal as well as total energy output, and of the energy necessary for growth. Thus, the recommendations of WHO concern not only how much energy out to be ingested, but also how much ought to be spent by exercise and physical activity so as to achieve healthy growth, and cardiovascular and muscular development. An adequate level of physical activity and nutrition is also considered as important factors in the prevention during early growth of noninfectious diseases later in life (WHO, Geneva 1980).

At the present time, in cities of industrially developed countries it is often more difficult to provide facilities needed for adequate physical activity and exercise for children than to provide them enough food. This applies especially for great urban agglomerations. But the situation may be inadequate even in smaller communities, due to an insufficient interest and attractive opportunity for exercise, which concerns both parents and children.

3 Preschool children

Already at preschool age it is important to provide good opportunities for play and exercise of children. This period is also characterised as a "golden age of motorics". Cardiorespiratory capacity of children from 3 to 6 years of age improves significantly, which applies also to the development of physical performance in running, jumping, throwing, muscle strength and skill (Parizkova et al. 1983). Repeated research of all these parameters in our country showed the trends of development during the past 18 years, and also helped to specify the impact of various environmental variables such as nutrition and regular exercise.

Recent measurements of 1005 preschool children in 1988 showed that body size does not increase due to acceleration trends so much as before (Table 1). The level of motor performance showed a trend for better results as compared to the measurements several years ago (Table 2). Also skill tests showed good results; body posture, however, showed a trend for slight deterioration, mostly in boys.

Simultaneously, the impact of the situation in the family, e.g. of the education level of parents was examined in 9,572 children as regards their enrolment in exercise. Children of the parents with higher level of education tended to be taller, with lower body mass index, and were significantly more often enrolled in regular physical education of all forms suitable for this age period (e.g. the physical education classes of the children with one of the parents and/or grandparents, or gymnastics, skiing). Regular exercise always improved significantly the parameters of growth and physical performance already during preschool age.

Longitudinal observations of spontaneous levels of physical activity using pedometers in 34 children in the last year of kindergarten and later during the first year of primary school showed a significant decrease (98.8 + 14.1 km and 52.5 + 7.5 km per week respectively) which concerned the activity during weekdays, and during weekends.

Several examinations of usual dietary intake showed an increased energy intake mainly due to high amount of fat in the diet of urban children (Parizkova et al. 1983, 1986).

Table 1. Characteristics of somatic development in preschool children (boys n=506, girls n=499).

Age (years)		I		II		III	
		3	4	4	5	5	6
		boys	girls	boys	girls	boys	girls
Height (cm)	X	107.6	104.2	114.2	113.1	118.0	116.6
	SD	5.7	5.0	5.8	5.2	4.8	4.4
Weight (kg)	X	18.1	17.7	20.2	19.8	22.0	21.2
	SD	2.6	2.3	3.0	3.0	4.2	2.9
BMI	X	14.6	14.4	13.6	13.7	13.3	13.4
	SD	1.8	1.5	1.5	1.9	2.0	1.7
Chest	X	56.0	55.3	57.8	56.5	59.2	57.4
circumf. (cm)	SD	4.1	3.4	3.0	3.8	4.9	3.9
Waist	X	52.7	51.9	53.7	52.5	54.3	52.4
circumf. (cm)	SD	4.7	3.5	3.6	4.2	5.5	3.7
Hips	X	58.4	58.6	54.4	60.9	62.0	62.7
circumf. (cm)	SD	4.5	3.7	4.1	4.2	5.0	3.9
Birth	X	3389	3252	3413	3302	3402	3324
weight (g)	SD	611	450	531	482	512	527

4 Obesity in childhood

The impact of overweight and obesity on physical performance was not as obvious in preschool children as later on in early school age and adolescence. Only broad jump was shorter in overweight children; performances in running and throwing were not significantly different.

But obese children in later years show significantly lower levels of aerobic power and performance in most physical fitness tests. Therefore, the reduction therapy using both monitored diet and exercise not only decreased body mass, body mass index and the amount of depot fat, but also improved functional parameters, e.g. decreased the oxygen consumption during the same work load, increased vital capacity and improved performance in most fitness tests. Aerobic power increased significantly, and the oxygen ceiling was achieved after a greater work load on a treadmill, i.e. after longer duration and higher velocity of treadmill running (Parizkova and Hainer 1989).

Table 2. Development of physical performance in preschool children.

		I		II		III	
		boys	girls	boys	girls	boys	girls
20 m dash	X	6.63	6.90	6.30	6.25	5.70	5.80
	SD	1.80	1.70	1.70	1.61	1.40	1.40
500 m run	X	219.21	231.30	201.03	208.10	183.30	188.70
(s)	SD	41.10	44.74	47.35	45.70	40.40	32.23
broad jump	X	87.8	84.00	100.4	95.5	110.65	106.20
(cm)	SD	17.6	18.3	20.2	19.8	17.0	17.4
ball throw	X	618.5	467.3	800.7	600.6	938.9	639.4
(right) (cm)	SD	232.2	148.3	308.6	229.5	304.9	146.7
ball throw	X	444.3	372.6	560.6	462.2	638.2	523.8
(left) (cm)	SD	187.2	122.6	216.9	162.7	239.8	193.6

5 Body composition, blood lipids and physical activity in early childhood

An adequate regime of nutrition and exercise appears thus as an indispensable factor, in optimal mutual relationship, for achieving and preserving desirable development of the growing organism from the morphological, functional and health points of view. This was apparent moreover from the observations of preschool children with both high and low levels of spontaneous physical activity during the preschool period. Children with high levels of activity tended to be slimmer with a trend for higher dietary intake, higher level of cardiorespiratory efficiency (as shown by the results of modified step test). Such children had also significantly higher levels of HDL as compared to children who were spontaneously much less active (Parizkova et al. 1986).

6 Nutrition and physical training during growth and adolescence

6.1 Gymnastics

The impact of nutrition is also apparent when following adolescents enrolled in some sort of sport training. Very special case are e.g. girl gymnasts who ought to preserve a particular physique corresponding to the needs of this sport. Short girls are primarily selected, and their weight and body composition development are carefully monitored. These girls are usually below the 50th percentile of the national growth grids in stature; the same applies to body weight, body mass index and fatness. When they continued to grow in their particular growth channels, they trained and performed without particular problems; when they fell below their particular growth channel, they had problems concerning both physical performance and sometimes health.

The monitoring of dietary intake in gymnastic training has been most necessary for girls (Parizkova 1986), and not so much for boys who need more muscle strength for their performance. Their energy intake may therefore be relatively higher, even when in comparison with other sport disciplines (e. g. swimming, track-and-field etc.) it has been always lower (Tables 3, 4)

However, when gymnasts changed their energy output as e.g. in the mountains where their training also included skiing, their intake of energy and other food components increased significantly to much higher levels. The evaluation of the energy output as related to the energy input during six days of ski training in the mountains was performed. The energy output was estimated from heart rate using Sporttesters, with the help of a three-compartmental linear model based on the relationship (regression lines) between heart rate and oxygen uptake established individually for each subject. The energy balance was well established during six days of ad libitum food intake. The aerobic power of these gymnasts was also on an adequate level (i.e. 60. 2 $\pm$ 5. 1 ml O_2/ kg body weight/min (Heller et al. 1989).

The mechanical efficiency was 26.03 $\pm$ 1.4% : in normal untrained subjects the mechanical efficiency under the same conditions is usually 20 -21% (Heller et al. 1989; Parizkova and Heller, in press).

Under such conditions, no energy deficit was apparent; but in girl gymnasts it seemed that some economization of energy output occurs, as theoretical estimations of their energy output did not correspond well to their energy intake. Improved mechanical efficiency and adaptation to lower levels of energy intake resulting in better energy efficiency obviously occurrred, as was also shown in other cases such as agricultural workers in East Java (Edmundson 1977). Satisfactory health and desirable levels of physical performance may exist in well adapted individuals even under such conditions.

Table 3. Mean values of somatic indices, body composition and of the daily intake of energy, nutrients, minerals and vitamins in boy swimmers (n=10) (V_X = coefficient of variation).

	X	SD	V_X
Age (years)	16.55	2.08	12.5
Height (cm)	180.1	5.4	2.9
Weight (kg)	67.0	5.2	7.7
Body mass index	20.6	1.0	4.8
Depot fat (%)	11.4	2.8	24.5
Lean body mass (kg)	59.3	4.7	7.9
Intake of energy (MJ/day)	15.77	3.58	22
Intake of proteins(total-g/day)	116	17	14
Intake of proteins (animal-g/day)	81	15	18
Intake of proteins (plant-g/day)	35	6	17
Intake of fats (total-g/day)	179	40	22
Intake of fats (animal-g/day)	101	22	21
Intake of fats (plant-g/day)	78	24	30
Intake of carbohydrates (g/day)	435	126	28
Intake of minerals : Ca (mg/day)	898	351	39
Fe (mg/day)	19	4	21
Intake of vitamins : A (µg/day)	1568	504	32
B_1 (mg/day)	2.5	0.3	12
B_2 (mg/day)	1.6	3	11
PP (mg/day)	27	3	11
C (mg/day)	54	19	35

Table 4. Mean values of somatic indices, body composition and of the daily intake of energy, nutrients, mineral and vitamins in girl track-and-field athletes (n=9) (V_X = coefficient of variation).

	X	SD	V_X
Age (years)	17.78	0.43	2.4
Height (cm)	167.16	1.64	1.0
Weight (kg)	52.7	1.76	3.3
Body mass index	18.8	0.3	1.5
Depot fat (%)	7.6	3.4	46.2
Intake of energy (kJ/day)	14328	3688	25.7
Intake of proteins (total-g/day)	110	27	25.1
Intake of proteins (animal-g/day)	71	16	22.7
Intake of proteins (plant-g/day)	39	17	45.8
Intake of fats (total-g/day)	140	31	22.3
Intake of fats (animal-g/day)	96	31	32.5
Intake of fats (plant-g/day)	44	2	6.0
Intake of carbohydrates (g/day)	446	124	27.9
Intake of minerals : Ca (mg/day)	1682	577	34.3
Fe (mg/day)	14.7	4.5	25
Intake of vitamins : A (µg/day)	1969	386	19.6
B_1 (mg/day)	1.6	0.57	35.5
B_2 (mg/day)	2.7	0.4	16.2
PP (mg/day)	20.3	9.1	44.7
C (mg/day)	95	42	44.9

6.2 Diving
Another exemple of adolescents in training who had to watch their body weight and fatness were girl divers (Table 5). Their energy intake does not differ much from that for normal girls without any intensive training.

This applies both to energy and individual food components. The comparison of the intake of the main food components, i.e. energy and proteins with both normal population and other exercising groups of adolescents showed only slightly increased values (Parizkova and Heller, in press).

6.3 Skiing, track-and-field
Observations of groups training in dynamic sport disciplines such as cross-country skiing and track-and-field show much higher values of dietary intake (Tables 6, 7). Training of this character has high energy demands; food intake ad libitum is therefore possible which also ensures a higher supply of proteins, fats, carbohydrates, vitamins and minerals. Body weight and fatness do not increase when energy needs are met by an adequate energy intake.

7 Importance of diet monitoring and weight-watching

However, it is necessary to monitor in growing subjects the dietary intakes when the intensity and character of training are changing during various parts of the training cycle. Unwanted increased deposition of fat can occur (e.g. during a period of interrupted training, or illness or injury when the dietary intake is not well monitored due to the regulations mentioned above).

Recommended dietary allowances for adolescent athletes therefore have to be carefully controlled the same as for the normal population. Reduction of weight during growth is always a problem, especially in adolescents who undergo intensive training. At the present time this has become a topic of special interest as more and more of athletes with unfinished growth and development take part in top level sport. Recommended dietary allowances (RDA) have been established for adult athletes in many countries; however, as regards training children and adolescents, very few data are available up to now in spite of the fact that adequate nutrition is even more important for the growing organism than for the adult.

8 Interindividual variations in dietary intake

Similarly to adult athletes (Parizkova 1989), there has always appeared a marked interindividual variability in dietary intakes under the same conditions of training in relatively very homogeneous groups of adolescent athletes. "Nutritional individualities" exist since the beginning of life, as shown e.g. in infants during the first year of life. Dietary guidelines are indispensable, but the individual approach ought to be

Table 5. Mean values of somatic indices, body composition and of the daily intake of energy, nutrients, mineral and vitamins in girl divers (n=8) (V_X = coefficient of variation).

	X	SD	V_X
Age (years)	17.35	2.44	11.8
Height (cm)	164.1	2.14	1.3
Weight (kg)	56.6	5.43	9.5
Body mass index	21.0	1.65	7.8
Depot fat (%)	12.5	4.0	32.0
Intake of energy (kJ/day)	8770	1979	22
Intake of proteins (total-g/day)	74	14	19
Intake of proteins (animal-g/day)	48	9	18
Intake of proteins (plant-g/day)	26	6	23
Intake of fats (total-g/day)	80	21	26
Intake of fats (animal-g/day)	54	14	26
Intake of fats (plant-g/day)	26	14	53
Intake of carbohydrates (g/day)	272	74	27
Intake of minerals : Ca (mg/day)	576	241	41
Fe (mg/day)	11.9	3	25
Intake of vitamins : A (µg/day)	855	253	29
B_1 (mg/day)	1.2	0.3	25
B_2 (mg/day)	1.4	0.3	21
PP (mg/day)	17.2	4.2	24
C (mg/day)	105	102	97

respected when monitoring dietary regimes for growing athletes. The most important criteria are satisfactory health, optimal functional capacity level and achievement of high athletic performance. However, it was shown that individuals can get along well, achieving good results, with very differing dietary intakes.

Table 6. Mean values of somatic indices, body composition and of the daily intake of energy, nutrients, mineral and vitamins in female skiers (during school year) (n=10) (V_X = coefficient of variation).

	X	SD	V_X
Age (years)	15.66	1.32	15.7
Height (cm)	164.7	5.73	3.4
Weight (kg)	50.03	7.29	14.7
Body mass index	18.44	0.5	2.7
Depot fat (%)	9.13	5.6	61.3
Intake of energy (kJ/day)	11682.3	1470.7	12.6
Intake of proteins (total-g/day)	84.8	13.3	13.3
Intake of proteins (animal-g/day)	44.6	6.9	15.6
Intake of proteins (plant-g/day)	40.2	6.3	15.8
Intake of fats (total-g/day)	117.6	17.7	10.9
Intake of fats (animal-g/day)	82.1	8.8	10.8
Intake of fats (plant-g/day)	35.5	8.9	25.0
Intake of carbohydrates (g/day)	366.8	64.7	17.6
Intake of minerals : Ca (mg/day)	878.6	184.2	20.9
Fe (mg/day)	12.1	2.0	16.8
Intake of vitamins : A (µg/day)	1581.2	297.9	18.8
B_1 (mg/day)	1.4	0.25	17.5
B_2 (mg/day)	1.8	0.35	19.0
PP (mg/day)	16.9	3.5	20.5
C (mg/day)	80.43	27.2	33.9

Nevertheless great care must be applied to diet when preparing young athletes for top level sport; deficiencies have often been found, concerning e.g. minerals (Ca, Fe), vitamins (C, PP factor etc.) and fiber in those who did not adopt adequate nutritional habits early in life (Parizkova 1989; Parizkova and Keller, in press). This happens much more often than is

Table 7. Mean values of somatic indices, body composition and of the daily intake of energy, nutrients, mineral and vitamins in female skiers (training camp; n=10) (V_X = coefficient of variation).

	X	SD	V_X
Age (years)	15.7	1.37	8.4
Height (cm)	165.2	5.1	3.1
Weight (kg)	50.03	7.00	13.9
Body mass index	18.3	1.5	8.1
Depot fat (%)	11.0	3.2	29.2
Intake of energy (kJ/day)	17369.6	2939.0	16.9
Intake of proteins (total-g/day)	115.6	19.8	16.8
Intake of proteins (animal-g/day)	61.7	10.3	16.7
Intake of proteins (plant-g/day)	53.9	9.4	17.5
Intake of fats (total-g/day)	165.4	46.4	25.7
Intake of fats (animal-g/day)	117.5	39.1	33.3
Intake of fats (plant-g/day)	47.9	7.3	15.2
Intake of carbohydrates (g/day)	570.2	78.7	13.8
Intake of minerals : Ca (mg/day)	1100.8	227.1	20.6
Fe (mg/day)	19.1	3.2	16.6
Intake of vitamins : A (µg/day)	2202	494.6	22.4
B_1 (mg/day)	2.13	0.3	14.0
B_2 (mg/day)	2.77	0.5	18.05
PP (mg/day)	27.0	3.8	14.1
C (mg/day)	129.5	15.9	12.6

realized, and applies mostly to those sport disciplines in which weight watching is necessary even during growth. In such cases permanent supervision of dietary intakes is indispensable, supplying to young individuals all of the recommended dietary allowances for their age groups.

97

9 Conclusions

The monitoring of dietary intakes during growth may be of the same importance as the monitoring of work load in training. The results of good training can be negated by unsatisfactory dietary regimes. This applies not only to those who are enrolled in regular training, but to the whole of growing population.

Energy intake and output must be considered in mutual relationship; so that not only the actual health level and physical development can be assured, but also the predisposition for future status as adults can be guaranteed. Health and physical performance of children and adolescents are the key to the health, economic productivity and physical fitness of adults; optimal balance between diet and exercise is of the utmost importance for that.

10 References

Edmundson, W. (1977) Individual variations in work output per unit energy intake, in **East Java. Ecol. Food Nutr.** , 8, pp. 147-151.

Heller, J. Novotny, I. Bunc, V. Parizkova, I. Dlouha, R. Tuma, 5. (1989) Energy expenditure during training of Junior gymnasts. **Trener**, 33, 686-688 (in Czech).

Parizkova, J. (1986) Body compositon and nutrition in different types of athletes, in **Proceedings of the XIII International Congres of Nutrition**, (eds T.G. Taylor and N.K. Jenkins), John Libbey, London and Paris, pp. 309-311.

Parizkova, J. (1987) Growth, functional capacity and physical fitness in normal and malnourished children, in **Nutrition in health and disease** (ed G. H. Bourne), Wld. Rev. Nutr., Karger, Basel, pp. 1-44.

Parizkova, J. (1989) Age dependent changes in dietary intake related to work output. **Amer. J. Clin. Nutr.** 89, 962-967.

Parizkova, J. Adamec, A. Berdychova, J. Cermak, J. Horna, J. Teply, J. (1983) **Growth, fitness and nutrition in preschool children.** Universitas Carolina, Prague.

Parizkova, J. Hainer,V. (1989) Exercise in growing and adult obese individuals, in **Current therapy in sports medicine** (eds J. S. Torg, R. P. Welsh and R. J. Shephard), B. C. Decker Inc., Toronto and Philadelphia.

Parizkova, J. Mackova, E. Kabele, J. Mackova, J. and Skopkova, M. (1986) Body composition, food intake, cardiorespiratory fitness, blood lipids and psychological development in highly active and inactive preschool children. **Hum. Biol.** , 58, 261-273.

- , **Energy and protein requirements** (1985). Report of a Joint FAO / WHO / UNO Expert Consultation. Technical Report Series 724, World Health Organization, Geneva.

6

WINDSURFING: EFFECTS OF YOUTH-SPECIFIC CHANGES IN MATERIALS AND TECHNIQUES CONCERNING THE LOAD ON THE LOWER BACK DURING THE LIFTING OF THE SAIL

D. DE CLERCQ, N. DEBO and R. CLAEYS
Institute of Physical Education, State University of Gent, Belgium

Keywords: Windsurfing, Youth sport, Lumbar spine.

1 Introduction

1.1 Youngsters in windsurfing

During the last decade windsurfing has known a spectacular growth. Both in leisure and in competitive windsurfing, a lot of youngsters are involved. It's difficult to have an exact idea about the number of windsurfing adherents. Most of them practise their sport in family or with friends, on holiday or combined with other leisure activities.
The federal Windsurfing Federation of Flanders (LWF) estimates the "known" windsurfers, who are member of club, as less than 10% of the total number of practitioners. The data in Table 1 give an idea about the number of youngsters involved.

Based on these data we can estimate the number of youngsters who are practising windsurfing in Flanders on a more or less regular basis, around

Table 1. Youth windsurfing in Flanders in 1989.

Members of a Windsurfing club (LWF)	
12y - 13y : 352	
14y - 15y : 645	TOT. 2371
16y - 17y : 740	
18y - 19y : 634	

Participants in Windsurfing classes (LWF and BLOSO°)	
age < 14y : 4796	TOT. 9616°°
20y > age > 14y : 4820	

°BLOSO : Flemish Administration for Sports and Open Air recreation
°°An overlap between the LWF members and the participants in
   windsurfing classes could exist

100,000. The competitive youth circuit is growing every year. The federal and national school championships give access to European and even World finals. Youth windsurfing will also be a part of the World Gymnasiade in Bruges in 1990.

In the Netherlands, the Royal Dutch Water Sports federation (KNWV) estimates the number of youngsters in windsurfing between 100,000 and 200,000. In competition the minimal age limit is 12 years in Flanders and 13 years in the Netherlands.

1.2 Low back pains in windsurfing
Only a few studies report on injuries caused by windsurfing (e.g. Boydens 1983). Low back pains are the most frequent injury. These findings are in conformity with the everyday experiences when teaching windsurfing. The lifting of the sail is always pointed out as the main malefactor. Despite improvements in materials and technical guidelines in windsurfing books, low back pains remain the windsurfing injury n°1. A biomechanical study was conducted to examine the lifting of the sail under different conditions.

2 Method

To control all external influences, the lifting of the sail was executed in the swimming pool. With the sail lying in the water, the subject was standing on the border of the swimming pool. The kinematics in the saggital plane were studied by 16 mm film analysis at 60 sec^{-1}. Ground reaction forces were measured at 850 sec^{-1} with a built-in Kistler force plate. In a previous study (De Clercq 1983), a perfect correlation between the ground reaction forces and the force exerted on the pull up rope was found. Twelve college students (6 males and 6 females) aged 19 ± 1.5 years participated in the new study. All results were calculated proportional to the individual's length and weight. The following conditions were alternated: two different movement techniques, the speed of lifting and the material characteristics of the rigg. The rigg consists of the sail, the mast and the wishbone.

3 Results

3.1 First condition: the movement technique.
In the "old" technique, which is still frequently used, the surfer starts in a deep position and bends the knees maximally. Most of the time the back is in kyphosis, although the subjects are instructed to keep the back

upright during the whole movement. The knees are stretched and the body leans backwards to lift the sail.

In the "new" counterbalance technique, the subject starts with the body in a nearly upright position. Then the subject leans backwards without a significant change in knee or hip angle. The back remains in the normal anatomic position.

The time history of the resulting ground reaction force on the feet during the lifting of the sail indicates where the force is at the highest level. In both techniques the load is maximal during the initial phase, namely the first degrees of lifting, because of the water which has to flow out of the sail.

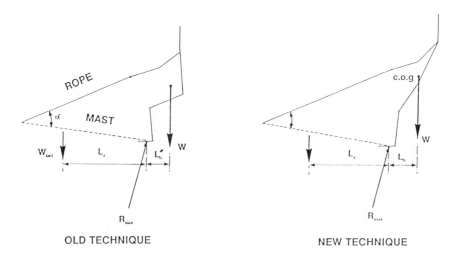

OLD TECHNIQUE   NEW TECHNIQUE

Fig.1. Stick figures representing the position of the subject and the rigg at the time when the maximal resulting ground reaction force is measured.

The rigg rotates out of the water around an axis through a fixation point (mast feet) which is located between the feet of the subject. In both movement techniques, this rotation in the dorsal direction is due to a moment in which the weight of the surfer (Wbody) plays an important role (Fig.1).

Some essential differences between the old and new techniques were found, however.

3.1a. Functional differences
The path of the center of gravity (c.o.g.) of the body is different (Fig. 2). In the old leg extension technique, the c.o.g. is travelling mainiy upwards. The displacement backwards is less important. In the new technique, the

c.o.g. displacement occurs exclusively in an antero-dorsal direction. Through that the force arm of the dorsal moment is longer (e.g. Fig. 1: at the time of Rmax L_b is 0.055 ± 0.015 m larger than L'_b). In the new technique the lift force is generated in a passive way by leaning backwards. In the old technique the leg extension contributes to the lifting of the sail.

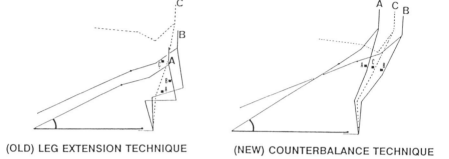

(OLD) LEG EXTENSION TECHNIQUE   (NEW) COUNTERBALANCE TECHNIQUE

Fig. 2. Path of the center of gravity (c.o.g.) of the subject illustrated withstick diagrams of some representative positions : A. starting position; B. position at maximal ground reaction force; C. ending position

In both techniques, the maximal ground reaction force occurs at 46 ± 5 % of the total lifting time. Although not significant, this maximal resulting ground reaction force (R_{max}) is smaller when performing the new technique: 1.24 ± 0.07 times body weight against 1.28 ± 0.09) B.W. for the old technique. This could be explained by the magnitude of the functional angle α (Fig.1) which is throughout the movement a few degrees larger when using the new counterbalance technique.

The evolution of the knee angle differs a lot in both techniques. In the old technique the knee angle remains the first part of the movement (68 ± 6% of the total lifting time) below 110°. In the new technique the knee angle is always larger than 140° and therefore the stress on the quadriceps and the patella will be much lower. This possitive effect of the larger knee angle is caused by the geometry of the forces acting around the knee articulation and is also due to the reinforcement of the knee extension action by a co-contraction of the harmstrings.

3.1b Differences in the load on the lumbar spine

A simplified free body technique for coplanar forces will be used to illustrate the quasi-static load conditions on the spine when the rigg is pulled out of the water. The free body diagram of the upper body is drawn in the position where the maximal ground reaction force is measured. In both techniques four forces are acting on the spine. The reaction force produced by the sail (Rsail) and the force produced by the weight of the upper body (W) are counteracted by the force produced by the contraction of the erector spinae muscles (M). These forces produce torques at the lumbo-sacral joint (L5-S1) and result also in a compression force (C) on L5.

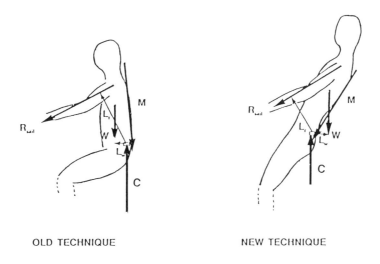

OLD TECHNIQUE   NEW TECHNIQUE

Fig. 3. Free body diagram to illustrate the quasi-static load conditions on the spine during the lifting of the sail: old knee extension technique and new counterbalance technique, both in the position where the maximal ground reaction force is measured.

The large forward bending moment ($R_{sail} \times L_R$) is counteracted by a moment ($M \times L_M$). As the lever arm L_M is small ($\pm$ 0.05m) the erector spinae muscles have to develop a very high tension. The frequent high stresses on those muscles are a first reason for the occurrence of low back pains after a windsurfing session. However, when using the new counterbalance technique to lift the sail, the intensity of the contraction of the erector spinae muscles will be much lower due to the positive

103

contribution of the moment produced by the upper body weight (W x L_W) and to the smaller negative lever arm L_R.

A second reason for low back pains are the large compressive forces which act on the lumbar spine. For the old technique, a maximal compressive force of 7.3 $\pm$ 1.2 times body weight was calculated (0° inclination of L5). Such values are in the same range of the compressive forces reported in a load (50 kg) lifting study from Jäger (1989). Based upon the literature, Jäger concludes that such large compressive forces, falling within the same range as the static strenght values of the lumbar spine, should be avoided.

Even when the compression is in the same order of magnitude for both lift techniques, the new technique is still an advantage. This counter-balance technique allows the surfer to stand in an upright position. The spine will stay more or less in its normal anatomical position with a good dispersion of the compressive loads on the intervertebral discs. When using the old technique, the trunk bends forward, which causes a kyphosis of the spine. The intervertebral disc is subjected to an uneven distribution of stress. The disc bulges on the compressive side which results in an increased stress on the dorsal ligaments of the spine.

Concerning the load on the spine we can conclude that the position of the trunk, forwards in the old technique and backwards in the new technique, makes the main difference.

3.2 Second condition: the speed of lifting the sail
The speed of pulling out the sail influences the load drastically. Increasing the speed by 10% resulted in much larger ground reaction forces on the feet. A rise of more than 30% was measured. A certain amount of water has to flow out of the emerged sail. Therefore, the first phase of the movement should be slow.

3.3 Third condition: characteristics of the rigg
The weight of the sail, the mast or the wishbone influence the load significantly. The dimensions and the shape of the sail are even more important. When lifting a large sail (6.5 m^2) instead of a small sail (4.1 m^2), especially designed for beginners, the maximal ground reaction forces exceeded in both movement techniques 1.45 times body weight. When the emerged part of the sail enlarges or when the distribution is further away from the mast feet, the weight (W_S) or the lever arm (L_S) increase (Fig. 1).

3.4 Conclusions
The new counterbalance technique is more effective by creating in a passive way a dorsal moment to turn the sail out of the water. Due to a backwards position of the trunk, the new technique combines a smaller

load with a better posture of the spine. In order to keep the load as low as possible a slow performance and an adapted rigg are recommended.

4 Youth-specific guidelines concerning the movement technique and the characteristics of the rigg

4.1 Movement technique
It has been demonstrated in the biomechanical approach that the new counterbalance technique should be taught. The pupils should be instructed to lean backwards in a passive way, without bending the arms or the legs and with the back and the head in an upright position. Hyperextension of the back should not occur. The speed of movement is of major importance: the slower, the better.

When an appropriate light-weight rigg is used, the child should grasp the pull-up rope with one hand. This allows the free arm to hang downwards thus reinforcing the dorsal moment. After the initial phase, when the sail has turned $\pm$ 60 degrees out of the water, the arms can raise the rigg further.

4.2 Characteristics of a rigg adapted for children
First of all a youth rigg has to be light. A maximal weight of 3.5 kg is recommended. This light weight can be achieved by smaller dimensions and adapted light materials. The area of the sail measures between 2 and 3 m^2. The mast, $\pm$ 3.2m long, and the wishbone, with a length of $\pm$ 1.4 m, can be made out of thin aluminum tubes. All pieces must be watertight. A little ball attached to the top of the mast can prevent it from sinking. The pull-up rope should be long enough to allow the surfer to lean backwards with stretched arms when lifting the sail. The pull-up rope should be partially connected with the top of the mast in order to create a long force arm.

4.3 Other recommendations
When teaching windsurfing, especially with children, it makes sense to limit the number of falls as much as possible. Easy, stable boards should be used. The weather conditions should be appropriate for beginners i.e. low winds (<10 knots or <3Bft) and smooth water. For initiation, a minimal age limit of 10 years is suggested.

5 References

Boydens, E. De Clercq, D. (1983) Enkele medische en biomechanische aspecten van het windsurfen, in **Congresboek van de 2de Sportgeneeskundige dagen van het AZ St-Jan**, Brugge.

De Clercq, D. (1983) Bewegingsanalyse van het optrekken van het zeil bij windsurfing, in **Congresboek van de 2de Sportgeneeskundige dagen van het AZ St-Jan**, Brugge.

Farke, U. Schröder, D. (1985) **Ich will auch Surfen**. Delius Klassing, Bielefeld.

Jäger, M. Luttmann, A. (1989) Biomechanical analysis and assessment of lumbar stress during load lifting using a dynamic 19 - segment human model, in: **Ergonomics**, vol. 32, pp. 93-112

Nordin, M. Frankel, V. (1989) **Basic Biomechanics of the Musculoskeletal System**. Lea and Febiger, Philadelphia, 183-207

7

SKELETAL RUGGEDNESS AS A FACTOR IN PERFORMANCE OF OLYMPIC AND NATIONAL CALIBRE SYNCHRONISED SWIMMERS

M.R. HAWES and D. SOVAK
The University of Calgary, Alberta, Canada

Keywords: Kinanthropometry, Density, Proportionality, Muscle mass, Bone mass, Segmental volumes.

1 Introduction

The successful performer in synchronised swimming combines athletic ability in executing complex figures with an easy grace and attractive performance. Factors such as strength, endurance, aerobic and anaerobic capacity have been reported as important characteristics that contribute to the success of elite synchro swimmers. However, it has been suggested that another factor that may be of considerable significance in the graceful performance of complex movements at and above the surface of the water is the ease of flotation (Roby et al 1989) or buoyancy characteristics of the competitor. Buoyancy is determined through the interplay of body tissues of greater or lesser density than water and thus the monitoring of the body composition of synchronised swimmers takes on additional importance. Synchronised swimming coaches may use body composition data to chart progress in conditioning but they may also use the data to understand why an athlete may have difficulty performing certain skills. It is the purpose of this paper to examine body composition data determined by standard anthropometric methods for evidence of increased buoyancy in synchronised swimmers of national and Olympic calibre.

Various estimates of the density of human tissues have been suggested. The value of 0.900 g/ml reported by Fidanza et al. (1953) is well accepted as the density of human fat while recognising that small amounts of lipid are found in the brain with slightly higher density. The density of fat free muscle is reported by Allen (1959) as 1.070 g/ml and Martin (1984) estimated the density of fat free bone at 1.431 g/ml and residual tissue at 1.039 g/ml. It is evident (Martin et al. 1985) that there is considerable variation in the proportion, and in the case of bone, density of human tissues and thus the contribution of individual tissues to buoyancy can at best only be estimated. It is clear that positive buoyancy may be enhanced by a proportionate increase of adipose tissue or by a proportionate reduction of adipose tissue free muscle, bone or residual tissue. The density of bone is much further removed from the density of water than fat, muscle or residual and small changes in skeletal mass will have a proportionately greater effect on buoyancy than the other tissues. Bone mass may be altered by changes in bone density or in shape (primarily breadth).

2 Methods

Anthropometric analysis of the body composition of Canadian national and international calibre synchronised swimmers has routinely been conducted in the Sport Anthropology Laboratory at the University of Calgary since 1986. The initial assessment consisting of 56 directly measured parameters many of which are subsequently used to compute secondary variables describing overall body composition and active tissue (muscle+bone) diameters, volumes and masses in the upper and lower extremities has been described by Sovak and Hawes (1987). On subsequent testing 38 directly measured parameters are recorded yielding 17 secondary variables which are anticipated to respond to short term training or dietary regimes. All measurements are taken on the right side of the body using anthropometric procedures according to Ross and Marfell Jones (1982), Parizkova (1978) and Ulbrichova (1977). The data for this study were collected by the same investigator (DS) whose reliability of repeated measurement had previously been established beyond the 0.01 level of confidence.

3 Subjects

Two groups of subjects and one case study are included in this study - a world and Olympic synchronised swimming champion (OCHAMP), 14 members of the Canadian national synchronised swimming team as of September 1989 (NATSS) and 77 female university students (REF). Anthropometric assessments had been conducted on the synchro swimmers on a regular basis for several years, for the purposes of this study the last test date (OCHAMP Sept. 1988; NATSS Sept. 1989) was assumed to reflect their peak condition. All subjects were Caucasian and their mean age (± S.D.) at the last test date was 22.37yrs, 18.96 ± 1.20yrs, 20.2 ± 3.3yrs for OCHAMP, NATSS and REF respectively. All subjects provided informed consent prior to participation. The mean and standard deviation of the REF and NATSS scores was determined for all variables and the Student t test at a level of 0.05 was accepted as statistically significant. T scores were computed to compare the case study to group means and a difference of 10 points was accepted as an indication of disproportionality.

Table 1. Mean and SD of anthropometric variables for REF, NATSS and OCHAMP.

Variable	Reference Group n = 77		National Team n = 14		Olympic Champion
	X	S.D.	X	S.D.	
Age (yr)	20,20	3,30	18,96	1,20	22,37
Height (cm)	165,05	5,54	165,22	6,47	169,00
Body mass (kg)	60,50	6,77	58,72	4,33	56,60
Leg length (cm)	88,30	4,60	87,89	4,51	90,40
Trunk length (cm)	46,10	3,20	45,76	1,94	45,90
ITL	52,20	3,50	52,15	2,65	50,77
Body composition					
Sum of 10 skinfolds (mm)	132,07	42,23	117,49	18,36	104,30
Fat (%)	21,83	5,44	20,49	2,68	17,58
Skeleton (%)	13,88	1,73	14,51	0,76	13,33
Muscle (%)	35,58	3,66	*37,88	3,09	37,60
F:M ratio (g fat/kg muscle)	729,75	227,75	*548,1	109,76	467,58
Corrected diameters (cm)					
CDU (upper arm)	6,91	0,70	*7,26	0,50	7,46
CDF (forearm)	6,58	0,36	6,74	0,19	6,69
CDT (thigh)	13,47	1,06	13,50	0,69	12,87
CDC (calf)	9,00	0,52	8,84	0,58	8,19
Segment lengths (cm)					
Upper arm proximal	13,67	0,48	13,56	0,88	}
Upper arm distal	13,08	1,06	*13,97	0,89	}26.60
Forearm proximal	3,08	0,46	*2,53	0,47	}
Forearm distal	18,96	0,88	*20,53	1,55	}22.80
Thigh proximal	19,68	0,78	*21,14	1,07	}
Thigh distal	20,03	0,93	*20,93	1,09	}42.80
Calf proximal	12,16	1,16	*11,35	0,85	}
Calf distal	26,42	1,35	*27,74	2,47	}40.10
Segment fat free volumes (l)					
FF vol UA	1,20	0,22	*1,4	0,17	1,39
FF vol F	0,52	0,05	*0,57	0,04	0,57
FF vol T	5,89	0,64	*6,32	0,59	5,99
FF vol C	1,85	0,20	1,93	0,22	1,72
Bone breadths (cm)					
Biepicondylar humerus	6,15	1,40	6,12	0,23	5,90
Bistyloideus	4,89	0,30	4,90	0,18	4,50
Biepicondylar femur	8,76	0,60	8,86	0,30	8,30
Bimaleolare	6,28	0,40	6,31	0,27	5,70

* $\alpha = 0.05$

109

4 Results

The mean and standard deviation of the anthropometric data for the three groups are shown in Table 1. It is evident that REF and NATSS are closely matched in age, height and leg and trunk lengths. OCHAMP is slightly older and taller than the other two groups with slightly longer legs and a lower ratio of trunk length to leg length (ITL). As would be expected the body composition parameters reflect the intensive nature of the synchronised swimming training regime and the sum of 10 skinfolds (S10SF) and % Fat are lower for NATSS and lower still for OCHAMP.

Estimation of relative skeletal mass indicates higher values for the NATSS than the REF and lower values for OCHAMP. Estimated relative muscle mass is greater for NATSS ($\alpha = 0.05$) and OCHAMP than REF. This is particularly evident in the skinfold corrected diameters of the upper arm (CDU) and forearm (CDF) where both NATSS and OCHAMP have greater values than the REF. Equally significant is the observation that skinfold corrected diameters in the lower extremities (CDT and CDC)

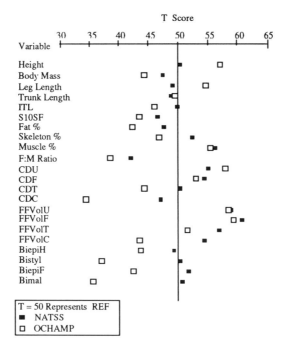

Fig. 1. T-score values of selected anthropometric variables for REF, NATSS and OCHAMP.

are equal or less than that for REF for NATSS and substantially less for OCHAMP. The fat free volumes (FFvol) estimated from the corrected diameters and length of arm and leg segments again illustrate greater muscle mass in the upper extremities for OCHAMP and NATSS ($\alpha = 0.05$) compared to REF, larger thigh ($\alpha = 0.05$) and calf volumes for NATSS over REF and lower calf volume for OCHAMP than NATSS or REF.

The values of selected anthropometric variables are expressed as T scores in fig. 1 where a deviation of 10 points from the mean or individual heights is accepted as an indication of disproportionality. The T score plot graphically illustrates that in most parameters the NATSS have similar proportionate values to the REF group. The exceptions are a trend towards a reduced adipose tissue to muscle ratio (F:M) and a strong tendency towards disproportionately greater adipose tissue free volume in the upper arm and forearm. The OCHAMP, for her height, is disproportionately smaller in ITL, body mass, adipose tissue mass, skeletal mass, F:M, CDT, CDC, FFvolC and all four bony breadths.

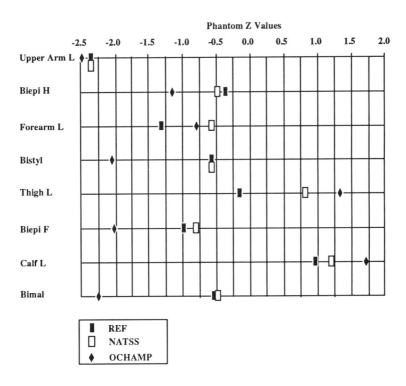

Fig. 2. Phantom Z values for segment lengths and breadths.

The OCHAMP has proportionately less estimated skeletal mass which is evident from narrow bony breadths at the elbow, wrist, knee and ankle. Since the OCHAMP is somewhat taller than both REF and NATSS groups these values were scaled to a unisex reference phantom (Ross and Wilson 1974)) to examine these differences without the influence of size (fig. 2). This figure illustrates that when scaled to a common height the extremity lengths of the three groups are very similar but there is a clear indication that the OCHAMP has narrower bones than either the REF or NATSS groups.

5 Discussion

The purpose of this paper was to examine body composition factors in synchronised swimmers that might contribute to enhanced buoyancy. The evidence suggests that there are very few differences between national calibre synchronised swimmers and a control group of university students. As one would expect S10SF is less, muscle mass is slightly greater and this is located on the upper extremities which are the predominate locomotor limbs in synchronised swimming. The lower extremities of the NATSS group is no different than that of the reference group. These results confirm the observations of Ross et al (1977) who suggested that there were no distinguishing anthropometric features for national calibre synchronised swimmers when compared to a reference group of non-swimming peers. The results of the study by Ross et al. and the current study suggest that up to the level of national competition enhanced buoyancy as evaluated by anthropometry is not a factor in successful competition. However, the case study of an Olympic champion suggests that there may be differences in body composition which enhanced her possibilities of success. The OCHAMP has proportionately less body mass, adipose tissue mass, skeletal mass and bony breadths than either the REF group or her peers on the national team. The reduced adiposity would mitigate against advantageous buoyancy but this may be offset by an inherently slighter skeleton. The use of the unisex phantom to compare the bone breadths of the three groups illustrates that the proportionately narrower bones of the OCHAMP are not a reflection of her increased height and almost certainly improved her buoyancy.

6 Conclusion

Roby et al (1989) have suggested that performance at the national level in synchronised swimming may be enhanced by reduced bone density contributing to above average buoyancy or flotation which implies higher elevation out of the water and a more attractive presentation of skills and figures. It is evident from this case study that positive flotation characteristics may be achieved through narrower bones but the interplay of reduced adipose tissue and increased muscle tissue in elite athletes may only allow them to achieve buoyant characteristics close to those of a reference population.

7 References

Allen, T.H. Krzywicki, H.J. and Roberts, J.E. (1959) Density, fat, water and solids in freshly isolated tissues. **J. Appl. Physiol.,** 14 (6), 1005-1008.

Fidanza, F. Keys, A.and Anderson J.T. (1953) Density of body fat in man and other animals. **J. App. Physiol.,** 6, 252-256.

Martin, A.D. (1984) **An anatomical basis for assessing human body composition: evidence from 25 dissections**. PhD Thesis, Simon Fraser University, pp 77.

Martin, A.D. Ross, W.D. Drinkwater D.T. and Clarijs J.P. (1985) Prediction of body fat by skinfold caliper: assumptions and cadaver evidence. **Int. J. of Obesity**, 9, suppl. 1, 31-39.

Matiegka J. (1921) The testing of physical fitness **Am. J. Phys. Anthropol.,** 4, 223-230.

Mineral content in synchronised swimmers, in **Proceedings of First IOC World Congress on Sport Sciences**, Colorado Springs pp. 198-199.

Parizkova, J. (1978) Lean body mass and depot fat during ontogenesis in humans, in **Nutrition, Physical Fitness and Health.** (eds J. Parizkova and V.A. Rogozkin), International Series on Sport Sciences, 7, University Park Press, Baltimore, pp. 24-51.

Roby, F.B. Atwater, A.E. Going, S.B Lohman, T.G. Puhl, J.L. and Tucker, M. (1989) Bone mineral content in synchronised swimmers, in **Proceedings of First IOC World Congress on Sport Sciences**, Colorado Springs pp. 198-199.

Ross W.D. and Marfell-Jones M.J. (1982) Kinanthropometry, in **Physiological Testing of the Elite Athlete** (eds J.D. MacDougall, H.A.Wenger and H.J. Green), CASS, Ottawa, pp. 75-115.

Ross W.D. and Wilson, N.C. (1974) A stratagem for proportional growth assessment. Children in Exercise (eds M. Hebbelinck and J. Borms), **Acta Paed.,** Suppl. 28, 169-182.

Ross W.D. Corlett J. Drinkwater D. Faulkner R. and Vajda A. (1977) Anthropometry of synchronised swimmers. **Can. J. Appl. Sp. Sc.,** 2, 4 227 (abstract).

Sovak, D. and Hawes M.R. (1987) Anthropological status of international calibre speed skaters. **J. of Sport Sci.,** 5, 287-304.

Ulbrichova, M. (1977) The parameters of body segments. **Dilci zav. zprava DU** VII-5-1313, Praha, VUT FTVS UK, 35-42.

8

APPLICATIONS OF SPINAL SHRINKAGE TO SUBJECTS WITH LOW BACK PAIN

G. GARBUTT, M.G. BOOCOCK, T. REILLY and J.D.G. TROUP
School of Pharmacology, Sunderland Polytechnic, England

Keywords: Spinal loading, Stature, Distance running, Exercise intensity.

1 Introduction

Chronic low back pain affects between 9% and 12% of distance runners (Devereaux and Lachmann 1980; Lutter 1980). It has been suggested that compressive loading which is unavoidable in running, is a possible cause of low back pain (Hirch 1955). Changes in vertebral dimensions are reflected in changes in stature. Therefore decreases in stature have been used to indicate the load on the spine in exercise (Corlett et al. 1987).

In order to use shrinkage as a measure of spinal loading, posture must be controlled during successive measurements. This is done using a purpose built stadiometer, similar to that described by Boocock et al. (1986). The apparatus is interfaced with a BBC microcomputer for data capture, control of procedures and analysis.

De Puky (1935) drew attention to the role of the intervertebral disc in the oscillation of body length. He stated that the pressure of the body weight on the intervertebral discs caused them to flatten which resulted in people being taller in the morning than in the evening. Further he suggested that exercise and spinal loading would increase shrinkage. Both of these suggestions have since been verified (Corlett et al. 1987).

Greater deformation in response to loading has been demonstrated in motion segments from cadavers with degenerated discs (Taylor and Twomey 1980). It is therefore possible that low back pain in runners may be associated with increased spinal shrinkage. The study reported by Garbutt et al. (1990) failed to confirm this.

De Puky (1935) first identified the problems of measuring stature in subjects with low back pain. He attempted unsuccessfully to demonstrate that stature increased after bed-rest in patients on a surgical ward. His lack of success was attributed to 'defensive rigidity' in the muscles as a result of pain.

The purpose of this report is to examine : (1) the effects of shrinkage responses to running in athletes with and without low back pain; (2) the circadian variation in shrinkage in patients with severe low back pain.

2 Methods

2.1 Shrinkage responses to running

Male marathon runners (n=14) were used as subjects in this experiment. The mean ($\pm$ SD) height, weight and age for the group were 176.7 ($\pm$ 6.6) cm, 69.07 ($\pm$ 8.59) kg and 31 ($\pm$ 9) years respectively. Seven of the runners had a history of chronic low back pain, and still had symptoms at the time of testing. Chronic low back pain was defined as pain between the mid-back and buttocks occuring more than once a month, the first episode being at least 12 months prior to testing. The remaining seven were asymptomatic.

Loading was induced by subjecting the runners to two consecutive 15 min bouts on a motor driven treadmill. Measurements on the stadiometer were taken before the first run, after the first run and after the second run. Subjects performed the protocol on three separate occasions and were randomly assigned to either 70%, 85% or 100% of marathon performance speed. Each visit was at 09:00 hours to control for circadian variation in stature (Tyrrell et al. 1985). Subjects were requested to follow their normal daily routine on the morning of the experiments. When this involved a morning run or other strenuous exercise they were asked to refrain from such activity.

2.2 Measurement procedure

To ensure that reliable and accurate data were recorded, each subject underwent a period of training on the stadiometer. They were required to produce 10 consecutive measurements with a standard deviation of less than 0.5 mm. All subjects achieved the target, the average deviation being 0.42 (range 0.26 - 0.49) mm.

The mean of five consecutive, discrete measures was recorded, between which the subjects moved away from the stadiometer to break contact with the posture controlling microswitches (Boocock et al. 1986). Measurement took 4.4 ($\pm$ 0.8) min which included time to allow heel compression to stabilize. This is a modification to the previously reported protocol allowing time for heel compression to occur which could affect shrinkage measurements (Foreman 1989). The possibility that soft tissue compression could affect stature had previously been denied (De Puky 1935).

2.3 Chronic low back pain and diurnal variation

Subjects were eight male patients, aged 32-57 years, on an orthopaedic ward awaiting surgery for chronic low back pain. During this study the same training and measurement criterion as reported for the previous study applied.

The first measurement of stature was made at 07:15 hours immediately on rising from bed. Subsequent measurements were taken and 08:15, 09:15, 10:15, 12:15, 14:15, 18:15 and 22:15 hours.

3 Results

3.1 Shrinkage responses to running

Table 1 shows the results of shrinkage measures taken during treadmill running in the symptomatic and asymptomatic groups. The ANOVA revealed that there was no significant difference in shrinkage response between the two groups ($P>0.05$). There was an effect of running speed, the 100% condition causing greater shrinkage than the other two conditions ($P<0.05$). Significantly greater shrinkage occured in the first 15 min running compared with the second 15 min running ($P<0.05$).

Age was not significantly correlated with shrinkage incurred during running. This applied to all running speeds, both groups of subjects and to the complete sample ($P>0.05$).

3.2 Chronic low back pain and diurnal variation

Difficulty was experienced in training patients with severe chronic low back pain to use the stadiometer. Only 5 of the 8 patients were able to meet the acceptable reliability level - an SD < 0.05 mm over 10 consecutive measures. Diurnal variation in the trained subjects was 7.2 ($\pm$ 4.8 mm) from peak to trough. The range was from 3.1 mm to 13.1 mm.

Table 1. Changes in stature during a 30 min treadmill run in runners with and without low back pain.

Speed	Time (min)	Low Back Pain (n = 7) Shrinkage (mm $\pm$ SD)	Non-low Back Pain (n = 7) Shrinkage (mm $\pm$ SD)
70%	15	3.6 (3.1)	0.8 (2.1)
	30	4.9 (1.4)	1.9 (1.2)
85%	15	3.2 (0.8)	2.8 (3.3)
	30	4.7 (1.4)	5.5 (2.0)
100%	15	4.3 (2.5)	5.0 (3.0)
	30	7.2 (1.3)	8.1 (1.3)

4 Discussion

The reported studies illustrate some of the potential limitations of measuring changes in stature as an index of spinal loading. Although spinal shrinkage is increased by an elevation in running speed when duration is held constant, no differences were found in spinal shrinkage between back pain sufferers and non-back pain sufferers. This suggests that shrinkage induced by running was independent of low back pain symptoms. However, at the time of carrying out the tests all the runners were still training and competing. Therefore, the absence of a difference in spinal shrinkage attributable to low back pain symptoms could be explained by the relatively mild level of pain suffered by the runners. Runners with pain severe enough to curtail training have not been studied and this should be an area of future investigation.

A reduced amount of shrinkage was observed in the second 15 min of the run; this may render the disc more vulnerable to injury as it stiffens during a long run. Increased stiffness and vulnerability to damage is associated with a slowing in rate of height loss in the disc (Kazarian 1975; Brinckmann 1988). The present data are insufficient to predict the amount of shrinkage likely to occur in a complete marathon run, or the variation in rate of shrinkage with time. Further research is required to determine the effect of longer duration runs on spinal shrinkage.

Shrinkage incurred was unrelated to the age of the subjects for any of the running conditions. This result may not apply to subjects older than the current range of subjects studied, and in whom the disc response to loading might be attenuated (Kazarian 1975).

Some patients awaiting surgery were unable to maintain a relaxed posture on the stadiometer whilst measurements were taken due to pain. A peak to trough variation in stature of 7.2 mm was recorded on 5 patients. This is approximately 40% of the 19.3 mm previously recorded for normal subjects (Tyrrell et al. 1985). Part of this discrepancy was due to the daily routine being interrupted by bouts of bed rest and other activities which patients adopted to alleviate their pain. Direct comparison between the two studies is also made difficult by the significantly different ages of the two groups. The chronic low back pain patients were aged 32-57 years whereas the normal subjects were aged 19-21 years. Age affects the structure of the spine and hence its dynamic response characteristics. Nevertheless, the likelihood is that back pain patients in this age group will have a depressed amplitude of the normal circadian variation.

Patients with severe chronic low back pain were unable to relax on the stadiometer, suggesting that the shrinkage technique may have limited use in this group of subjects. The usefulness of spinal shrinkage as an index of spinal loading in subjects with low back pain is as yet unclear. The two groups analysed in this work were extreme examples : those who could still run and those debilitated by pain and awaiting surgery. The runners with mild low back pain were capable subjects for experimental studies of shrinkage whereas those awaiting surgery were not. More useful data may be obtained from a population with symptoms in between the examples studied to date.

5 Acknowledgements

This research project was supported by a grant from the Health Promotion Research Trust. Thanks are also given to the collaborting establishment, the Department of Orthopaedic and Accident Surgery, Royal Liverpool Hospital, University of Liverpool, P.O. Box 147, Liverpool L69 3BX, England.

6 References

Boocock, M.G. Reilly, T. Linge, K. and Troup, J.D.G. (1986) Fine measurements of stature for measuring spinal loading, in **Kinanthropometry III** (eds T. Reilly, J. Watkins and J. Borms) E & F.N. Spon, London, pp. 98-103.

Brinckmann, P. (1988) Stress and strain of human lumbar discs. **Clin. Biomech.**, 3, 232-235.

De Puky, P. (1935) The physiological oscillation of the length of the body. **Acta Orthop. Scand.**, 6, 338-347.

Devereaux, M.D. and Lachmann, S.L. (1980) Athletes attending a sports injuries clinic - a review. **Brit. J. Sports Med.**, 17, 137-142.

Corlett, E.N. Eklund, J.A.E. Reilly, T. and Troup, J.D.G. (1987) Assessment of workload from measurement of stature. **Appl. Ergon.**, 18, 65-71.

Foreman,T.K. (1989) **Low back pain prevalence, work activity analysis and spinal shrinkage.** Doctoral Thesis, University of Liverpool.

Garbutt, G. Boocock, M.G. Reilly, T. and Troup, J.D.G. (1990) Running speed and spinal shrinkage in runners with and without low back pain. **Med. Sci. Sport. Exer.**, (in press).

Hirch, C. (1955) The reaction of intevertebral discs to compression forces. **J. Bone Joint Surg.**, 37-A, 1188-1196.

Kazarian, L.E. (1975) Creep characteristiscs of the human spinal column. **Orthop. Clin. North. Am.**, 6, 3-18.

Lutter, L. (1980) Injuries to runners and joggers. **Minnesota Medicine** , 63, 45-51.

Taylor, J.F. and Twomey, T.F. (1980) Sagittal and horizontal plane movement of the lumbar vertebral column in cadavers and in the living. **Rheumatol. Rehabil.**, 19, 223-232.

Tyrrell, A.R., Reilly, T. and Troup, J.D.G. (1985) Circadian variations in human stature and the effects of spinal loading. **Spine**, 109, 161-164.

9

FLEXIBILITY, WARM-UP AND INJURIES IN MATURE GAMES PLAYERS

T. REILLY and A. STIRLING
Liverpool Polytechnic, Liverpool, England

Keywords: Flexibility, Games players, Injury, Warm-up.

1 Introduction

The intensive competitiveness of contemporary games play and the arduous nature of training regimens used by players have led to a concern for the injuries incurred by players. Injury may hamper players both in training and competition and prevent them from realising their playing potential. Although in games play injury causation may be due to factors extraneous to the individual, there is evidence that kinanthropometric factors predispose towards injury. Ekstrand and Gillquist (1982), for example, estimated that 42% of soccer injuries were due to player factors such as joint stability, muscle tightness, inadequate rehabilitation or lack of training. In further work Ekstrand (1982) reported that 67% of soccer players had tight muscles and such players were vulnerable to injury. A programme of flexibility training was found to reduce the injury rate. It seems that the degree of flexibility is an important protective factor against injury. It is thought also that warm-up exercises which improve flexibility short-term are also beneficial in preventing injury (Reilly 1981). It is questionable whether flexibility is a general whole-body factor or specific to each joint. Reviews in the literature cite evidence of its specificity (Reilly 1981; Hebbelinck 1988). The joints most relevant for examination in games players are back, hip and knee, encompassing the region most susceptible to injury.
The aims of this study were to: (a) investigate a range of flexibility measures among games players; (b) relate such measures to training practices and injuries sustained by the players.

2 Methods

Forty adult male games players agreed to participate in the study. Mean values were 21.5 years, 175 cm and 74.5 kg, for age, height and body mass respectively. Each subject participated regularly in match-play in either rugby, soccer, hockey or handball.

A battery of 25 flexibility tests was applied to subjects after first confirming their feasibility and reliability on 5 subjects in a pilot study. Measurements were performed using the principle of Cave and Roberts (1936). For the lower limb, measurements were made on both sides of the body; three measurements were made on each variable and the mean of these recorded. On the day of testing physical exercise was prohibited prior to measurement.

Flexibility tests included sit and reach, lateral flexion of the spine, trunk rotation, hip abduction, hip adduction straight leg raise, hip flexion, hip extension, thoracic and lumbar spine extension, hip rotation in flexion, hip rotation in extension, dynamic whole-body flexibility according to Fleishman (1964). The equipment consisted of a sit-and-reach box, and two large (1 m in diameter) protractor-style goniometers.

Subjects also completed a questionnaire containing 10 items. These were designed to establish profiles for training, warm-up and injury occurrence.

The flexibility measures were examined using principal components analysis for data reduction; this incorporated an analysis of the correlations between variables. Multiple discriminatory analysis was employed to examine differences between groups. This multivariate procedure was used in an attempt to distinguish between frequently injured and infrequently injured players on the basis of their flexibility components and warm-up practices.

3 Results

From the 25 flexibility measures, six principal components were extracted. These accounted for 79% of the total variance. The components were identified from loadings on the oblique factor structure matrix (Table 1).

Component 1 loaded highly on five tests, including straight leg raise (left and right legs), hip flexion (left leg) and hip abduction (left and right). This was identified as relating to hip flexion and abduction. Component 2 loaded highly on five tests which included trunk rotation, lateral flexion of the spine (right and left) and sit-and-reach. It was named 'trunk rotation'. Component 3 had high loadings on four tests representing inward hip rotation in flexion and extension. It was referred to as hip rotation. The remaining components were identified as hip extension with rotation, dynamic flexibility and a general flexibility factor. Discriminant analysis, using all the six principal components combined, failed to significantly separate players more frequently injured (n=20) from those infrequently injured (n = 20). Components 3 and 4 on their own were found to discriminate between the injured and uninjured players (P<0.01). According to univariate t-tests, individual flexibility measures best distinguishing between the frequently injured and

Table 1. Significant factor loadings for flexibility measures on the principle components extracted.

Flexibility measure	Principal components' factor loadings					
	1	2	3	4	5	6
Sit and reach		0.20				-0.34
Dynamic flexibility					0.43	0.55
Lateral flexion: spine (L)		0.44				0.29
Lateral flexion: spine (R)		0.40				0.29
Trunk rotation (L)		0.36				
Trunk rotation (R)		0.28	-0.30			
Extension (spine)			-0.42			
Straight leg raise (L)	-0.24					
Straight leg raise (R)	-0.22					
Hip flexion (L)	-0.24					
Hip flexion (R)					0.33	
Hip extension (L)				0.30		-0.28
Hip extension (R)				0.38		
Hip abduction (L)	-0.26					
Hip abduction (R)	-0.29					
Hip adduction (L)						
Hip adduction (R)						
Hip rotation (fl. inw. L)			0.27			
Hip rotation (fl. inw. R)			0.25			
Hip rotation (fl. out L)				0.40		
Hip rotation (fl. out R)				0.44		
Hip rotation (ext. inw. L)			0.25			
Hip rotation (ext. inw. R)			0.27			
Hip rotation (ext. out. L)						
Hip rotation (ext. out. R)						

infrequently injured were hip extension (right leg), hip extension (left leg) and outward hip rotation in flexion (right leg).

Of the total injuries incurred 33% were to rugby footballers, 24% to soccer players, 24% to hockey players and 19% to handballers. The lower limbs and hips suffered 62% of the overall injuries, the trunk region accounting for a further 14%. Match-play accounted for 64% of injuries, training 36%.

Ascribed causes of injury were chance (47%), lack of warm-up (19%), inadequate rehabilitation (17%) and foul play (17%). In no case was the injury causation attributed to equipment, inadequate lighting, weather or playing surface. The injury-prone players spent less time jogging ($P<0.01$), on technique work ($P<0.01$) and on lower body exercises ($P<0.05$) in warming-up compared to non-injured. Attention to upper body exercises, fast running and sport-specific exercises in warming-up was not significantly different between the frequently injured and less frequently injured players. Nor did the total duration of warm-up practices differ between the groups ($P<0.05$).

4 Discussion

The principal components analysis of the flexibility measures successfully extracted components that were largely movement specific, for example Components 2 and 3 (trunk and hip rotation respectively). Other components incorporated high loadings for combinations of movements such as the contributions of hip flexion, hip abduction and straight leg raising to Component 1. Nevertheless there was some evidence of a general factor in flexibility, especially Component 6. Lower back movements were common among the tests loading highly in this component, although there was variability in the movements between tests. The fifth component was deemed unique to the dynamic flexibility test : this entailed repeated whole-body movements touching alternately the floor and a mark on the wall located behind the back of the subject as frequently as possible in 30 s.

Although six principal components were extracted from the flexibility matrix, correlations between individual test variables were generally low. It seems rather that particular groups of movements are interrelated. This supports the view that flexibility is not common to all joints but is joint-specific or at least specific to groups of movements.

A degree of heterogeneity may have been introduced into the flexibility data by considering games players as a group. The present intention was not to explore differences between the sports but rather to examine commonalties among them. The training and warm-up practices showed broad similarities between the groups. The main difference between them was in injury occurrence. The injury risk was greatest in rugby football and least in handball : a majority of the injuries occurred during match-play in all the games, except for handball.

Although the data reduction process helped to identify general and specific flexibility factors, further analysis of the six components as a set failed to discriminate between the injured and non-injured (or infrequently injured) players. Two of the six components did show relations with injury occurrence, as did individual flexibility tests. Individual measures related to injury occurrence were movements at the hip, whose flexibility is relevant for games play. The value of these tests in pinpointing predisposition to injury would need to be further examined in a prospective study. This would obviate the difficulty in interpretation of present observations where loss of flexibility may have been in part caused by injury and not fully restored subsequently.

The observations support the view that warm-up has a role to play in injury prevention. In about 1 in 5 cases players felt that lack of warm-up was the cause of the injury. The training and practice profiles showed that the injured players paid less attention to jogging, technique work and lower body exercise than did the less frequently injured subjects. In consequence they would fail to elevate body temperature sufficiently, rehearse games skills or mobilise the joints most vulnerable to injury.

5 References

Cave, E.F. and Roberts, S.M. (1936) A method of measuring and recording joint function. **J. Bone Joint. Surg.**, 18, 455.

Ekstrand, J. (1982) **Soccer injuries and their prevention**. Medical dissertation No. 130, Linköping University.

Ekstrand and Gillquist, J. (1982) The frequency of muscle tightness and injuries in soccer players. **Am. J. Sport. Med.** , 10, 75-78.

Fleishman, E.A. (1964) **The Structure and Measurement of Physical Fitness**. Prentice-Hall, Englewood Cliffs.

Hebbelinck, M. (1988) Flexibility, in **The Olympic Book of Sports Medicine** (eds A. Dirix, H.G. Knuttgen and K. Tittel), Blackwell Scientific, Oxford, pp. 212-217.

Reilly, T. (1981) **Sports Fitness and Sports Injuries**. Faber and Faber, London.

10

DAILY PHYSICAL ACTIVITY AND ITS RELATIONSHIP WITH HEALTH RELATED AND PERFORMANCE RELATED FITNESS IN 30 YEAR-OLD MEN

C. VAN DEN BOSSCHE, G. BEUNEN, R. RENSON, J. LEFEVRE,
A. CLAESSENS, R. LYSENS, H. MAES, J. SIMONS, B. VANDEN EYNDE
and B. VANREUSEL
Center for Physical Development Research, K.U.Leuven, Belgium

Keywords: Daily physical activity, Health related fitness, Performance related fitness.

1 Introduction

The health benefits of regular physical activity are not limited to structural and functional characteristics but also include psychosocial factors. Whereas definitive evidence of a cause-and-effect relationship between an increase in habitual physical activity or exercise and many specific health benefits is still lacking, there is sufficient evidence that physical activity and physical fitness are inversely associated with morbidity and mortality from several chronic diseases, such as coronary heart disease, some forms of cancer, diabetes and osteoporosis (Hollozy 1990; Meredith 1988). The effect of physical activity on the incidence of cardiovascular diseases is established: physical activity may directly help prevent hypertension (Paffenbarger et al. 1983; Leon et al. 1987) and may indirectly affect the risk of hypertension by producing weight loss and by influencing health behaviours such as overeating, smoking, substance abuse, stress management, risk taking and others (Blair et al. 1985; Bruce 1984; Slattery and Jacobs 1987). There is also a longstanding debate about whether exercise extends longevity. Physical activity and fitness are reported in an inverse relationship with mortality (Paffenbarger 1986; Blair 1990).

If physical activity is beneficial, the question arises about the intensity and the required amount of exercise so that the desired changes in health are produced and also the question about how to assess daily physical activity then becomes considerable. In other words, who is an active adult and who is a non-active adult and how can daily physical activity be measured? The assessment of daily physical activity by direct or indirect calorimetry in studies with a large number of subjects is very difficult to carry out because of the practical aspects of these measurement methods. Large surveys concentrate therefore on the estimation of the daily physical activity by questionnaire, observation of behaviour or by job-

Table 1. Comparison of active versus non-active adults during work activity (full line : active; dashed line : non-active).

	P3	P10	P25	P50	P75	P90	P97
Somatic dimensions:							
Weight (kg)	60.2	63.9	68.2	72.8	79.4	85.4	91.5
Height (cm)	167	169.3	173.6	178.0	181.8	184.5	187.1
Biacromial width (cm)	36.8	37.9	38.8	39.8	40.7	41.8	42.9
Circ. fl. upper arm (cm)	27.5	28.7	30.0	31.5	33.2	34.8	36.8
Circ. of forearm (cm)	24.8	25.3	26.1	27.0	28.2	28.8	29.9
Biceps skf (cm)	9.9	6.8	5.6	4.4	3.4	2.8	2.4
Supra-iliac skf (mm)	28.0	23.0	17.8	10.6	7.8	5.9	4.7
Triceps skf (mm)	19.4	16.1	13.2	9.8	7.5	5.8	4.8
Scapula skf (mm)	24.8	19.2	15.3	12.0	9.6	7.8	6.9
Calf skf (mm)	7.1	13.6	10.2	7.4	5.4	4.6	3.8
Endomorphy	50	45	40	40	30	25	20
Mesomorphy	30	30	35	40	45	50	55
Ectomorphy	15	20	20	30	40	50	50
Quetelet index	1.9	2.0	2.2	2.3	2.5	2.6	2.8
Physiological characteristics:							
Pulse at rest (/min)	92	82	74.5	65.5	57.5	51	47
Pulse after 60"(/min)	122	110	98	82	70	60	58
Pulse after 120" (/min)	116	104	90	74	66	58	50
Heart freq. at VT(/min)	169	164	156	146	136	124	110
O_2 uptake (l/min)	1.04	1.22	1.47	1.93	2.18	2.37	2.50
Work VT (Watt)	108	128	148	179	210	222	249
Heart freq. peak (/min)	196	190	187	182	178	162	148
O_2 uptake peak (l/min)	2.02	2.35	2.72	3.11	3.47	3.8	4.36
Work peak (Watt)	177	207	236	276	299	340	370
Sum pulses (/min)	236	212	180	156	136	120	108
Blood pressure measurements:							
Systolic BP	180	165	160	140	130	120	115
Diastolic BP	100	100	90	80	80	75	70

Table 1 (cont'd)

	P3	P10	P25	P50	P75	P90	P97
Health related fitness:							
Sit and reach (cm)	10	14	19	25	30	34	39
Bent arm hang (sec)	10.0	13.6	22.2	33.7	43.8	56.3	64.3
Leg lifts (/20 sec)	14	16	17	18	19	20	22
VO$_2$ peak (l/min)	2.02	2.35	2.72	3.11	3.47	3.8.0	4.36
Sum of skfs	80.8	72.1	57.8	44.8	33.2	27.4	22.4
Performance related fitness:							
Arm pull (kg)	60.5	70.0	76.0	83.5	95.0	104.5	120.5
Shuttle run (sec)	23.7	22.7	21.6	20.7	19.9	19.1	18.6
Plate tapping (/20 sec)	81	89	94	102	106	110	112
Flamingo (att./min)	21	18	14	11	7	4	3
Vertical jump (cm)	40	44	47	50	56	61	64

classification. The aim of the study was to investigate if adults active during leisure time have better results on health and performance related fitness variables than adults not active during leisure time and than adults active during work activity.

2 Methods

2.1 Sample
The data are from a longitudinal study of Flemish boys who were followed from 12 through 18 years of age and who were re-measured as adults at the age of 30. A total of 588 boys were followed longitudinally over six years and 173 of these 588 boys were re-measured in 1986. At that time their ages varied between 29.5 and 31.5 years. The somatic and motor characteristics and sociocultural background of the 173 subjects enrolled in the second part of the study did not significantly deviate from the characteristics of the total Flemish sample at the age of 18 (data from 1984). It can thus be concluded that the 173 men are a representative sample of the boys who were followed longitudinally through adolescence.

Table 2. Comparison of active versus non-active adults during leisure time activity (full line : active; dashed line : non-active).

	P3	P10	P25	P50	P75	P90	P97
Somatic dimensions:							
Weight (kg)	60.2	63.9	68.2	72.8	79.4	85.4	91.5
Height (cm)	167.0	169.3	173.6	178.0	181.8	184.5	187.1
Biacromial width (cm)	36.8	37.9	38.8	39.8	40.7	41.8	42.9
Circ. fl. upper arm (cm)	27.5	28.7	30.0	31.5	33.2	34.8	36.8
Circ. of forearm (cm)	24.8	25.3	26.1	27.0	28.2	28.8	29.9
Biceps skf (cm)	9.9	6.8	5.6	4.4	3.4	2.8	2.4
Supra-iliac skf (mm)	28.0	23.0	17.8	10.6	7.8	5.9	4.7
Triceps skf (mm)	19.4	16.1	13.2	9.8	7.5	5.8	4.8
Scapula skf (mm)	24.8	19.2	15.3	12.0	9.6	7.8	6.9
Calf skf (mm)	7.1	13.6	10.2	7.4	5.4	4.6	3.8
Endomorphy	50	45	40	40	30	25	20
Mesomorphy	30	30	35	40	45	50	55
Ectomorphy	15	20	20	30	40	50	50
Quetelet index	1.9	2.0	2.2	2.3	2.5	2.6	2.8
Physiological characteristics:							
Pulse at rest (/min)	92.0	82.0	74.5	65.5	57.5	51.0	47.0
Pulse after 60"(/min)	122	110	98	82	70	60	58
Pulse after 120" (/min)	116	104	90	74	66	58	50
Heart freq. at VT(/min)	169	164	156	146	136	124	110
O_2 uptake (l/min)	1.04	1.22	1.47	1.93	2.18	2.37	2.50
Work VT (Watt)	108	128	148	179	210	222	249
Heart freq. peak (/min)	196	190	187	182	178	162	148
O_2 uptake peak (l/min)	2.02	2.35	2.72	3.11	3.47	3.80	4.36
Work peak (Watt)	177	207	236	276	299	340	370
Sum pulses (/min)	236	212	180	156	136	120	108
Blood pressure measurements:							
Systolic BP	180	165	160	140	130	120	115
Diastolic BP	100	100	90	80	80	75	70

Table 2 (cont'd)

	P3	P10	P25	P50	P75	P90	P97
Health related fitness:							
Sit and reach (cm)	10	14	19	25	30	34	39
Bent arm hang (sec)	10	13.6	22.2	33.7	43.8	56.3	64.3
Leg lifts (/20 sec)	14	16	17	18	19	20	22
VO$_2$ peak (l/min)	2.02	2.35	2.72	3.11	3.47	3.8	4.36
Sum of skfs	80.8	72.1	57.8	44.8	33.2	27.4	22.4
Performance related fitness:							
Arm pull (kg)	60.5	70	76	83.5	95	104.5	120.5
Shuttle run (sec)	23.7	22.7	21.6	20.7	19.9	19.1	18.6
Plate tapping (/20 sec))	81	89	94	102	106	110	112
Flamingo (att./min)	21	18	14	11	7	4	3
Vertical jump (cm)	40	44	47	50	56	61	64

2.2 Assessment of daily physical activity tests and measurement

Daily physical activity was assessed by means of a standardized questionnaire, an adapted version of the structured interview protocol used for the Tecumseh study (Reiff et al. 1967). Because of the size of this longitudinal study a retrospective method was adopted. By means of a structured interview an inventory was made of the physical activity of an average week of last year. The intensity of an activity during work or leisure time is given by the proportion of work metabolic rate (WMR) and basal metabolic rate (BMR). Somatic dimensions included weight, stature, biacromial width, circumference of flexed upper arm and of forearm, skinfolds (biceps, supra-iliac, triceps, sub-scapular and sum of skinfolds). Somatotype and Quetelet index were also calculated. Eight motor tests were administered (Simons et al. 1969, 1990) : flamingo balance (balance), plate tapping (speed of limb movement), sit and reach (flexibility), vertical jump (explosive strength), arm pull (static strength), leg lifts (trunk strength), bent arm hang (functional strength), shuttle run (running speed agility). During a standardized bicycle ergometer test and during a step test physiological characteristics were recorded: pulse at rest, pulse after 60 seconds and after 120 seconds, heart frequency at ventilatory threshold and at VO$_2$ peak, oxygen uptake at ventilatory threshold and at VO$_2$ peak, work at ventilatory threshold and at VO$_2$ peak. Also the blood pressure at rest was observed.

2.3 Statistics

In order to compare 'active' with 'non-active' adults the extreme quartiles were selected on the basis of the intensity and duration of the activity. For activity on the job the extremes were WMR/BMR < 1.815 and < 39.6 hours/week (P=25, N=9) and WMR/BMR > 2.695 and > 48.85 hours/week (P=75, N=10). For active leisure time the extremes were WMR/BMR < 3.97 and < 5.05 hours/week (P=25, N=8) and WMR/BMR > 5.64 and > 14.9 hours/week (P=75, N=9). Differences between the means of active and non-active adults were tested with the Student t-test.

3 Results

3.1 Energy expenditure

The average energy expenditure during work was 51.9 KJ/kg body weight/day during work (SD = 21.8), 25.5 KJ/kg body weight/day during active leisure time (SD = 19.7) and 157 KJ/kg body weight/day during a whole day (SD = 31.8).

3.2 Comparison of active and non-active adults

For job activity, only a few significant differences were found. Active adults had smaller skinfolds and better results on the flamingo balance than the non-active (see Table 1).

For active leisure time, active adults differed significantly from the non-active for height, subcutaneous skinfolds and mesomorphy. The active adults were smaller, had smaller skinfolds and a higher mesomorphy score than the non-active. For the health and performance related fitness characteristics differences were found for bent arm hang (functional strength of the upper body), leg lifts (trunk strength), pulse recovery after the step test, oxygen consumption and work at peak (see Table 2).

4 Discussion

Some of the results of this study are in agreement with those of studies in which the relationship between daily physical activity and somatic, health and performance related variables was also investigated. Blair et al. (1985) reported that the more active individuals of the Tecumseh Community Health Study had a lower sum of four skinfold measurements than the less active persons (p < 0.05). Also Slattery and Jacobs (1987) found that active men had smaller skinfolds than sedentary men (p < 0.01). This is in agreement with the results of this study where active adults during work and during leisure time have less adiposities. Although Epstein and

Wing (in Blair et al. 1985) characterize overweight persons as underexercised rather than overfed, we do not find significant differences between active and non-active adults for weight. Nevertheless, active adults show both for leisure time and for work a tendency to weigh less than the non-active adults.

In agreement with the findings of Bruce (1984) that physical exercise increases the aerobic metabolism and associated ventilatory, respiratory and circulatory responses, we found that active adults during leisure time had significantly higher maximal oxygen uptake (p < 0.01) and recovered significantly better. Bruce (1984) found that the longitudinal rate of decline in VO_2max in sedentary men is twice that of active men.

Although it has been found in several studies that vigorous exercise is associated with lower blood pressure, there were no significant differences in systolic and diastolic blood pressure between active and non-active adults during work and during leisure time.

More studies about the influence of leisure time activity have reported an inverse relationship between physical activity and the risk of coronary heart disease than studies about the influence of work related activity (Meredith 1988). Also in this study more significant differences were found between active and non-active adults during leisure time than during work activities and most health related fitness variables (maximal oxygen uptake, pulse recovery, adiposity, functional strength of the upper body and trunk strength) show significant differences between active and non-active adults during leisure time. These findings indicate that the intensity and the duration of a leisure time activity seem to be more important than the intensity and the duration of job activities.

5 Acknowledgements

This study was supported by grants from the Research Fund K.U. Leuven and by the National Scientific Foundation (Fund for Medical Research).

6 References

Blair, S.N. Jacobbs, D.R and Powell, K.E. (1985) Relationships between exercise or physical activity and other health behaviors. **Public Health Rep.,** 100(2), 172-180.
Blair, S.N. Kohl, H.W Paffenbarger, R.S. Clark, D.G. Cooper, K.H. and Gibbons, L.W. (1990) Physical fitness and all-cause mortality: a prospective study of healthy men and women. **J. Am. Med. Assoc.**
Bruce, R.A. (1984) Exercise, functional aerobic capacity, and aging - another viewpoint. **Med. Sci. Sport. Exer.,** 16 (1), 8-13.

Haskell, W.L. Montoye, H.J. and Orenstein, D. (1985) Physical activity and exercise to achieve health-related physical fitness components. **Public Health Rep.**, 100(2), 203-212.

Holloszy, J.O. (1990) The roles of exercise in health maintenance and treatment of disease in middle and old age, in **Fitness for the aged disabled, and industrial worker** (ed M. Kaneko), Human Kinetics Books, Champaign, Ill., pp. 1-8.

Leon, A.S. Connett, J. Jacobs, D.R. and Rainer, R. (1987) Leisure-time physical activity levels and risk of coronary heart disease and death. **J. Am. Med. Assoc.**, 258(17), 2388-2395.

Meredith, M.D. (1988) Activity or fitness: is the process or the product more important for public health? **Quest**, 40, 180-186.

Paffenbarger, R.S. Wing, A.L. Hyde, R.T. and Jung, D.L. (1983) Physical activity and incidence of hypertension in college alumni. **J. Epidem.**, 117(3), 245-257.

Paffenbarger, R.S. Hyde, R.T. and Wing , A.L. (1986) Physical activity, all-cause mortality and longevity of college alumni. **New Engl. J. Med.**, 314(10), 605-613.

Siconolfi, S.F. Lasater, T.M. McKinlay, S. Boggia, P. and Carleton, R.A. (1985) Physical fitness and blood pressure: the role of age. **Am. J. Epidem.**, 122(3): 452-457

Simons, J. Beunen, G. Ostyn, M. Renson, R. Swalus, P. Van Gerven, D. and Willems, E. (1969) Construction d'une batterie de tests d'aptitude motrice pour garçons de 12 à 19 ans par la methode d'analyse factorielle, **Kinanthropologie**, 1, 323-362.

Simons, J. Beunen, G. Renson, R. Claessens, A. Vanreusel, B. and Lefevre, J. (1990) **Growth and fitness of Flemish girls. The Leuven Growth Study.** HKP Sport Science Monograph series, Vol 3. Human Kinetics, Champaign, Ill.

Slattery, M.L. and Jacobs, D.R. (1987) The inter-relationships of physical activity, physical fitness and body measurements, **Med. Sci. Sport. Exer.**, 19, 564-569.

Steens, G. Vanreusel, B. Renson, R. Beunen, G. Simons, J. Lysens, R. Claessens, A. Lefevre, J. and Vanden Eynde, B. (1987-1988) Levensstijl en physical-fitness permanentie: dagelijkse fysieke activiteit. **Hermes,** K.U.Leuven, Leuven, XIX, 311-320.

11

THE EFFECTS OF CONTINUOUS AND INTERMITTENT TRAINING ON THE VENTILATORY THRESHOLD TWO AND MAXIMUM EXERCISE CAPACITY OF MIDDLE-AGED MEN

P.S.C. GOMES [1] and Y. BHAMBHANI [2]
[1] School of Physical Education, University of São Paulo, São Paulo, Brazil
[2] Faculty of Rehab. Medicine, University of Alberta, Edmonton, Canada

Keywords : Threshold of anaerobic metabolism, Body composition, Densitometry, Skinfolds, Continuous and interval training.

1 Introduction

Exercise alone (Skinner et al. 1964; Ribisl 1969; Pollock et al. 1969, Carter and Phillips 1969, Wilmore et al. 1970; Wilmore et al. 1980; Depres et al. 1985) and exercise combined with food restriction (Passmore et al. 1958; Buskirk et al. 1963; Zuti and Golding, 1976) have been shown to be effective in reducing body weight and/or body fat.

Several exercise modes have been reported to cause changes in body composition of male and female non-athletes. Among these were walking/jogging/running (Carter and Phillips 1969; Pollock et al. 1971; Getchell 1975; Pollock et al. 1976), bicycle/cycle ergometry (Johnson et al. 1972; Pollock et al. 1975; Wilmore et al. 1980) and circuit training/circuit weight training/weight training (Fahey and Brown 1973; Girandola and Katch 1973; Wilmore et al. 1978).

Surprisingly, very few studies have made use of interval training methods (Bhambhani, Singh and Gomes 1987; Thomas et al. 1984), as specific stimulus for their body weight and/or fat reduction exercise training schemes. These studies however, did not assess the subject's nutritional intake during the course of their training programmes.

The purpose of the present study was to compare the effects of one intermittent and two continuous training programmes on the body density of active middle-aged males after a twelve week period.

2 Methodology

Thirty-three male volunteers with a mean age of 36 years, were ranked in descending order according to their initial VO_2 (ml.kg $^{-1}$. min $^{-1}$), assessed by means of a progressive maximal exercise capacity test (Bhambhani and Singh 1985) on an electromagnetically braked cycle ergometer Uniwork

Model 845 (Quinton Instruments, U.S.A.). The subjects were subsequently randomly assigned to one intermittent and two continuous training groups. Six non-exercising male volunteers were also tested and used as controls (CG). Gas exchange measurements were continuously monitored during all exercise tests with an automated Horizon Metabolic Measurement Cart (SensorMedics, Anaheim, CA), programmed to output data every 30 seconds. During the test, the ventilatory threshold (VT_2) was identified, as the VO_2 ($l.min^{-1}$) and the power output (P.O.) at which the V_E/VCO_2 reached a minimum and F_ECO_2 reached a maximum (Reinhard et al., 1979, Bhambhany and Singh 1985; Bhambhani, Singh and Gomes 1987). All subjects were submitted to the same test protocol at weeks zero (PRE) and thirteen (POST). The test/retest reliability of VT_2 was determined prior to the beginning of the study, in seven male subjects who did not participate in the training study. They were tested twice, a week apart, with VT_2 being identified by the same investigator in both occasions. Intraclass correlation coefficients for the variables measured at VT_2 were the following : P.O. = .96; VO_2 ($l.min^{-1}$) = .87; VO_2 (as a % of VO_2 max) = .69; HR = .88; HR (as % of HR max) = .78.

During the 12-week study all subjects participated in three training sessions per week with at least a 24 hour interval between the sessions. The subjects exercised continuously at a P.O. requiring a VO_2 similar to that observed at either the VT_2 (VTG) or 15 % below VT_2 (BVTG). Subjects in the interval training (ITG) group exercised at 100 % of the VO_2 max (1:1). Training was performed with the same equipment used for testing. The total amount of work performed per training session was calculated in the three experimental groups. Each subject in the VTG exercised for 20 minutes every session. The total amount of work performed for each subject was calculated by multiplying the P.O. in kpm/min times 20 minutes. The duration of the training for the subject of the same rank order in the BVTG and ITG groups was calculated by dividing the total amount of work of the subject in the VTG by the P.O. at which the subjects of the same rank order in BVTG and ITG were supposed to train. At training sessions nine, eighteen and twenty-seven, all subjects in the experimental groups were tested in order to adjust the training work loads to their new physical conditioning. As a result, all training loads and times were recalculated on the new values obtained.

Hydrostatic weighing following the procedure described by Wilmore (1963) was performed in all subjects at week zero (PRE), six (MID) and twelve (POST). Body density was then calculated using the equation proposed by Sloan et al (1962). Standing height, body weight and seven skinfolds (triceps, biceps, subscapular, suprailiac, abdominal, front thigh and medial calf) were also measured at the three testing times, by the same technician, following the procedure described by Ross and Marfell-Jones (1982).

During the course of the study a nutritional assessment was conducted on all subjects by means of nutritional recall diaries. The total caloric intake was analyzed by utilizing the Kellogs/University of Alberta (Canada) database. In order to establish a baseline, all subjects were asked to record their dietary intake twice, for three consecutive days (Thursday, Friday and Saturday) in the two weeks preceding the study (PRE). The participants were reassessed at weeks six (MID) and twelve (POST) for comparison purposes.

Two-way Anova with repeated measures and Duncan multiple range test (Keppel, 1973) were used for comparisons. The computer package SPSSX (SPSS Inc, 1986) with the user procedure UANOVA written by Terry Taerum (unpublished) at the University of Alberta, were used for data analyses. The .05 level of significance was used for all Anova and post-hoc comparisons.

3 Results and discussion

At the end of 12 weeks of training, eight subjects, all from the experimental groups, were forced to drop out of the study for reasons not related to the programme (Table 1).

Anova results showed significant alterations in body composition (body weight, and density, percent fat, absolute fat and sum of seven skinfolds) as a result of training below the VT_2. No changes were observed for the VTG and ITG groups in any of the structural variables studied (Tables 2 and 3). These changes are well within the values reported in the literature, as reviewed by Wilmore (1983), for a wide variety of exercise modes. The present data supports previous reports that exercise alone can reduce body fat (Bjorntorp 1980; Thompson et al. 1982; Leon et al. 1979 Glick and Kaufmann 1976; Wilmore et al. 1970) with no necessity of controlling over caloric intake. Considering that there were no significant changes in total caloric intake (Table 4), the observed structural modifications can be attributed to the training intensity at which the subjects were exposed. Total caloric intake values were within the normal range recommended for Canadians and Americans in the same age group (Goodhart and Shils 1980).

The present data showed that exercising intermittently at 100 % of the VO_2 max and continuously at the threshold did not promote any significant changes in body composition. These training intensities, however, did promote a significant increase in absolute and relative VO_2 at the maximum exercise capacity and at the VT_2.

Table 1 : Characteristics (mean and SD) of the participants who completed the study (n=31).

Group	Age (yr)	Height (cm)	Weight (kg)	VO$_2$ Max (ml.kg^{-1}. min^{-1})
VTG	36.1	180.9	87.9[1]	41.0
(n=8)	7.24	4.56	9.93	7.12
BVTG	42.4[1]	175.4	84.3[1]	39.3
(n=10)	9.51	3.98	8.47	7.59
ITG	39.9[1]	172.8	77.4	41.6
(n=7)	7.55	3.10	9.66	9.44
CG	27.8	178.6	78.5	45.3
(n=6)	5.96	3.10	3.97	5.59

[1] sig. different from CG (p<.05)

Table 2 : Changes in body density (g.ml^{-1}) as a result of different exercise intensities : means and standard deviations.

Group	PRE	MID	POST
VTG	1.04359[1]	1.04578	1.04349[2]
(n=8)	0.01720	0.01691	0.01803
BVTG	1.03725[1]	1.03836	1.04283[ab2]
(n=10)	0.00950	0.01201	0.01140
ITG	1.05041	1.05044	1.05356
(n=7)	0.00836	0.01176	0.01140
CG	1.06542		1.06595
(n=6)			

[a] sig. different from   PRE (p<.05)
[b]   MID
[1]   CG at PRE
[2]   CG at POST

Table 3 : Changes in the sum of seven skinfolds (mm) as a result of training at different exercise intensities : means and standard deviations.

Group	PRE	MID	POST
VTG	105.8	108.0	108.1
(n=8)	43.5	44.7	44.5
BVTG	121.0[1]	118.2	111.9[ab]
(n=10)	24.3	23.8	25.2
ITG	96.7	97.1	100.3
(n=7)	30.3	30.3	33.2
CG	69.0		75.7[a]
(n=6)	19.7		32.4

[a] sig. different from   PRE (p<.05)
[b]   MID (p<.05)
[1]   CG at PRE

Table 4 : Total caloric intake (Kcal) for the three experimental groups at the different phases of the training programme : means and standard deviations.

GROUP	PRE	MID	POST
VTG	2770.4	2513.2	2524.2
(n=8)	848.2	875.4	837.4
BVTG	2882.7	2529.3	3001.6
(n=10)	312.9	395.1	599.7
ITG	2377.3	2348.4	2510.1
(n=7)	694.8	567.7	450.2

The observed modifications in body composition could be associated with an elevated metabolic rate after the training session. As reported by Chad and Wenger (1988), VO_2 values during the post-exercise phase increase with time (i.e. duration of the training session). In the present study, duration of exercise in BVTG was significantly higher than in the other experimental groups.

Changes in body density were not related to the alterations in the sum of seven skinfolds, leading to the belief that the use of skinfolds may not be appropriate to determine small alterations in body fat.

Based on the present findings, and within the limitations of this investigation, the use of continuous training programmes with exercise intensities being set below the VT_2, should be preferred if body fat reduction is the main goal. However, if the improvement in aerobic capacity is also the purpose of the exercise stimulus, training continuously above the threshold or intermittently at 100 % of VO_2 max should be preferred.

4 References

Bhambhani, Y. and Singh, M. (1985) Ventilatory threshold during a graded exercise test. **Respiration**, 47, 120-128.

Bhambhani, Y. Singh, M. and Gomes, P. (1987) Equivalent changes in VO_2 max and percent body fat subsequent to continuous and interval training. **Med. Sci. Sport. Exerc.**, 19(2), S88.

Buskirk, E.R. Thompson, R.H. Luttwak and L. Whedon, G.O. (1963) Energy balance in obese patients during weight reduction : influence of diet restriction and exercise. **Ann. N. Y. Acad. Sci.**, 110, 918-940.

Carter, J.E.L. and Phillips, W.H. (1969) Structural changes in exercising middle-aged males during a 2-year period. **J. Appl. Physiol.**, 27, 787-794.

Chad, K.E. and Wenger, H.A. (1988) The effects of exercise duration on the exercise and post-exercise oxygen consumption. **Can. J. Appl. Sport Sci.**, 13(4), 204-207.

Despres, J.P. Bouchard, C. Tremblay, A. Savard and R. Marcotte, M. (1985) Effects of aerobic training on fat distribution in male subjects. **Med. Sci. Sport. Exerc.**, 17(1), 113-118.

Fahey, T.D. and Brown, C.H. (1973) The effects of anabolic steroid on the strength, body composition, and endurance of college males when accompanied by a weight training programme. **Med. Sci. Sport.**, 5, 272-296.

Getchell, L.H. and Moore, J.C. (1975) Physical training comparative responses of middle-aged adults. **Arch. Phys. Med. Rehabil.**, 56, 250-254.

Girandola, R.N. and Katch, V. (1973) Effects of nine weeks of physical training on aerobic capacity and body composition in college men. **Arch. Phys. Med. Rehabil.**, 54, 521-524.

Goodhart, R.S. and Shils, M.E. (1980) **Modern Nutrition in Health and Disease. 6th Edition**, Lea & Febiger, New York.

Keppel, G. (1973) **Design and Analysis : A Researcher Handbook**. Prentice-Hall Inc., Englewood Cliffs, New Jersey.

Passmore, R. Strong, J.A. and Ritchie, F.J. (1958) The chemical composition of the tissue lost by obese patients on a reducing regimen. **Brit. J. Nutr.**, 12, 113-122.

Pollock, M.L. (1973) The quantification of endurance training, in **Exercise and Sport Science Reviews**, (ed J.H. Wilmore), New York : Academic Press, Vol. 1, pp. 155-188.

Pollock, M.L. Cureton, T.K. Greninger, L. (1969) Effects of frequency of training on working capacity, cardiovascular function, and body composition of adult mens. **Med. Sci. Sport.**, 1, 70-74.

Pollock, M.L. Miller, J.S. Jr. Janeway, R. Linnerud, A.C. Robertson, B. and Valentino, R. (1971) Effects of walking on body composition and cardiovascular function of middle-aged men. **J. Appl. Physiol.**, 30, 126-130.

Pollock, M.L. Dimmick, J. Miller, H.S. Kendrik, Z. and Linnerud, A.C. (1975) Effects of mode of training on cardiovascular function and body composition of adult men. **Med. Sci. Sport.**, 7(2), 139-145.

Pollock, M.L. Dawson, G.A. and Miller, H.S. Jr. (1976) Physiologic responses of men 49 to 65 years of age to endurance training. **J. Am. Geriatry Soc.**, 24, 97-104.

Reinhard, V. Muller, P.H. and Schmulling, R.M. (1979) Determination of anaerobic threshold by the ventilation equivalent in normal individuals. **Respiration**, 38, 36-42.

Ribisl, P.M. (1969) Effects of training upon the maximal oxygen uptake of middle-aged men. **Int. Z. Angew. Physiol.**, 27, 151-160.

Ross, W.D. and Marfell-Jones, M.J. (1982) Kinanthropometry, in Physiological Testing of the Elite Athlete (eds J.D. MacDougall, H.A. Wenger and H.J. Green). **Canadian Association of Sport Sciences and Sport Medicine Council of Canada**, 75-115.

Skinner, J.S. Holloszy, J.O. and Cureton, T.K. (1964) Effects of endurance exercises on physical work capacity and anthropometric measurements of 15 middle-aged men. **Am. J. Cardiol.**, 14, 747-752.

Sloan, A.W. (1962) Estimation of body fat in young men. **J. Appl. Physiol.**, 17, 967-970.

Thomas, T.R. Adeniran, S.B. and Eltheridge, G.L. (1984) Effects of different running s on VO2 max, percent fat and plasma lipids. **Can. J. Appl. Sport Sci.**, 9(2), 55-62.

Thompson, J.K. Jarvie, G.J. Lahey, B.B. and Cureton, K.J. (1982) Exercise and obesity : etiology, physiology, and intervention. **Psychol. Bull.**, 91, 55-79.

Wilmore, J.H. (1963) The use of actual, predicted, and constant residual volumes in the assessment of body composition by underwater weigh. **Med. Sci. Sport.**, 1, 87.

Wilmore, J.H. Royce, J. Girandola, R.N. Katch, F.I. and Katch, V.L. (1970) Body composition changes with a 10-week of jogging. **Med. Sci. Sport.**, 2; 113-117.

Wilmore, J.H. (1974) Alterations in strength, body composition and anthropometric measurements consequent to a 10-week training. **Med. Sci. Sport.**, 6, 133-138.

Wilmore, J.H. Parr, R.B. and Girandola, R.N. (1978) Physiological alterations consequent to circuit training. **Med. Sci. Sport.**, 10, 79-84.

Wilmore, J.H. Davis, J.A. O'Brien, R.S. Vodak, P.A. Wlader, G.R. and Amsterdam, E.A. (1980) Physiological alterations consequent to 20-week conditioning of bicycling, tennis, and jogging. **Med. Sci. Sport.**, 12, 1-8.

Wilmore, J.H. (1983) Body composition in sport and exercise : directions for future research. **Med. Sci. Sport. Exerc.**, 15(1), 21-31.

Zuti, W.B. and Golding, L.A. (1976) Comparing diet and exercise as weight reduction tools. **Physic. Sports Med.**, 4(1), 49-53.

12

HERITABILITY OF HEALTH- AND PERFORMANCE-RELATED FITNESS
Data from the Leuven Longitudinal Twin Study

H. MAES[1], G. BEUNEN[1], R. VLIETINCK[2], J. LEFEVRE[1], C. VAN DEN BOSSCHE[1], A. CLAESSENS[1], R. DEROM[3], R. LYSENS[1], R. RENSON, J. SIMONS and B. VANDEN EYNDE[1]
[1] Institute of Physical Education, K.U.Leuven, Belgium
[2] Centre for Human Genetics, K.U.Leuven, Belgium
[3] Department of Obstetrics, R.U.Gent, Belgium

Supported by Research Fund K.U.Leuven and National Bank of Belgium

Keywords: Heritability, Health, Performance, Fitness, Genetic factors, Environmental factors.

1 Introduction

A considerable amount of research has been done on the estimated heritability of anthropometric characteristics, especially of height and weight and to a lesser degree skinfolds and circumferences. In contrast there are relatively few studies on the genetic determination of motor ability, while the heritability of cardio-vascular endurance has been studied more frequently. Health related fitness and performance related fitness have not been explicitly studied in the genetic context.

Heritability estimates vary with age and sex of subjects, population and methods used to derive them. Heritability estimates derived from twin studies are almost always higher than those calculated when data from other relationships such as parent-child and sib-sib are included. Based on estimates reported in literature (Bouchard 1983; Bouchard 1986; Malina 1986; Kovar 1981) the heritability of skinfolds varies between .50 and .70 while those for cardio-vascular endurance (VO_2 max) span the whole range of heritability estimates. Estimated variation of motor characteristics due to genetic factors is highest for flexibility, followed by different strength factors : explosive, static, functional and trunk strength. Running speed appears to be more genetically determined than speed of limb movement and balance.

This study focuses on univariate genetic analysis of health and performance related fitness using maximum likelihood estimation in path analysis. This technique has only recently been used in this field (Bouchard 1980; Byard 1984; Pérusse 1987). Results of these studies show a lesser degree of heritability of all the anthropometric and motor ability characteristics. The heritability coefficients for skinfolds vary between .0

and .55 while those for some motor tests and for cardiorespiratory endurance are around .30.

2 Material and methods

In a longitudinal project a variety of physical fitness data are collected from 110 twins and their parents and siblings. The twins are being followed from prepuberty to postpuberty with annual investigations. This paper only reports on the data of the first visits of 91 twins, all measured at the age of 10 years ($\overline{X}$ = 10.3, SD = .3) and equally subdivided according to zygosity and sex (21 female monozygotic pairs (MZFF), 20 male monozygotic pairs (MZMM), 13 like-sexed female dizygotic pairs (DZFF), 20 like-sexed male dizygotic pairs (DZMM), 17 unlike-sexed dizygotic pairs (DZFM). The zygosity of the twins was determined at birth.

The physical fitness characteristics include measures of health- and performance related fitness. Health-related fitness is measured by the sum of 6 skinfolds (biceps, supra-iliacal, triceps, subscapular, calf medial and lateral), VO_2 max (maximal exercise test on the treadmill), flexibility (sit and reach, SAR), trunk strength (leg lifts, LEL) and functional strength (bent arm hang, BAH). Performance related fitness is tested by explosive strength (vertical jump, VTJ), static strength (arm pull, ARP), speed (shuttle run, SHR), speed of limb (plate tapping, PLT) and balance (flamingo balance, FBA). A logarithmic transformation was performed on the sum of 6 skinfolds and the bent arm hang results to normalize the distribution.

Model fitting was used to estimate the contribution of genetic and environmental factors to the physical fitness characteristics. This technique assumes linear relationships between dependent and independent variables. A structural equation model is set up to specify causal and correlational relationships. Two alternative models will be tested to explain the observed variation and covariation among the measured dependent variables of the twins. The simple model estimates the effect of genetic (H) and environmental (E) factors. In the second model, the significance of environmental factors common to both twins apart from the influence of specific environmental factors is tested.

Alternative models were compared by subtracting their chi-squares and their respective degrees of freedom. This results in another chi-square which is evaluated by its degrees of freedom. In this study, the HCE-model in which one extra parameter (C) was estimated had one degree of freedom less than the HE-model. It will be tested whether the addition of a parameter resulted in a statistically significant increase in the goodness-of-fit statistic. If the inclusion of this parameter (C) did not result in a significantly better fit, the simpler of the two models, the HE model, was preferred (Heath et al. 1989; Neale et al. 1989).

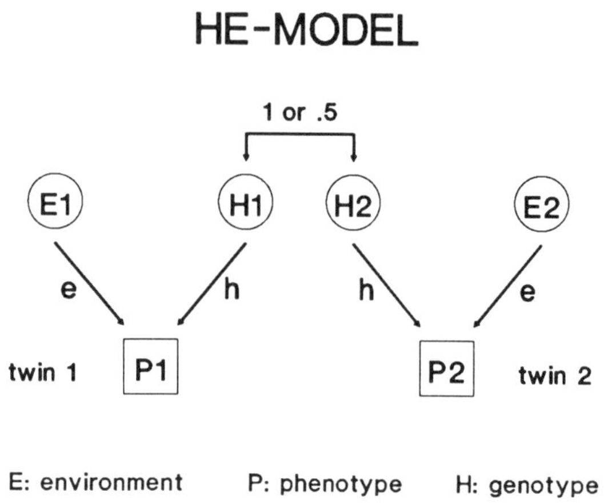

HE-MODEL

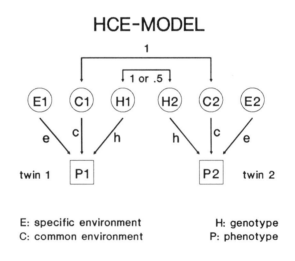

Fig. 1. Path diagram for the genotype-environment model (HE-model).

HCE-MODEL

Fig. 2. Path diagram for the genotype-common-and-specific-environment model (HCE-model).

The path diagram shown in Figures 1 and 2 illustrate the different models. The correlation between the genetic factors of both twins is 1 for MZ twins and .5 for DZ twins. The correlation between common environmental factors is 1 for both MZ and DZ twins, there is no correlation between specific environmental factors because they are assumed to be unique to the individual twins. The path coefficients are estimated using the maximum likelihood function of LISREL, a program to analyze linear structural relationships (Jöreskog 1988). A chi-square goodness-of-fit statistic is obtained as well by LISREL. The input covariance matrices were calculated using PRELIS, a preprocessor for LISREL (Jöreskog 1986).

3 Results

Means and standard deviations for all variables are listed in Table 1. There are no significant differences between means and standard deviations of twins as compared to singletons. There are no significant differences between the means of MZ and DZ twins, except for shuttle run (p<.05). However the variances of MZ and DZ twins are significantly different (p<.05) for the sum of skinfolds and (p<.01) for leg lifts, the bent arm hang and for shuttle run. The means of males and females differ significantly for most of the motor variables : balance, plate tapping, sit and reach, arm pull, bent arm hang, sum of skinfolds and VO_2 max (p<.01). Girls perform better in balance, plate tapping, sit and reach and leg lifts, while boys do better in arm pull, bent arm hang and VO_2 max. Variances differ as well for bent arm hang and sum of skinfolds.

Table 2 shows the within pair correlations for MZ and DZ twins. The MZ correlations are always higher than the DZ correlations but the correlations between MZ and DZ twins differ significantly only for the sum of skinfolds, the vertical jump and arm pull. Correlations for the different variables in DZ twins do not differ. However, some differences between the correlations for different variables in MZ twins are significant. The MZ correlation for plate tapping is significantly different (p<.05) from MZ correlations for all the health-related fitness variables, except leg lifts and shuttle run. The MZ correlation for balance also differs from the MZ correlation for three of the health-related fitness variables (p<.05). Despite the significant differences in means for boys and girls for most variables, no significant difference could be noted between the total DZ correlation (DZMM, DZFF and DZMF) and the same sex DZ correlation (DZSS).

The results of model fitting (Table 3 and 4) show that (with the exception of leg lifts) all the goodness-of-fit tests are non-significant (p<.01), which means that there is a good agreement between the observed and the predicted covariances. No significant differences are apparent between the

Table 1. Means and standard deviations for health- and performance-related fitness variables in MZ and DZ twins.

	$\overline{X}_{MZ}$	SD_{MZ}	$\overline{X}_{DZ}$	SD_{DZ}
Health Related Fitness				
Sum of 6 skinfolds	48.4	17.2	46.0	12.9*
VO$_2$ max (l/min/kg)	47.9	10.6	48.3	9.9
SAR (cm)	21.4	6.2	20.3	6.0
LEL (N/20sec)	14.3	2.2	14.4	2.8**
BAH (sec)	14.0	14.0	12.0	10.7**
Performance Related Fitness				
VTJ (cm)	29.2	4.5	28.3	4.0
ARP (kg)	25.8	4.1	24.7	4.4
SHR (sec)	23.3	1.9	22.7*	1.5**
PLT (N/20sec)	64.3	5.6	62.9	6.7
FBA (N/1min)	16.3	5.6	16.9	6.4

* p<.05
** p<.01

Table 2. Within pair correlations for health- and performance-related fitness variables in MZ, DZ and DZSS twins.

	r_{MZ}	r_{DZ}	r_{DZSS}
Health Related Fitness			
Sum of 6 skinfolds	.894	.479*	.583
VO$_2$ max (l/min/kg)	.845	.557	.591
SAR (cm)	.824	.528	.645
LEL (N/20sec)	.558	.394	.308
BAH (sec)	.651	.458	.311
Performance Related Fitness			
VTJ (cm)	.673	.240*	.319
ARP (kg)	.714	.244*	.240
SHR (sec)	.756	.435	.257
PLT (N/20sec)	.373	.208	.360
FBA (N/1 min)	.440	.377	.397

* p<.05

genotype-environment model (EG-model) and the genotype-common-and-specific-environment model (ECG-model) for either the health-related fitness or the performance-related fitness variables. For most health-related fitness variables, the ECG-model is slightly better than the EG-model, but the difference is not significant. For the performance-related fitness variables, there is no indication for a common environmental influence, the observed covariation can be fully explained by genetic and specific environmental factors. Omitting the opposite-sex DZ twins did not result in a significant different fit of the models. A more detailed analysis of possible sex effects will be done when larger sample sizes are available.

Under the EG-model, the percentage of the variance explained by genetic factors for the health-related fitness variables varies between 86.5 % for VO_2 max and 63.4 % for trunk strength. For performance-related fitness variables, the percentage of explained genetic variance varies from 42.5 % for speed of limb movement to 71.7 % for static strength. With larger sample size, the inclusion of a common environmental factor might result in a significantly better fit for health-related fitness variables (Martin 1977). The percentage of explained variance by genetic factors would then decrease by approximately 25 % which would be explained by common environmental factors.

4 Discussion

Path analysis has not often been used to study genetic versus environmental influences on physical fitness variables. No path analysis studies are available for most of the variables under consideration. Our results are compared to heritability coefficients, calculated based upon classical methods.

Correlations for skinfolds between MZ and DZ twins in the present study are consistent with data from other twin studies (Després 1984; Sharma 1984). The heritability estimates calculated using path-analysis, however, are much higher (.82) than those reported by Bouchard (1980), Byard (1983) and Pérusse (1987). The latter vary between .03 and .55, but a different path-analysis model was used. Comparable results would probably have been obtained with larger sample sizes.

Many studies on the genetic contribution of cardiovascular endurance, mostly measured by VO_2 max, are available in the literature but in most cases sample sizes are very small and different ages are included. Further, results of these studies are very contradictory. Komi et al. (1973) state that there is no significant genetic effect on VO_2max, while Klissouras (1973, 1977) and Crielaard and Pirnay (1982) report very high heritabilities. More recent studies and studies with larger sample sizes (Engstrom and

Table 3. Measures of fit, Heritability (h^2) and Environmentability (e^2) from fitting the model in Fig. 1.

	CHI^2	Prob	h^2	e^2
Health Related Fitness				
SSK	4.22	.377	.865	.135
VO_2	3.24	.518	.834	.166
SAR	2.62	.624	.818	.182
LEL	12.30	.015	.645	.355
BAH	2.47	.649	.634	.366
Performance Related Fitness				
VTJ	5.21	.267	.625	.375
ARP	2.12	.714	.717	.283
SHR	5.85	.211	.709	.291
PLT	7.95	.094	.425	.575
FBA	9.35	.053	.515	.485

Table 4. Measures of fit, Heritability (h^2), Common Environmentability (c^2) and Environmentability (e^2) from fitting the model in Fig. 2.

	CHI^2	Prob	h^2	e^2	c^2
Health Related Fitness					
SSK	3.43	.329	.660	.207	.133
VO_2	1.14	.768	.522	.310	.168
SAR	1.31	.727	.566	.250	.184
LEL	12.27	.007	.600	.400	.360
BAH	.70	.873	.274	.335	.391
Performance Related Fitness					
VTJ	5.21	.157	.625	.000	.375
ARP	2.12	.548	.717	.000	.283
SHR	4.47	.215	.396	.306	.299
PLT	7.95	.047	.425	.000	.575
FBA	8.86	.031	.300	.183	.517

Fischbein 1977; Bouchard 1986) indicate a moderate genetic effect of about .40. Only one study used path analysis (Pérusse 1987) and noted a transmissibility of .28 for PWC150. The MZ and DZ correlations in the present study are similar to those in the literature. They are slightly higher than those in the most recent studies, as is the case for heritability estimated by maximum likelihood. These estimates would probably decrease as well with larger sample sizes.

Only a few studies are available on the heritability of other health-related fitness variables. Flexibility is highly heritable (.90) (Kovar 1981), which is confirmed in our study, where a different test (sit and reach) is used. Kovar reports a heritability coefficient of .69 for trunk strength, measured with sit-ups. Pérusse (1987) reports a lower coefficient for sit-ups (.21) using path analysis. Our estimate for leg lifts, however, is comparable to that of Kovar. For functional strength, measured by the bent arm hang test, the heritability estimate of Kovar (1981) (.35) is much lower than the present study (.65).

For performance-related fitness variables, static and explosive strength have been studied most often. Explosive strength, tested by the vertical jump, has a high genetic component (around .85) according to Kovar (1981) and Crielaard & Pirnay (1982-83). Similar results are found for running speed, using the shuttle run test, with coefficients varying from .72 to .90 (Kovar 1981). The mean heritability estimate for static strength measured with different strength tests is somewhat lower (.65) (Kovar 1981; Crielaard & Pirnay 1982-83; Engstrom & Fischbein 1977). Pérusse (1987) reports an even lower coefficient for static strength (.30) with path analysis. Our results however, suggest a higher heritability for static strength and running speed (.71) than for explosive strength (.63). In contrast to the high heritability (around .80) reported for speed of limb movement reported by Kovar (1981), a lower estimate (.47) was found in our study. This estimate is comparable to that for balance (.51), for which no unambiguous results are reported in the literature. Most of the studies are reviewed by Malina (1986).

In general there is a fairly good agreement between our results and those in the literature. However, the heritability estimates are slightly higher for most of the health-related fitness variables in the present study. When looking at the model fitting results, the model including a common environmental factor, fits better for these variables, but the differences between this model and the genotype-environment model are not significant so that the simpler model is preferred. The data suggest, however, that common environmental factors explain part of the observed covariances for these health-related fitness variables which might prove significant with larger sample sizes. The percentage of variance which would be contributed to these family environmental factors is now added to the percentage of the variance explained by genetic factors. This could be an explanation for the somewhat higher heritability estimates in our study. On the other hand, the model fitting results for performance-related fitness variables show no evidence for common environmental influences. The goodness-of-fit statistics are the same for both models so that the model with the fewest parameters, genetic and specific environmental factors, is preferred.

In summary a genotype-environment model fits best for health-and performance-related fitness variables. This suggests that the observed covariances for these variables in twins can be fully explained by genetic and specific environmental factors. No evidence was found for a difference in heritability of health-related fitness and performance-related fitness variables.

5 References

Bouchard, C. Demirjian, A. and Malina, R.M. (1980) Path analysis of family resemblance in physique. **Studies in Physical Anthropology** , 6, pp. 61-70.

Bouchard, C. and Malina, R.M. (1983) Genetics of physiological fitness and motor performance, in **Exercise and sports sciences reviews** (American College of Sports Medicine Series 11) (ed R.L. Terlung), Franklin Institute Press, Philadelphia, pp. 306-309.

Bouchard, C. (1986) Genetics of aerobic power and capacity, in, **Sport and Human Genetics**, (eds R.M. Malina and C. Bouchard), Human Kinetics Publishers, Champaign, Ill., pp. 59-88.

Byard, P.J. Sharma, K. Russel, J.M. Rao, D.C. (1984) A family study of anthropometric traits in a Punjabi community, II. An investigation of familial transmission, **Am. J. Phys. Anthrop.**, 64, 97-104.

Crielaard, J.M. Pirnay, F. (1982) Déterminisme Génétique de l'Aptitude Physique, **Travaux de la Société Francophone de la Médicine et des Sciences du Sport**, vol. 31, 136-144.

Després, B.J. Bouchard, C. Savard, R. Prud'homme, D. Bukowiecki, L. Thériault, G. (1984) Adaptive changes to training in adipose tissue lipolysis are genotype dependent. **Int. J. Obesity**, 8, 87-95.

Engstrom, L.M. Fischbein, S. (1973) Physical capacity in twins. **Acta Genet. Med. Gemellol.** , 26, 159-165.

Heath, A.C. Neale, M.C. Hewitt, J.K. Eaves, L.J. Fulker, D.W. (1989) Testing structural equation models for twin data using LISREL, **Behav. Genet.**, 19 (1), 9-36.

Jöreskog, K.G. Sörbom, D. (1986) **PRELIS : A preprocessor for LISREL.** Scientific Software, Inc., Mooresville.

Jöreskog, K.G. Sörbom, D. (1988) **LISREL : A guide to the program and applications.**, SPSS Inc., Chicago.

Klissouras, V. (1973) Genetic aspects of physical fitness, **J. Sports Med.** , 13, 164-170.

Klissouras, V. (1977) Twin studies on functional capacity, in **Physiological Variation and its Genetic Basis** (ed J.S. Weiner), (Symposia for the Society for the Study of Human Biology, vol. 17), Taylor and Francis, London, pp. 43-55.

Komi, P.V. Klissouras, V. Karvinen, E. (1973) Genetic variation in neuromuscular performance, **Int. Z. Angew. Physiol.** , 3, 289-304.

Kovar, R. (1981) **Human variation in motor abilities and its genetic basis.** Charles University, Prague, 178 p.

Malina, R.M. (1983) Genetics of motor development and performance, in **Sport and Human Genetics** (ed R.M. Malina and C. Bouchard), Human Kinetics Publishers, Champaign, Ill. , pp. 23-58.

Martin, N.G. Eaves, L.J. Kearsey, M.J. Davies, R. (1978) The power of the classical twin study. **Heredity**, 40 (1), 97-116.

Neale, M.C. Heath, A.C. Hewitt, J.K. Eaves, L.J. Fulker, D.W. (1989) Fitting genetic models with LISREL : Hypothesis testing. **Behavior Genetics**, 19 (1), 37-50.

Pérusse, L. Lortie, G. Leblanc, C. Tremblay, A. Thériault, G. (1987) Genetic and environmental sources of variation in physical fitness. **Ann. Hum. Biol.**, 14, 425-434.

13

ERGOMETRIC ASSESSMENTS OF KAYAK PADDLERS

S. DERHAM and T. REILLY
Centre for Sport and Exercise Sciences, Liverpool Polytechnic, England.

Keywords: Ergometry, Kayak, Maximal oxygen uptake, Peak lactate, Specificity.

1 Introduction

Specificity is recognised as an important principle in sports training. Specific adaptations accrue long-term as athletes gain expertise and technical skills in their chosen sport. This specificity reflects the unique demands of the sport and the training drills performed in preparation for competition. It should be reflected also in the choice of ergometer used for assessment of the training status. To this end ergometers are now designed to match as far as possible the muscle groups and type of activity involved in the particular sport (Reilly and Lees 1984; Dal Monte 1988).

Flatwater kayaking entails competitive racing from 500 m to 10,000 m. Typical times range from 1 min 45 s (500 m) to 45 min (10,000 m). Except for the 500 m race, the other competitive events predominantly tax aerobic power. As kayaking engages arm, shoulder and trunk muscles, their actions should be mimicked when measuring aerobic power of competitors. Campagna et al. (1982) modified a swim bench to allow the paddler to assume the same anatomical position on the ergometer as would occur in the kayak. Film analysis providing traces of the paths of joint centres, showed a similar pattern for on-water kayaking and for actions on the dry-land ergometer. This validated the ergometer for fitness assessment and conditioning of kayak paddlers.

For success of the paddler, the maximal aerobic power is more critical than body mass. The slightly greater resistance caused by friction of the craft in the water due to any extra body mass is significant. Although trunk and shoulder muscles are engaged in the paddling technique, the major part of the work is performed by the arms. This would suggest that a high peak oxygen uptake in arm exercise may be an important requirement of kayakers.

The purpose of this study was to examine peak aerobic power and physiological responses to maximal exercise in kayak specialists. The intention was to compare responses to exercise on arm ergometry, leg ergometry and two specific kayak paddling ergometers. It was hypothesised that values on the kayak ergometer would attain higher fractional utilisation of responses to leg exercise than would values for arm ergometry.

2 Methods

2.1 Subjects

Ten male kayak paddlers from clubs in the North West region of England volunteered to participate in the study. They were grouped into a regional elite squad (n = 5; aged 20.2 ± 0.8 years; height 176.8 ± 5.3 cm; body mass 74.8 ± 2.9 kg) and a ranked group (n = 5; aged 22.3 ± 2.7 years; height 179.4 ± 11.5 cm; body mass 79.0 ± 7.5 kg). The elite group consisted of paddlers engaged in regular systematic training once or twice daily who had competed to a high standard in national regattas. The 'ranked' group consisted of paddlers at a lower level of the divisional racing system. The ten subjects were tested just prior to and during the early part of the racing season, these tests being conducted in March and April 1989.

2.2 Tests

Four tests of maximal effort were carried out in the laboratory and one on-water in order to determine the physiological characteristics of the kayak paddlers. These exercise bouts were performed in random order on separate days between 1-7 days apart.

A friction braked cycle ergometer (Monark) was used to assess maximal oxygen uptake (VO_2 max) during leg exercise and peak oxygen uptake of the arms (VO_2 peak(a)). This entailed an incremental test to voluntary exhaustion. For leg exercise the protocol started at 120 W for 5 min, followed by 30 W increments every 2 min until volitional exhaustion. The cycling frequency was maintained at 60 rev min^{-1}. The arm exercise protocol consisted of a 5 min warm-up at 80 W followed by a 5 min rest. The test was resumed at 110 W for 3 min, and the work-rate then increased by 15 W every 2 min. Arm cycling frequency was maintained at 50 rev min^{-1}. During both tests exhaled air was analysed continuously to determine VO_2 using an online system (P.K. Morgan, Gillingham). Heart rate was monitored using short-range radio telemetry (Sport-tester). Pre-exercise and post-exercise blood samples were obtained for measurement of lactate concentration using an enzymatic method (Bergmeyer, 1974).

The kayak ergometer trials consisted of 4 min all-out exercise bouts. The 4 min exercise bout was chosen after a pilot study which showed that further durations did not produce a higher VO_2. This time also approximates to time taken by elite paddlers to race 1000 m. The speed settings on the two ergometers were also determined from pilot investigations. The ergometers were a 'biokinetic swim bench' (Isokinetics Inc; Albany, Ca.) modified for use by paddlers (Fig. 1) and an isokinetic kayak training device (Isosport Training System: Hand M. Engineering, Gwent). In the modified 'swim bench' the paddler sat on a separate seat bench with foot-rest and used a paddle shaft connected with two wires, via pulleys, to the resistance generator of the ergometer. This allowed the paddler to execute a smooth and uninterrupted style as performed in the kayak.

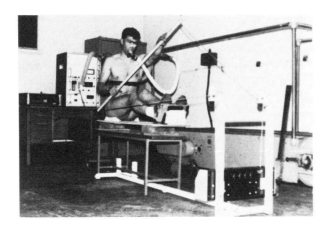

Fig. 1. Paddler using the 'Biokinetic' kayak ergometer.

The on-water test was carried out using the subject's own racing kayak (K1) over a relatively flat and still course. A 10 min warm-up was followed by a 5 min rest, then 1 min easy paddling preceding a 4 min effort of maximal propelling. Heart rate was recorded during the maximal effort using short-range radio telemetry (Sport-tester), the recorder being worn on the wrist by the subject. Blood samples were obtained prior to warm-up and post-exercise for analysis of blood lactate concentration.

As subjects raced over distances above and below 1000 m, their relative performances were ranked by an expert coach. This provided a basis for correlating performance levels with the physiological responses using Spearman's rank order correlation (Siegel, 1956).

3 Results

The results for the whole sample (Table 1) indicated that highest values for VO_2, heart rate and blood lactate were noted for leg cycling ($P < 0.01$). The VO_2 peak during specific kayak ergometer paddling was significantly greater than that during maximal arm cycling ($P < 0.05$). There was no difference between the two kayak simulators in the peak VO_2 values attained. The VO_2 peak(a) for arm work was 78% of that obtained for leg exercise VO_2 max. Values reached on the two kayak simulators were highly correlated ($r = 0.97$ according to the Pearson Product method) and reached 87% of the VO_2 max.

Heart rates during leg exercise were significantly higher than in the other conditions, with the exception of the isokinetic kayak ergometer (P 0.05). The lowest values were observed on-water. Blood lactates were highest following the VO_2 max test employing leg exercise: significantly lower values were observed for arm cycling and for the on-water tests than for the other conditions ($P < 0.05$).

Table 1. Physiological responses (mean $\pm$ S.D.) of kayak paddlers (n = 10) to ergometric tests.

	Cycle ergometer		Kayak ergometer		On-water
	Legs	Arms	Swim-bench	Isosport	Kayak
VO_2 (1 min^{-1})	4.36 ± 0.61	3.37 ± 0.44	3.68 ± 0.63	3.71 ± 0.59	-
Heart rate (beat min^{-1})	186 ± 8	183 ± 8	182 ± 9	183 ± 9	179 ± 10
Blood lactate (mM)	8.6 ± 2.0	6.1 ± 1.2	7.6 ± 1.6	7.5 ± 1.2	6.2 ± 1.6

The VO_2 values were significantly correlated with competitive performance for all the ergometer tests. The highest correlation with performance was obtained for the isokinetic ergometer ($r = 0.87$; $P < 0.01$), the lowest with leg pedalling on the cycle ergometer ($r = 0.77$; $P < 0.01$).

When subjects were divided into elite and ranked categories, the elite paddlers had significantly higher oxygen uptake values in all four ergometry tests ($P < 0.05$). Measures of heart rate and blood lactate did not differ between the groups on any of the tests ($P > 0.05$). The VO_2 peak values obtained on the simulator were 88% of values obtained in leg exercise for the elite group. These values were highly correlated with competitive performance levels, the correlation coefficient being 0.973 for both simulators. These high correlations with performance were not evident in the elite group for the conventional arm and leg exercise tests.

Table 2. Highest VO_2 values for elite and ranked kayak paddlers on all four ergometer tests (mean $\pm$ S.D.).

	Cycle ergometer		Kayak ergometer	
	Legs	Arms	Swim bench	Isosport
Elite (n = 5) :				
VO_2 (l min^{-1})	4.76 $\pm$ 0.51	3.75 $\pm$ 0.14	4.18 $\pm$ 0.45	4.17 $\pm$ 0.43
(ml kg^{-1} min^{-1})	63.2 $\pm$ 4.2	50.1 $\pm$ 3.8	55.8 $\pm$ 4.8	55.8 $\pm$ 4.6
Ranked (n=5) :				
VO_2 (l min^{-1})	3.97 $\pm$ 0.42	3.08 $\pm$ 0.22	3.18 $\pm$ 0.20	3.23 $\pm$ 0.20
(ml kg^{-1} min^{-1})	51.1 $\pm$ 4.6	38.6 $\pm$ 4.4	40.8 $\pm$ 2.7	41.6 $\pm$ 1.8

4 Discussion

It is generally held that paddlers have a higher aerobic power in arm exercise relative to leg exercise than other groups (Reilly and Secher 1990). The mean arm-leg ratio of 77% for the whole group of paddlers is higher than the fractional oxygen uptakes of about 70% found in physically active but not specifically arm-trained men (Davis et al. 1976). The arm-leg ratio noted among elite paddlers is not as high as reported in previous studies of international calibre Scandinavian paddlers (Tesch et al. 1976; Larsson et al. 1988). It is likely that a very high fractional utilisation of VO_2 max is achieved by successful international competitors, the elite group in this study being successful at a domestic level.

Higher peak VO_2 values were attained on the kayak simulators than in arm cycling. Nevertheless the 88- fractional utilisation of VO_2 max in this group was lower than that observed for Danish internationals exercising on a wind-braked kayak ergometer (Larsson et al. 1988). The fractional utilisation of the Danish internationals was 97% of the VO_2 max determined whilst pedalling with the legs on a cycle ergometer. It is likely that a higher ratio would have been obtained by the present subjects if testing were conducted later in the competitive season.

In addition to the specificity of actions, the greater muscle mass involved in performance on the simulator may have contributed to the higher VO_2 values compared to responses during arm work on the cycle ergometer. This was reflected also in the blood lactate results, values being highest after leg exercise and lowest after the arm ergometry test. Values for lactate were well below the 14 mM level observed following competitive races (Tesch and Karlsson 1984), the low concentrations following the on-water test reflecting its time-trial nature. Nevertheless, results compare favourably with the figure of 7.2 $\pm$ 2.2 mM cited by Shephard (1987) for ergometric paddling. The attainment of near-maximal heart rates on the kayak ergometers is comparable with previous findings on kayak specialists (Reilly and Secher 1990).

The validity of the kayak ergometer was partly confirmed by the high correlations between peak VO_2 and competitive performance. The two simulators were equal in this respect. As the two devices were designed essentially for training purposes, a further validation would investigate the extent to which supplementary training on the devices enhances competitive performance. Results of this study suggest that both dry-land kayak ergometers do provide a reasonable physiological representation of kayak paddling and an appropriate mode for assessing kayak specialists.

5 References

Bergmeyer, H.U. (1974) **Methods of Enzymatic Analysis**. Academic Press, New York.

Campagna, P.D. Brien, D. Holt, L.E. Alexander, A. and Greenberger, H. (1982) A biomechanical comparison of Olympic flatwater kayaking and a dry land kayak ergometer. **Can. J. Appl. Sport Sci.,** 7, 242.

Dal Monte, A. (1988) Exercise testing and ergometers, in **The Olympic Book of Sports Medicine** (eds A. Dirix, H.G. Knuttgen and K. Tittel), Blackwell Scientific, Oxford, pp. 121-150.

Davis, J.A. Vodak, P. Wilmore, J.H. Vodak, J. and Kurtz, P. (1976) Anaerobic threshold and maximal aerobic power for three modes of exercise. **J. Appl. Physiol.,** 41, 544-550.

Larsson, B. Larsen, J. Modest, R. Serup, B. and Secher, N.H. (1988) A new kayak ergometer based on wind resistance. **Ergonomics,** 31, 1701-1708.

Reilly, T. and Lees, A. (1984) Exercise and sports equipment; some ergonomic aspects. **Appl. Ergon.,** 15, 259-279.

Reilly, T. and Secher, N.H. (1990) Physiology of sports: overview, in **Physiology of Sports** (eds T. Reilly, N.H. Secher, P. Snell and C. Williams), E. & F.N. Spon, London, pp. 466-485.

Shephard, R.J. (1987) Science and medicine of canoeing and kayaking. **Sports Med.,** 4, 19-33.

Siegel, S. (1956) **Nonparametric Statistics for the Behavioural Sciences.** McGraw-Hill, Tokyo.

Tesch, P.A. and Karlsson, J. (1984) Muscle metabolite accumulation following maximal exercise: a comparison between short term and prolonged kayak performance. **Europ. J. Appl. Physiol.,** 52, 243-246.

Tesch, P.A., Piehl, K., Wilson, G. and Karlsson, J. (1976) Physiological investigations of Swedish elite canoe competitors. **Med. Sci. Sport. Exerc.,** 8, 214-218.

Part Three

Performance and Anthropometry

.

14

PHYSICAL ACTIVITY AND BONE

D.A. BAILEY [1] and R.G. McCULLOCH [2]
[1] College of Physical Education, University of Saskatchewan, Saskatoon, Canada
[2] Faculty of Physical Activity Studies, University of Regina, Regina, Canada

Keywords: Physical activity, Osteoporosis, Bone mass, Bone density, Bone mineral content.

1 Introduction

The present interest in osteoporosis has resulted in considerable research to identify factors underlying age-related bone loss. Skeletal fragility in the elderly represents a tremendous public health problem, economically and clinically. Two hypotheses have been put forward to explain the cause of dangerously reduced bone mass in the senior population; a) unusually accelerated loss in later years; or b) failure to attain a sufficient level of peak bone density in young adulthood. It is probable that reduced bone mass in elderly patients results from some combination of these factors.

Virtually all the research to date has been directed at understanding the mechanisms of, and providing strategies for, reducing the rate of bone loss in the adult and senior populations. There is considerable knowledge about bone density loss in the elderly and very little about bone density gain when the skeleton is growing and developing. Longitudinal studies are lacking and there are few norms available for the adolescent years. It has been suggested that one of the most important determinants of whether or not a person is going to develop osteoporosis in later life is how large and dense the bones are at the time of skeletal maturity. Clearly, more information is needed about the determinants of bone gain in childhood and peak bone mass in young adults. The aim of the present paper is to provide insight into the mechanisms of bone density gain during the growing years, and to evaluate the effects of differing levels of physical activity on bone mineralization.

Bones provide more than just a structural framework for the body. In reality, bone is a multifunctional tissue dependent on, and sensitive to, a wide variety of biological, biochemical and biomechanical stimuli. This complex system is highly responsive to the mechanical stresses imposed by gravity and muscular contractions. Animal studies as well as human cross-sectional and longitudinal studies all point to the importance of weight-bearing physical activity and mechanical loading as the prime modalities in the preservation of skeletal integrity. Lack of weight-bearing activity is extremely harmful to the skeleton. Loss of skeletal density in individuals subjected to various types of immobilization or under conditions of weightlessness is well documented. The role of physical activity in the maintenance of skeletal integrity is a topic of considerable current concern when the increasing incidence of skeletal fragility in the elderly is taken into account. The aim of the present paper is to provide insight into the mechanisms of bone density gain during the growing years, and to evaluate the effects of differing levels of physical activity on bone mineralization in the adult years.

2 Bone Mass Changes Through the Lifespan

Skeletal tissue is in a constant state of change throughout life. Two processes are involved in this dynamic condition, modeling and remodeling. Modeling is a process most active during growth and results in the alteration of size and shape through formation on one surface and resorption on another surface. Remodeling is a renewal process resulting in the continual breakdown and reformation of bone, even in old age, to maintain blood calcium at a constant level and to replace old microfractured bone with new bone. This process allows a bone to change its shape and structure in response to the mechanical circumstances of the tissue (Lanyon et al. 1982). Bone remodeling is influenced by a feedback mechanism which operates to maintain strain levels at optimal values (Lanyon et al. 1976). In the adult, it is estimated that 10% to 30% of the skeleton is replaced by remodeling in each year (Aloia 1989).

Bone density status of the skeleton at any time during the life span is dependent on bone gained during the growing and early adult years and bone lost with advancing years. Total bone mass and bone density increase during the growing years (Wardlaw 1988), reaching a maximum in early adulthood (Kaplan 1987). Approximately 48% of total skeletal mass is attained during adolescence (Benson et al. 1985). Cross-sectional studies (Atkinson and Weatherall 1967; Garn et al. 1967; Klemm et al. 1976) have indicated that the increase in bone density during growth follows a positive and nearly linear path until approximately age 20, after which, the rate of increase slows until peak bone density is reached (Wall et al. 1979). Others report a bone density spurt during puberty (Gilsanz et al. 1988). There is significant individual age and sex variation in bone mass and density (Christiansen et al. 1975) with the greatest variation occurring during late adolescence (Krabbe et al. 1979). Bone mass lags behind linear growth during adolescence (Kaplan 1983; Bailey et al. 1989) and reaches its peak after linear growth has ceased. Some women may increase skeletal mass 10% to 15% after the closure of the epiphyseal plates (Aloia 1989).

160

Peak bone mass and bone density is determined by genetic, mechanical, nutritional and hormonal forces (Wahner et al. 1984). It is generally agreed that peak bone parameters are lower in women than in men (Nilas and Christiansen 1987). Mazess (1982) reported that women had 15% lower peak bone density and 30% lower peak bone mass than men after completion of skeletal growth. The National Institute of Health (NIH) Consensus Conference on Osteoporosis in 1984 (Peck 1984) adopted a statement indicating that peak bone mass is approximately 30% less in women than men. However, two research groups have found that young women and men had similar values for vertebral bone density (Gilsanz et al. 1988; Riggs et al. 1981).

After a transient period of stability at peak bone density, an incessant, age-related loss of bone begins (Riggs and Melton 1986). The involution of bone with advancing age is observed in both men and women, but the rate of loss is greater in women (Nilas and Christiansen 1987). Over their lifetime, women lose about 35% of their cortical bone and 50 to 60% of their trabecular bone, whereas men lose about one third less (Mazess 1982; Riggs et al. 1981). In men, the decline of bone density with age appears to be largely due to a decrease in bone formation (Nordin et al. 1981); whereas postmenopausal bone loss in women apparently results from an increase in bone resorption (Heaney et al. 1978).

After age 35, the average rate of cortical bone loss for both sexes is about 0.3% to 0.5% of peak adult bone density per year. In women, the loss of cortical bone can be as high as 2 to 3% per year for the first 8 to 10 years after menopause (Lindsay et al. 1980; Mazess 1982)

The onset of trabecular bone loss can occur several years before cortical loss begins in both men and women (Riggs and Melton 1986) and can begin as early as age 20 in some individuals, with variable rates of loss (Hansson et al. 1980; Riggs et al. 1981). Age-related trabecular bone loss in women ranges from a linear decrease of 0.6% per year in the appendicular skeleton (distal radius) (Riggs et al. 1981) to a curvilinear decline as high as 2.4% per year in the axial skeleton (vertebrae) (Cann et al. 1985; Krolner and Nielsen 1982). On average, women lose approximately 1.2% per year of vertebral trabecular bone density (Riggs et al. 1986). Riggs and Melton (1986) suggest that the extent of trabecular bone loss for women in the first few years after menopause is much greater than cortical loss in the same years, but the duration of accelerated loss is shorter. On the other hand, Hansson and Roos (1986) have stated that there is no clear acceleration of axial bone loss around the usual time of menopause. The loss of vertebral trabecular bone for men ranges from 0.5% per year to 1.2% per year (Meier et al. 1984).

The loss of bone in later life has severe consequences since bone strength is closely related to bone density (Bartley et al. 1966; Frost 1985; Horsman and Currey 1983). In many people, the absolute decrease in the amount of bone progresses to frank osteoporosis and places segments of the skeleton at or near the fracture threshold in later life. While the etiology of age-related osteoporosis is still unclear, there is general agreement that three factors acting alone or in combination are pre-eminent in terms of maintenance of bone integrity; endocrine status, nutritional factors and physical activity. The relative contribution of each of these factors has not been established, but clearly, physical activity is a dominant player. In the absence of weight-bearing activity, no amount of nutritional or endocrine intervention can or will maintain bone density (Mazess and Whedon 1983).

3 Physical Activity and Bone

It takes mechanical forces on bone to bring about increased mineralization. This was partially recognized by Galileo in 1638 who noted the relationship between body weight and bone size. A Berlin anatomist, Julius Wolff in 1892 is given credit for first recognizing that changes in bone mass accompanied changes in mechanical loading through a process of remodeling. He noted that bone remodeling is driven by mechanical forces and that bone tissue reorganizes when mechanical forces change (Wolff 1892). Wolff's seminal work in German, 'Das Gesetz der Transformation der Knochen', has recently been translated into English (Maquet and Furlong 1986) and Wolff's Law, as it is has come to be known, can be re-stated as follows : the general form of a bone being given, alterations of the internal architecture and external form occur as a consequence of primary changes in mechanical stressors according to mathematical rules.

Muscular contraction and gravity are the two primary mechanical forces applied to bone. If either of these forces is reduced, eliminated, or increased, bone density is affected. Each skeletal segment appears to have its own threshold of mechanical stimuli necessary for response (Smith and Raab 1986). With a sufficient increase in loading, the bone tissue hypertrophies and reorganizes to reduce internal mechanical strains to optimum levels. The rate of change in the density of weight-bearing bones is primarily determined by factors related to physical activity (Martin and McCulloch 1987). As the dynamic nature of bone is better understood, the role of the mechanical factors related to physical activity is seen to be increasingly important in maintaining bone density throughout the adult years (Block et al. 1986; Simkin et al. 1987).

4 Animal Studies

The remodeling of bone after changes in mechanical load resulting from weight-bearing activity has been observed in many situations. Animal

162

studies have shown that bone mass, density and shape, rather than the quality of bone tissue, change in response to prolonged physical activity (Woo et al. 1981). Regimes of weight-bearing physical activity increase bone density in animal species ranging from rats (Saville and Whyte 1969) and mice (Bell et al. 1980) to pigs (Goodship et al. 1979) and dogs (Martin et al. 1981).

In addition, studies in various animal species have shed light on the relationship between stress variation and subsequent bone remodeling activity. Hert et al. (1971) were the first to show that static loads, regardless of magnitude, have no effect on bone remodeling. On the other hand, the animal skeleton demonstrated remarkable sensitivity to dynamic loading. For example, Lanyon and Rubin (1984) subjected avian ulna, in vivo, to 0, 4, 36, 360 or 1800 consecutive loading cycles per day at 0.5 Hz for 6 weeks. The 36-cycle regime increased bone mineral content by approximately 40%, a value that was not improved upon by increasing the cycles to 360 or 1800. The influence of functional strain as a determinant of bone remodeling has been discussed by Lanyon (1984), Rubin (1984) and Rubin and Lanyon (1985). Bone density does not change with low intensity exercise, but increases under higher intensity regimens (King and Pengelly 1973). Applying these results to humans, Martin and McCulloch (1987) suggest that the greatest increase in bone density may come from activities with high loading, but with few repetitions.

5 Cross-sectional Studies

Studies in humans are more difficult to carry out, but here as well, evidence is strong in support of the relationship between physical activity and skeletal integrity (Martin and Houston 1987).
Comparing the bone density of active subjects with that of sedentary or less active subjects is less costly and time consuming than experimental longitudinal studies, and the results are less conclusive (Montoye 1987). Nonetheless, cross-sectional studies generally indicate greater bone density in athletes and persons with higher levels of physical activity than in the average population (Smith and Raab 1986; Stillman 1987).

Most studies report that persons with high levels of physical activity have significantly higher bone density than less active persons (e.g., Bailey et al. 1986b; Dalen and Olsson 1974; Halioua 1986; Jacobsen et al. 1984; Sinaki and Offord 1988; Talmage and Anderson 1984). However, other studies have found no significant difference between the active and control groups (e.g., Johnell and Bilsson 1984; Montoye et al. 1976; Smith et al. 1976).

An inherent problem in cross-sectional research is subject bias, since the underlying genotype for bone density prior to participation in exercise is not known (Heaney 1986). Another difficulty in cross-sectional studies is quantifying levels of physical activity (Martin and Houston 1987).

The complicating effects of genetics, diet and metabolism usually encountered in cross-sectional reviews can be eliminated in sport studies involving unilateral activities such as tennis (Dalsky 1987). The preferred arm serves as the experimental limb and the contralateral arm as the control (Smith and Raab 1986). Muscle activity had a positive effect on cortical area (Martin et al. 1987) and bone density in the dominant limbs of the tennis players (Huddleston et al. 1980; Jones et al. 1977; Montoye et al. 1980). Jones et al. (1977) reported that men had 34.9% and women 28.4% greater cortical thickness in the dominant humerus compared to the nondominant humerus. The values for the nondominant arm were similar to those of age-matched controls. Montoye and co-workers (1980) found a 13% greater bone mineral content in the humerus and 7.9% greater bone mineral content in the radius in the dominant arm than in the contralateral limb. In a study of senior male tennis players with 25 - 74 years of experience, Huddleston et al. (1980) found a 13% greater bone mineral content for mid-radius region of the dominant arm. Again, the bone mineral content of the nondominant limb was similar to age predicted normal values in both the Montoye and Huddleston studies.

The specificity of bone mineralization in relation to the type of activity has been illustrated in cross-sectional sport studies. In a study conducted by Jacobsen et al. (1984), the bone mineral content of tennis players, swimmers and age-matched controls demonstrated a pattern relative to the level and distribution of force. The swimmers and tennis players had greater bone mineral content and bone width at the distal and mid-radius sites than did the control subjects. The metatarsal bone mineral content of the swimmers was 9% higher than the controls and the tennis players showed a 22% difference compared to the controls. Bone mineral content of the lumbar vertebrae was greater by 11% only in the tennis players over the controls.

Nilsson and Westlin (1971) compared top-ranked athletes from a variety of sports for bone mineral content at the distal femur. The amount of hypertrophy corresponded to the load of the activity on the lower limb. Weightlifters had the greatest bone density followed by throwers, runners and soccer players. The swimmers were not significantly different from the controls. It appears that swimming may provide a mechanical load adequate to cause hypertrophy in the upper limbs, but weight-bearing activity is required to generate adequate bone hypertrophy in the lower limbs and spine.

6 Longitudinal Studies

The longitudinal, experimental approach produces more definitive findings than in cross-sectional comparisons, but requires a considerable length of time before changes may be detected (Montoye 1987). Several recent longitudinal studies, measuring bone response to exercise at appendicular sites, have found significant change in bone status for the exercise group compared to the control group. These studies range from the most recent four year study by Smith et al. (1989) who found that exercise intervention can significantly slow the rate of bone loss in the radius and ulna of premenopausal and postmenopausal women, to a 1976 study by Smith and Reddan which was the first investigation to demonstrate that aging bone (subjects aged 69-95 years) is responsive to mechanical stimuli. The majority of these studies indicate a positive effect of physical activity on skeletal status. For example, the area density of the os calcis was measured by Williams et al. (1984) in male runners before and after a nine month training program. The runners were divided into two groups based on the consistency of training; the consistent runners averaged 141 km/month while the inconsistent runners averaged 57 km/month. The consistent runners averaged a 3% increase in area density, while the os calcis density of the inconsistent runners and control group remained constant. Margulies et al. (1986) reported the effect of high intensity physical training on the bone mineral content of the tibia in 268 young male infantry recruits. Significant increases in bone mineral content was achieved after only 14 weeks of training (8 hr/day, 6 days/week).

On the other hand, some investigations have found no significant change in bone density at appendicular sites following an exercise intervention (e.g., Sandler et al. 1987; Smith et al. 1976; White et al. 1984). White et al. (1984) reported on the effect of six months of walking and aerobic dancing on radius bone density in postmenopausal women. The controls and walkers lost bone at a greater rate compared to the dancers, suggesting that walking does not contribute appreciable stress to the radius.

The results of the longitudinal exercise studies measuring total body bone status and axial bone sites are mixed. The more recent studies (e.g. Chow et al. 1987; Dalsky et al. 1986; Dalsky et al. 1988) demonstrate a significant positive effect of exercise in women over the age of 50. Dalsky et al. (1988) reported that postmenopausal women participating in weight bearing exercise (walking, jogging, stair climbing) had significant increases above baseline in lumbar bone density compared to a control group. Other researchers report no statistically significant effect of exercise, although the subjects in the exercise group maintained bone density while the control subjects lost density (e.g., Aloia et al. 1978; Krolner et al. 1983; Sidney et al. 1977). More recently, Cavanaugh and Cann (1988) found that an exercise program of moderate brisk walking (three sessions per week for one year) did not stop spinal trabecular bone loss in postmenopausal women suggesting a possible intensity threshold.

In summary, longitudinal studies of bone at appendicular sites appear to confirm the generally positive effects of physical activity that were observed in the cross-sectional literature (Marcus and Carter 1988); as do the more recent studies at axial and total body sites. It would appear that the effectiveness of physical activity in abating bone loss in postmeno-pausal women is modest compared to the effectiveness of increased activity prior to menopause. While physical activity appears to have the potential to increase bone density or slow the rate of bone loss (Sinaki 1989), it is difficult to make specific recommendations for exercise prescription according to frequency, intensity, duration and type of activity (Dalsky 1987).

7 Inactivity and Bone

Under conditions of disuse, the case is clear that lack of weight-bearing activity is extremely detrimental to the skeleton (Bailey et al. 1986a). Bone loses density and size in response to a withdrawal of loading forces (Saville and Whyte 1969). A lack of adequate mechanical stimuli results in bone loss, mediated primarily by a proportionately greater increase in bone resorption without a concomitant increase in bone formation (Dalsky 1987).

Bone measurements conducted before and after space flights provide striking evidence regarding the role of the force of gravity in maintaining bone status. Astronauts in a gravity-free environment can lose bone at a monthly rate as high as 4% for trabecular bone and 1% for cortical bone (Mazess and Whedon 1983). The United States Skylab data also indicated that weight-bearing bones (ie., os calcis) are much more susceptible to loss and that trabecular bone is resorbed preferentially during weightlessness (Smith et al. 1977).

Bone atrophies when there is a substantial decrease in weight-bearing activity (Deitrick et al. 1948; Smith and Raab 1986). Rates of bone loss approaching 1% per week have been found in persons immobilized due to poliomyelitis (Whedon and Shorr 1957; Whedon 1984), muscular dystrophy (Walton and Warrick 1954), paraplegia (Abramson and Delagi 1961), bed rest (Krolner and Toft 1983; Mazess and Whedon 1983) and casting after sports injuries (Andersson and Nilsson 1979). Even stress protection through the use of implants can be shown to cause bone loss (Roesler 1987).

The average calcium loss from the os calcis of bedrest subjects was found to be 0%, 7% and 11.2% at 28, 59 and 84 days, respectively. Os calcis bone calcium losses of Skylab flight crew members paralleled those of bedrest subjects at the same periods with all values falling within one standard deviation of the bedrest group (Bundy 1989).

Lumbar vertebral density decreases by about 1% per week in patients confined to bed (Krolner and Toft 1983). With strict and prolonged rest such as recovery from scoliosis surgery, the loss of bone in the lumbar vertebrae can be as high as 2% per week (Hansson et al. 1975; Leblanc et al. 1987). In paraplegia, one-third of trabecular bone volume is lost during the first six to nine months following the causative spinal cord injury (Arnaud et al. 1986). It has been estimated that a loss of 30% of spine mineral could seriously compromise the mechanical strength of the vertebral column (Mazess and Whedon 1983).

Bone loss during immobilization is selective and much of the loss occurs in weight-bearing bones (Stillman 1987). In patients with paralysis of the upper extremity, bone demineralization in the arms may manifest itself after only eight months (Whedon 1984), while up to 25% of the bone density of the central os calcis can be lost following only 18 weeks of immobilization (Donaldson et al. 1970). Trabecular bone, because of its rapid remodeling, seems to be more sensitive to the cessation of mechanical loading (Stillman 1987). Since bone turnover in youth is higher than later in life, immobilization may have an even greater effect in younger people (Hattner and McMillan 1968).

Reambulation, with an increasing degree of gravity or muscular stress and strain, tends to reverse the decline in bone loss (Stillman 1987). The recovery period following reambulation appears to be several times longer than the period of loss, with a great deal of individual variation involved, and may not be complete in some people (Mazess and Whedon 1983). In a long term follow-up study of the Skylab experiments, Tilton et al. (1980) found a significant decrease in the os calcis bone mineral content of the nine crew members five years after the flights when compared to preflight values.

8 Conclusion

Animal studies as well as human epidemiological and intervention studies all point to the importance of weight-bearing physical activity and mechanical loading as the prime modalities in the preservation of skeletal integrity. Lack of weight-bearing is harmful to the skeleton. The rapid loss of bone in individuals subjected to weightlessness or various types of immobilization is well documented. Neither drug or diet treatment can prevent immobilization bone loss (Mazess and Whedon 1983).

From these and other experiments it can be generalized that remodeling of bone is dependent on individual strain and load history. The relationship between skeletal integrity, bone remodeling activity and increased external load is a fundamental assumption of bone biomechanics. The pre-eminent ingredient in the development and preservation of a healthy skeletal system is the mechanical stress imposed by physical activity. While it is recognized that bone is a multifunctional tissue dependent on, and sensitive to, a wide variety of biological, biochemical and biomechanical stimuli, the over-riding relationship between bone size, shape and mass and mechanical load has never been questioned. Indeed, in reading the historical literature on bone from Galileo onward, there has never been any doubt about the interrelationship between the physical stresses applied to bone and its resultant structure. What remains to be answered is what type of signal is created by the physical load on bone, and how is this signal translated by the cells thereby giving rise to a remodeled structure oriented to the new directions of stress imposed by the activity.

9 References

Abramson, A.S. and Delagi, E.F. (1961) Influence of weight-bearing and muscular contraction on disuse osteoporosis. **Arch. Phys. Med. Rehabil.,** 42, 147-151.

Aloia, J.F. (1989). **Osteoporosis : A Guide to Prevention and Treatment.** Champaign, Illinois : Leisure Press.

Aloia, J.F. Cohn, S.H. Ostuni, J.A. Cane, R. and Ellis, K. (1978) Prevention of involutional bone loss by exercise. **Ann. Int. Med.,** 89, 356-358.

Andersson, S.M. and Nilsson, B.E. (1979) Changes in bone mineral content following ligamentous knee injuries. **Med. Sci. Sport.,** 11, 351-353.

Arnaud, S.B. Schneider, V.S. and Morey-Holton, E. (1986) Effects of inactivity on bone and calcium metabolism, in **Inactivity : Physiological Effects** (eds H. Sandler and J. Vernikos), Academic Press,Toronto, pp. 49-76.

Atkinson, P.J. and Weatherall, J.A. (1967) Variation in the density of the femoral diaphysis with age. **J. Bone Joint Surg.,** 493, 781-788.

Bailey, D.A. Martin, A.D. Houston, C.S. and Howie, J.L. (1986a) Physical activity, nutrition, bone density and osteoporosis. **Aust. J. Sci. Med. Sport**, 18, 3-8.

Bailey, D.A. Martin, A.D. Houston, C.S. Simpson, C. Harrison, J.L. and Lee, E. (1986b) Bone density and physical activity in young women, in **Exercise, Nutrition and Performance** (eds P. Russo and G. Gass), Sydney, Cumberland College of Science, pp. 127-138.

Bailey, D.A. Wedge, J.H. McCulloch, R.G. Martin, A.D. and Bernhardson, S.C. (1989) Epidemiology of fractures of the distal end of the radius in children as associated with growth. **J. Bone Joint Surg. Am.,** 71-A, 1225-1231.

Bartley, M.H. Arnold, J.S. Haslam, R.K. and Jee, W.S. (1966) The relationship of bone strength and bone quality in health, disease and aging. **J. Gerontol.,** 21, 517-521.

Bell, R.R. Tzeng, D.Y. and Draper, H.H. (1980) Long-term effect of calcium, phosphorus and forced exercise on the bones of mature mice. **J. Nutr.,** 110, 1161-1167.

Benson, J. Gillien, P. Bourdet, K. and Loosli, A. (1985) Inadequate and chronic calorie restriction in adolescent ballerinas. **Physician Sportsmed.** 13(10), 79-90.

Block, J.E. Genant, H.K. and Black, D. (1986) Greater vertebral bone mineral mass in exercising young men. **West. J. Med.,** 145, 39-42.

Bundy, K.J. (1989) Composite material models for bone. in **Bone Mechanics.,** (ed S.C. Cowin), CRC Press, Boca Raton, Florida, pp. 197-210).

Cann, C.E. Genant, H.K. Kolb, F.O. and Ettinger, B. (1985) Quantitative computed tomography for prediction of vertebral fracture risk. **Bone,** 6, 1-7.

Cavanaugh, D.J. and Cann, C.E. (1988) Brisk walking does not stop bone loss in postmenopausal women. **Bone,** 9, 201-204.

Chow, R. Harrison, J.E. and Notarius, C. (1987) Effect of two randomized exercise programmes on bone mass of healthy postmenopausal women. **Br. Med. J.,** 295, 1441-1444.

Christiansen, C. Rodbro, P. and Thoger-Nielsen, C. (1975) Bone mineral content and estimated total body calcium in normal children and adolescents. **Scan. J. Clin. Lab. Inv.,** 35, 507-510.

Dalen, N. and Olsson, K.E. (1974) Bone mineral content and physical activity. **Acta Orthop. Scand.,** 45, 170-174.

Dalsky, G.P. (1987) Exercise : its effect on bone mineral content. **Clin. Obstet. Gynaecol.,** 30, 820-832.

Dalsky, G.P. Birge, S.J. Kleinheider, K.S. and Ehsani, A.S. (1986) The effect of endurance exercise training on lumbar bone mass in postmenopausal women. (Abstract). **Med. Sci. Sport Exerc.,** 18 (Suppl.), 96.

Dalsky, G.P. Stocke, K.S. Ehsani, A.A. Slatopolsky, E. Lee, W.C. and Birge, S.J. (1988) Weight-bearing exercise training and lumbar bone mineral content in postmenopausal women. **Ann. Intern. Med.,** 108, 824-828.

Deitrick, J.E. Whedon, G.D. and Shorr, E. (1948) Effects of immobilization upon various metabolic and physiologic functions of normal men. **Am. J. Med.,** 4, 3-35.

Donaldson, C.L. Hulley, S.B. Vogel, J.M. Hattner, R.S. Bayers, J.H. and McMillan, D.E. (1970) Effect of prolonged bed rest on bone mineral. **Metabolism,** 19, 1071-1084.

Frost, H.M. (1985) The pathomechanics of osteoporoses. **Clin. Orthop.,** 200, 198-225.

Garn, S.M. Rohmann, C.G. and Wagner, B. (1967) Bone loss as a general phenomenon in man. **Fed. Proc.,** 26, 1729-1736.

Gilsanz, V. Gibbens, D.T. Roe, T.F. Carlson, M. Senac, M.O. Boechat, M.I. Huang, H.K. Schuz, E.E. Libanati, C.R. and Cann, C.C. (1988) Vertebral bone density in children : effect of puberty. **Radiology,** 166, 847-850.

Goodship, A.E., Lanyon, L.E. and McFie, H. (1979) Functional adaptations of bone to increased stress. **J. Bone Joint Surg. Am.,** 61A, 539-546.

Halioua, L. (1986) High lifetime dietary calcium (Ca) intake and physical activity contribute to greater bone mineral content and bone density in healthy premenopausal women? (Abstract). **Fed. Proc.,** 45, 477.

Hansson, T. and Roos, B. (1986) Age changes in the bone mineral of the lumbar spine in normal women. **Calcified Tissue Int.,** 38, 249-251.

Hansson, T. Roos, B. and Nachemson, A. (1975) Development of osteopenia in the fourth lumbar vertebrae during prolonged bed rest after operation for scoliosis. **Acta Orthop. Scand.,** 46, 621-630.

Hansson, T. Roos, B. and Nachemson, A. (1980) The bone mineral content and ultimate compressive strength of lumbar vertebrae. **Spine,** 5, 46.

Heaney, R.P. (1986) Calcium, bone health and osteoporosis, in **Bone and Mineral Research/4** (ed W.A. Peck), Elsevier Science Publishers, Netherlands, pp. 255-301.

Heaney, R.P. Recker, R.R. and Saville, P.D. (1978) Menopausal changes in bone remodeling. **J. Lab. Clin. Med.,** 32, 964-970.

Hert, J. Liskova, M. and Landa, J. (1971) Reaction of bone to mechanical stimuli. Part 1 : Continuous and intermittent loading of tibia in rabbit. **Folia Morphol.,** 19, 280-300.

Horsman, A. and Currey, J.D. (1983) Estimation of mechanical properties of the distal radius from bone mineral content and cortical width. **Clin. Orthop. Relat. R.,** 176, 298-304.

Huddleston, A.L. Rockwell, D. Kulund, D.N. and Harrison, R.B. (1980) Bone mass in lifetime tennis players. **J. Am. Med. Assoc.,** 244, 1107-1109.

Jacobsen, P. Beaver, W. Grubb, S. Taft, T. and Talmage, R. (1984) Bone density in women : college athletes and older athletic women. **J. Orthop. Res.,** 2, 328-332.

Johnell, O. and Nilsson, B. (1984) Lifestyle and bone mineral mass in perimenopausal women, in **Osteoporosis** (eds C. Christiansen, C.D. Arnaud, B.E.C. Nordin, A.M. Parfitt, W.A. Peck and B.L. Riggs), Denmark : Glostrup Hospital, pp. 359.

Jones, H.H. Priest, J.D. Hayes, W.C. Tichenor, C.C. and Nagel, D.A. (1977) Humeral hypertrophy in response to exercise. **J. Bone Joint Surg. Am.,** 59A, 204-208.

Kaplan, F.S. (1983) Osteoporosis. **CIBA Clinical Symposia.,** 35(4).

Kaplan, F.S. (1987) Osteoporosis - pathophysiology and prevention. **CIBA-GEIGY Clinical Symposia.** No.4 (Canada).

King, D.W. and Pengelly, R.G. (1973) Effect of running on the density of rat tibias. **Med. Sci. Sp.,** 4, 55.

Klemm, T. Banzer, D.H. and Schneider, U. (1976) Bone mineral content of the growing skeleton. **Am. J. Roentgenol.,** 126, 1283-1284.

Krabbe, S. Christiansen, C. Rodbro, P. and Tranbon, J. (1979) Effects of puberty on rates of bone growth and mineralization. **Arch. Dis. Child.,** 54, 950-953.

Krolner, B. and Nielson, S.P. (1982) Bone mineral content of the lumbar spine in normal and osteoporotic women : cross-sectional and longitudinal studies. **Clin. Sci.,** 62, 329-336.

Krolner, B. and Toft, B. (1983) Vertebral bone loss, an unheeded side effect of therapeutic bed rest. **Clin. Sci.,** 64, 537-540.

Krolner, B. Toft, B. Nielsen, S.P. and Tondevold, E. (1983) Physical exercise as a prophylaxis against involutional vertebral bone loss : a controlled trial. **Clin. Sci.,** 64, 541-546.

Lanyon, L.E. (1984) Functional strain as a determinant for bone remodeling. **Calcif. Tiss. Int.,** 36, 556-561.

Lanyon, L.E. and Rubin, C.T. (1984) Static versus dynamic loads as an influence on bone remodeling. **J. Biomech.,** 17, 897-905.

Lanyon, L.E. Goodship, A.E. and Baggott, D.G. (1976) Mechanical function as an influence on the structure and form of bone. **J. Bone Joint Surg.,** 58B, 436-443.

Lanyon, L.E. Goodship, A.E. Pye, C.J. and MacFie, J.H. (1982) Mechanically adaptive bone remodeling. **J. Biomech.,** 15, 141-154.

Leblanc, A. Schneider, V. Krebs, J. Evans, H. Jhingran, S. and Johnson, P. (1987) Spinal bone mineral after 5 weeks of bed rest. **Calcif. Tiss. Int.,** 41, 259-261.

Lindsay, R. Hart, D.M. Forrest, C. and Baird, C. (1980) Prevention of spinal osteoporosis in oophorectomized women. **Lancet,** 2, 1151-1153.

Marcus, R. and Carter, D.R. (1988) The role of physical activity in bone mass regulation, in **Advances in Sports Medicine and Fitness** (ed W.A. Grana) Volume 1, Year Book Medical Publishers Inc., Chicago, pp. 63-82.

Margulies, J.Y. Simkin, A. Leichter, I. Bivas, A. Steinberg, R. Giladi, M. Stein, M. Kashtan, H. and Milgrom, C. (1986) Effect of intense physical activity on the bone mineral content in the lower limbs of young adults. **J. Bone Joint Surg. Am.,** 68A, 1090-1093.

Martin, A.D. and Houston, C.S. (1987) Osteoporosis, calcium and physical activity. **Can. Med. Assoc. J.,** 136, 587-593.

Martin, A.D. and McCulloch, R.G. (1987) Bone dynamics : stress, strain and fracture. **J. Sp. Sci.,** 5, 155-163.

Martin, A.D. Bailey, D.A. Leicester, J.B. and Gulka, I. (1987) Bone and muscle relationships in the forearms of lifetime tennis players. **Proceedings of International Symposium on Osteoporosis.** Aalborg, Denmark.

Martin, R.K. Albright, J.P. Clarke, W.R. and Niffenberger, J.A. (1981) Load-carrying effects on the adult beagle tibia. **Med. Sci. Sport Exerc.,** 13, 343-349.

Mazess, R.B. (1982) On aging bone loss. **Clin. Orthop.,** 165, 239-251.

Mazess, R.B. and Whedon, G.D. (1983) Immobilization and bone. **Calcified Tissue Int.,** 35, 265-267.

Meier, D.E. Orwoll, E.S. and Jones, J.M. (1984) Marked disparity between trabecular and cortical bone loss with age in healthy men : measurement by vertebral computed tomography and radial photon absorptiometry. **Ann. Int. Med.,** 101, 605-612.

Montoye, H.J. (1987) Better bones and biodynamics. **Res. Quart. Exercise Sport.,** 58, 334-348.

Montoye, H.J. McCabe, J.F. Metzner, H.L. and Garn, S.M. (1976) Physical activity and bone density. **Hum. Biol.,** 48, 559-610.

Montoye, H.J. Smith, E.L. Fardon, D.F. and Howley, E.T. (1980) Bone mineral in senior tennis players. **Scand. J. Sport Sci.,** 2, 26-32.

Nilas, L. and Christiansen, C. (1987) Bone mass and its relationship to age and the menopause. **J. Clin. Endoc. Metab.,** 65, 696-702.

Nilsson, B.E.C. and Westlin, N.E. (1971) Bone density in athletes. **Clin. Orthop. Relat. R.,** 77, 179-182.

Nordin, B.E.C. Marshall, D.H. Francis, R.M. and Crilly, R.G. (1981) The effect of sex steroid and corticosteroid hormones on bone. **J. Steroid B.,** 15, 171-174.

Peck, W.A. (1984) Osteoporosis consensus conference. **J. Am. Med. Assoc.** 252, 799-802.

Riggs, B.L. and Melton, L.J. (1986) Involutional osteoporosis. **N. Engl. J. Med.,** 314, 1676-1686.

Riggs, B.L. Wahner, H.W. Dunn, W.L. Mazess, R.B. Offord, K.P. and Melton, L.J. (1981) Differential changes in bone mineral density of the appendicular and axial skeleton with aging : relationship to spinal osteoporosis. **J. Clin. Inv.,** 67, 328-335.

Riggs, B.L. Wahner, H.W. Melton, L.J. III Richelson, L.S. Judd, H.L. and Offord, K.P. (1986) Rates of bone loss in the axial and appendicular skeletons of women : evidence of substantial vertebral bone loss prior to menopause. **J. Clin. Inv.,** 77, 1487-1491.

Roesler, H. (1987) The history of some fundamental concepts in bone biomechanics. **J. Biomech.,** 20, 1025-1034.

Rubin, C.T. (1984) Skeletal strain and the functional significance of bone architecture. **Calcified Tissue Int.,** 36, 511-518.

Rubin, C.T. and Lanyon, L.E. (1985) Regulation of bone mass by mechanical strain magnitude. **Calcified Tissue Int.,** 37, 411-417.

Sandler, R.B. Cauley, J.A. Hom, D.L. Sashim, D. and Kriska, A.M. (1987) The effects of walking on the cross-sectional dimensions of the radius in postmenopausal women. **Calcified Tissue Int.,** 41, 65-69.

Saville, P.D. and Whyte, M.P. (1969) Muscle and bone hypertrophy : a positive effect of running exercise in the rat. **Clin. Orthop. Related R.,** 65, 81-88.

Sidney, K.H. Shephard, R.J. and Harrison, J.E. (1977) Endurance training and body composition of the elderly. **Am. J. Clin. Nutr.,** 30, 326-333.

Simkin, A. Ayalon, J. and Leichter, I. (1987) Increased trabecular bone density due to bone-loading exercises in postmenopausal osteoporotic women. **Calcified Tissue Int.,** 40, 59-63.

Sinaki, M. (1989) Exercise and osteoporosis. **Arch. Phys. Med. Rehabil.,** 70, 220-229.

Sinaki, M. and Offord, K.P. (1988) Physical activity in postmenopausal women : Effect on back muscle strength and bone mineral density of the spine. **Arch. Phys. Med. Rehabil.,** 69, 277-280.

Smith, D.M. Khairi, M.R.A. Norton, J. and Johnston, C.C. (1976) Age and activity effects on rate of bone mineral loss. **J. Clin. Inv.,** 58, 716-721.

Smith, E.L. and Raab, D.M. (1986) Osteoporosis and physical activity. **Acta Med. Scand. Suppl.,** 711, 149-156.

Smith, E.L. and Reddan, W. (1976) Physical activity - a modality for bone accretion in the aged. (Abstract). **Am. J. Roentgenol.,** 126, 1297.

Smith, E.L. Gilligan, C. McAdam, M. Ensign, C.P. and Smith, P.E. (1989) Deterring bone loss by exercise intervention in premenopausal and postmenopausal women. **Calcif. Tissue Int.,** 44, 312-321.

Smith, M.C. Rambaut, P.C. Vogel, J.M. and Whittle, M.W. (1977) Bone mineral measurement - experiment M078, in **Biomedical Results from Skylab.** (eds R.S. Johnston and L.F. Dietlin), Washington, D.C. : U.S. Government Printing Office (NASA SP-377), pp. 183-190.

Stillman, R.J. (1987) Physical activity and skeletal health : a brief survey. **Med. Sport Sci.** 24, 1-12.

Talmage, R.V. and Anderson, J.J.B. (1984) Bone density loss in women : effects of childhood activity, exercise, calcium intake and estrogen therapy (abstract). **Calcif. Tissue Int.,** 36 (suppl. 2) , S52.

Tilton, F.E. Degioanni, J.J.C. and Scneider, V.D. (1980) Long-term follow-up of Skylab bone demineralization. **Aviat. Envir. Med.,** 51, 1209-1213.

Wahner, H.W. Dunn, W.L. and Riggs, B.L. (1984) Assessment of bone mineral. Part 1 and 2. **J. Nucl. Med.,** 25, 1134-1141 and 1241-1253.

Wall, J.C. Chatterji, S.K. and Jeffery, J.W. (1979) Age-related changes in the density and tensile strength of human femoral cortical bone. **Calcif. Tissue Int.,** 27, 105-108.

Walton, J.N. and Warrick, C.K. (1954) Osseous changes in myopathy. **Br. J. Radiol.,** 27, 1-15.

Wardlaw, G. (1988) The effects of diet and life-style on bone mass in women. **J. Am. Diet. A.,** 88, 17-25.

Whedon, G.D. (1984) Disuse osteoporosis : physiological aspects. **Calcif. Tissue Int.,** 36 (suppl.) , 146-150.

Whedon, G.D. and Shorr, E; (1957) Metabolic studies in paralytic acute anterior poliomyelitis. **J. Clin. Inv.,** 36, 941-1033.

White, M.K. Martin, R.B. Yeater, R.A. Butcher, R.L. and Radin, E.L. (1984) The effects of exercise on the bones of postmenopausal women. **Int. Orthop.,** 7, 209-214.

Williams, J.A., Wagner, J., Wasnich, R. and Heilbrun, L. (1984) The effect of long-distance running upon appendicular bone mineral content. **Med. Sci. Sport Exerc.,** 16, 223-227.

Wolff, J. (1892) **Das Gesetz der Tranformation der Knochen.** Berlin : A. Hirschwald.

Wolff, J. (1986) **The Law of Bone Remodeling.** (translators P. Maquet and R. Furlong). Springer, Berlin.

Wopo, S.L. Kuei, S. Amiel, D. Gomez, M.A. Hayes, W.C. White, F.C. and Akeson, W.H. (1981) The effect of prolonged physical training on the properties of long bone : a study of Wolff's Law. **J. Bone Joint Surg. Am.,** 63A, 780-786.

15

DISTINGUISHING ANTHROPOLOGICAL FACTORS IN FEMALE SPEED SKATERS WITH RESPECT TO THEIR SUCCESS IN THE 1988 WINTER OLYMPIC GAMES

D. SOVAK and M.R. HAWES
Faculty of Physical Education, The University of Calgary, Canada

Keywords: Kinanthropometry, Speed skating, Olympic athletes, Length proportionality, Muscle mass, Segmental volumes, Active tissues

1 Introduction

Studies of Olympic athletes support the validity of anthropological parameters as one of the possible predictors of success at the international level of competition (Hirata 1966; Carter 1982; De Garay et al. 1974; Pollock et al. 1982). Our previous research indicated that female speed skaters had absolutely and relatively shorter legs and longer trunks than the control group of female university students. The total muscle mass of speed skaters was significantly larger and specifically the active tissue (muscle and bone) component of the thigh distinguished them not only from controls but from elite female athletes in cross country skiing, figure skating and marathon running (Sovak and Hawes 1987). Pollock et al. (1982) in a study of American Olympic calibre speed skaters suggested that the FFM component of the thigh, modelled by a thigh girth/skinfold ratio, distinguished these athletes from average young men. The group of Olympians were found to be significantly older, taller and heavier in total body mass, weight and hydrostatically determined FFM when compared to non-selected speed skaters. A possible link between the upper and lower leg length proportionality and performance level in speed skating has been suggested by van Ingen Schenau et al. (1983). However, these authors expressed caution that this measure is probably just one of many factors which determine performance.

It has been hypothesized that there will be a difference in the length proportionality and total body muscular development which will be reflected mostly on the thigh, between the GDR and Canadian speed skaters.

2 Methods

2.1 Subjects
The subjects of the investigation were the entire complement of the GDR (N=7, mean age 25.01 ± 2.79 years) and Canadian (N=7, mean age 21.76 ± 2.17 years) female speed skating teams competing at the 1988 Winter Olympic Games. The control group consisted of non-competing generally active university students (N = 46, mean age 21.37 ± 3.7 years). The subjects provided written informed consent prior to participation in this study.

2.2 Measurements
The following anthropometric dimensions were measured: age, total body height and mass, 2 heights (anterior iliospinale height for calculation of leg length according to Herm (1975) and suprasternale height for calculation of trunk length = suprasternale height - leg length), 6 lengths (trochanterion - tibiale = thigh , tibiale - sphyrion fibulare = calf length, proximal and distal thigh and calf length), 7 girths (upper arm relaxed, max. forearm, subgluteal, mid thigh, knee, max. calf and max. ankle) and 8 skinfold sites (triceps, biceps, forearm volaris and lateralis, front thigh, patella, proximal and mid calf).

The body mass was taken using a medical beam scale to the nearest 0.1 kg , heights and length using a GPM anthropometer and girths with a retractable steel tape to the nearest 0.1 cm. Harpenden calipers were used to obtain skinfold measurements to the nearest 0.1 mm. All skinfold measurements were taken twice with an accepted tolerance up to 5 %. Muscle mass was estimated using the technique of Matiegka (1921) and fat free volumes of thigh and calf according to Ulbrichova (1977). The exact location of sites and calculation of secondary variables have been described by Sovak and Hawes (1987).

2.3 Statistical Analysis
Analysis of variance (ANOVA) was used to determine differences between speed skating teams and controls. Statistical significance was accepted at a confidence level of $P < 0.05$.

3 Results

3. 1 Length Proportionality
Table 1 shows the descriptive characteristics for total body height (TBH) and its components. The GDR speed skaters were the tallest with practically identical trunk to leg length ratio as controls and similar thigh to calf length ratio.

176

The Canadian team members were slightly taller than the control group with an increased share of trunk length in the total height (as indicated by higher trunk to leg length ratio). The proportionality of the lower extremity was significantly altered by an absolutely and relatively shorter calf (i.e. greater thigh to calf length ratio) when compared to the control group. None of the height, trunk to leg length or thigh to calf length ratios revealed significant differences between the GDR and Canadian teams.

Table 1. Length proportionality of GDR, Canada and control groups.

Variable	GDR		Canada		Controls	
	Mean	S.D.	Mean	S.D.	Mean	S.D.
THB (cm)	168.1	7.9	166.3	4.6	165.7	6.1
$\dfrac{\text{Trunk l.}}{\text{Leg l.}}\,100\;(\%)$	52.7	2.1	53.4	3.1	52.2	3.5
$\dfrac{\text{Thigh l.}}{\text{Calf l.}}\,100\;(\%)$	101.9	5.2	106.6*	3.0	103.7	3.0

* P < 0.05 (Team vs. Controls)

Table 2. Total body mass and estimated muscular component of GDR, Canada and control groups.

Variable	GDR		Canada		Controls	
	Mean	S.D.	Mean	S.D.	Mean	S.D.
TBM (cm)	64.8	5.1	60.0	2.4	62.6	7.5
Muscle Mass (kg)	27.9*+	2.9	24.7*	0.8	22.0	2.8
Relative Muscle	43.0*	1.7	41.1*	1.8	35.1	3.5

* P < 0.05 (Teams vs. Controls)
+ P < 0.05 (GDR vs. Canada)

3.2 Total Body Mass and Muscle Mass

Comparison of variables from Table 2 indicates significant differences in muscle mass in both absolute or relative terms between teams and controls. The GDR speed skaters had the greatest total mass followed by controls and the Canadian team. However, none of the differences were significant.

The GDR speed skaters were heavier and possessed significantly larger muscle mass than the Canadians. This advantage practically disappeared when their higher TBM was taken into consideration - the relative amount of muscle mass was comparable in both teams.

3.3 Regional Development of Active Tissues

Comparison of skinfold-corrected diameters (CD) of the upper arm (CDU), forearm (CDF), thigh (CDT) and calf (CDC) revealed significant differences between speed skating teams and controls in the lower extremity segments. The speed skaters of both teams possessed significantly larger CDT than the controls, but only the East German speed skaters had a significantly larger CD of the calf as well. These characteristics were further manifested in significantly larger fat free volumes of the thigh (FFVT) in both teams as compared to controls and significantly larger fat free volume of the calf (FFVC) in the GDR team exclusively.

The GDR speed skaters surpassed the Canadians in the active tissue development of the lower extremity by a significantly larger CD of the thigh (CDT) and calf (CDC). The CD of the forearm (CDF) followed the same trend thus suggesting that the active tissue development was not exclusively limited to the leg only. The FFVT of both teams were rather similar (7.8 l. vs. 7.4 l.) when the absolute height and segment length was considered but the GDR team members had significantly larger FFVC when compared to the Canadian speed skaters (2.9 l. vs 2.3 l.).

4 Discussion and conclusions

A review of anthropometric studies on female speed skaters by Sovak and Hawes (1987) indicates that they have previously been limited to an examination of either one team (national) or to various groups of skaters formed on the basis of their performance level. Van Ingen Schenau and de Groot (1983) discuss the impact of higher percentage body fat using a sample of 10 elite female speedskaters, participants in the 1982 all-round world championship. A comparison of other anthropological charac-teristics such as length proportionality, active tissue development and its regional distribution on Olympic calibre female speed skating teams has not previously been reported.

It has been suggested that speed skaters typically have relatively (with respect to total body height) and absolutely longer trunk and shorter legs when compared to control groups of non-competitors (Sovak and Hawes 1987). The data from the present study did not confirm this finding with respect to the GDR team whose length proportionality resembled the control group. Van Ingen Schenau et al. (1983) suggest that a relatively shorter upper leg (i.e. thigh) and thus moment arm, "can be advantageous in speed skating since a shorter upper leg will require less muscle force of the extensors of the hip and knee joint at the same skating angle during the gliding phase." If this concept is applied to each team the Canadians appeared to be at a disadvantage because their thigh segment constituted a larger proportion of the lower extremity than either the GDR team or the controls. This is shown by the index of thigh length (thigh length as a percent of calf length) with values of 106.6 $\pm$ 30%, 101.9 $\pm$ 52% and 103.7 $\pm$ 30% for Canada, GDR and controls, respectively. The GDR team closely resembles the proportion found by van Ingen Schenau et al. (1983) in a trained, although less accomplished group of speed skaters. Analysis of the individual scores however, indicated that 5 out of 7 GDR speed skaters had relatively short thighs when compared to leg length in a manner similar to the elite group studied by van Ingen Schenau et al. (1983).

The results of this study showed that there was a substantial difference between both teams and the control group and this was enhanced when the more and less accomplished teams were compared in muscular development and regional distribution of active tissue. The estimation of muscle mass presented a problem since the available equations (Matiegka 1921; Martin et al. 1990) were validated against older and less conditioned individuals than the present population. Recently published work by Martin et al. (1990) suggested that estimation of muscle mass in 50 to 94 year old cadavers by Matiegka's method reflected the dissected values but consistently understimated the absolute values. Thus the absolute values presented here should be viewed with caution although the relative values from sample to sample may provide important insights. The increase in the total muscle mass could be partially attributed to the overall greater height and mass of the GDR team and to a projected greater number of years in training. The absolute difference in muscle mass was reduced below significant levels when expressed as a percentage of the total body mass (GDR-43.0% muscle and Canada 41.1% muscle). Contrary to expectations the additional active tissue appeared to be located on the calf rather than the thigh of the speed skaters. The FFV of the calf was significantly greater for the GDR team as a result of a significantly larger skinfold corrected diameter of the calf and longer lower leg segment than the Canadians.

In conclusion it is possible to state that there are distinct differences between both teams in the lower extremity proportions, muscular development and distribution of active tissues of the leg. These were probably just one of many factors which contributed to the performance of the GDR team in the 1988 Winter Olympic Games.

5 References

Carter, J.E.L. (1982). **Physical structure of Olympic athletes: Part 1. The Montreal Olympic Games Anthropological Project.** Medicine and Sport, Vol. 16, Karger, Basel.

De Garay, A.L. Levine, L. and Carter J.E.L. (1974) **Genetic and Anthropological Studies of Olympic Athletes.** Academic Press, New York.

Herm, K.P. (1975). Vorschlag zum einheitlichen Beinlängenberechnung und Korrektur bei Sportanthropometrischen Langsschnitt-unter-suchungen. **Med. u. Sport,** 15, 2, pp. 60-71.

Hirata, K. (1966) Physique and age of Tokyo Olympic champions. **J. Sport. Med. Phys. Fit.,** 6 (4), 207-222.

Martin, A.D. Spents, L.F. Drinkwater, D.T. and Clarijs, J.P. (1990) Anthropometric estimation of muscle mass in men. **Med. Sci. Sport. Exer.,** 22, 5, 729-733.

Matiegka, J. (1921). The testing of physical fitness. **Am. J. of Phys. Anthrop.,** 4, pp. 223-230.

Pollock, M.L., Foster., C. Anholm, J., Hare, J. Farrell, P. and Maksud, M.G. (1982). Body composition of Olympic speed skating candidates. **Res. Quart. Exer. Sp.,** 53, pp. 150-155.

Sovak, D. and Hawes, M.R. (1987). Anthropological status of inter-national calibre speed skaters. **J. Sp. Sci.,** 5, pp. 287-304.

Ulbrichova, M. (1977). The parameters of body segments. **Dilci zaverecna zprava** DU VII-5-1313, Praha, VVT FTVS UK, pp. 35-42.

van Ingen Schenau, G.J., de Groot, G. and Hollander, A.P. (1983). Some technical, physiological and anthropological aspects of speed skating. **Eur. J. Appl. Physiol.,** 50, pp. 343-354.

van Ingen Schenau, G.J. and de Groot, G. (1983). On the origin of differences in performance level between elite male and female speed skaters. **Hum. Movement Sci.** 2, pp. 151-159.

16

SEXUAL DIMORPHISM IN FAT PATTERNING IN YOUNG TRACK AND FIELD ATHLETES

J. MAIA and A. COSTA
Faculda da Ciencias Desporto, Universida do Porto, Portugal

Keywords: Track and field, Fat patterning, Principal component analysis, Z-score, Sexual dimorphism.

1 Introduction

Sexual dimorphism and fat patterning in homo sapiens have been challenging questions for workers in several fields. Although sexual dimorphism in human species remains to be fully understood and explained (Hall 1982; Wilner and Martin 1985; Pickford 1986: Pickford and Chiarelli 1986), how body dimensions grow and vary within and between sexes at puberty is well documented (Tanner 1962, 1978; Lieberman 1982).

Human body fat and fat patterning are topics of concern not only for health/epidemiological reasons (Ashwell, McCall and Dixon 1985; Bjorntorp 1985; Mueller 1985), but also for performance purposes (Carter 1982; Malina et al. 1982; Mueller, Shoup and Malina 1982; Carter and Yuhasz 1984). If age, sex and ethnic differences in physique and body composition of senior athletes in a variety of sports is well documented, the same is not true for adolescent athletes. Little is known about their body fat and especially their fat patterning. Although the question of sexual dimorphism in body composition has been studied in depth by Bailey (1982), he did not consider the topic of fat patterning in young athletes.

Therefore, the purposes of this study are : (1) to demonstrate the presence of sexual dimorphism in fat patterning and (2) to evaluate the relationship between the chosen event of track and field and fat patterning of adolescent athletes.

2 Material and methods

The subjects were 140 boys and 135 girls finalists in a major competition of track field from the North of Portugal. The distribution of the sample by sex and event is shown in Table 1.

Five skinfold measurements (triceps, subscapular, iliac, mid-thigh and medial calf) were included in a series of anthropometric dimensions taken on the athletes according to the procedures outlined by Ross and

Table 1. Number of athletes by the chosen event.

	Male	Female
Sprinters	39	33
Jumpers	27	29
Throwers	23	24
M.D. Runners	44	42
Race Walkers	6	8

Marfell-Jones (1982). All the measurements were taken with a Harpender caliper and with an accuracy to the nearest 0.1 mm.

Principal component analysis of the five skinfolds was employed to identify components of fatness and anatomical distribution of fat (Mueller and Reid 1979; Mueller, Shoup and Malina 1982). Subsequent to principal component analysis, component scores were computed for each subject for each of the identified components, based on the loadings obtained from the analysis. Component scores were submitted to a two-way ANOVA to discover significant differences associated with sex and the chosen event. The method outlined by Garn (1955) for studying anthropometric fat patterning was used to establish absolute and relative profiles. The values in the relative profiles are standard scores (z-scores).

3 Results and Discussion

The results of the principal component analysis (unrotated) are shown in Table 2.

The two components are easy to interpret. The first component accounts for 60.7% of the total variance, and all subcutaneous sites are positively correlated with it. It is termed a component of fatness. The second component explains 17.3% of the variance, and extremity fat sites are correlated with it in a direction which is opposite to that of trunk sites. Hence, it has been termed an extremity-trunk component. These results confirm those of previous studies: Mueller and Wohlleb (1981) in a study of fat patterning of samples of all ages, in both sexes, and in various ethnic, racial and/or national groups, found two components. Malina et al. (1982), whose study concentrates on Olympic athletes, and Mueller, Shoup and Malina (1982) in a study of fat patterning related to ethnic origin and sport, furnished evidence of two components: one of fatness and another of extremity/trunk ratio. Nevertheless, when we performed separate principal component analyses to boys and girls, 2 principal components have also emerged. The first explained 53.7% of the

Table 2. Principal component analysis of five skinfold thicknesses for total boys and girls.

	Principal components	
	1	2
Triceps skinfold	0.913	0.019
Subscapular skinfold	0.701	- 0.552
Iliac skinfold	0.848	- 0.295
Mid-thigh skinfold	0.798	0.327
Medical calf skinfold	0.593	0.604
Eigenvalue	3.034	0.863
Proportion of variance	60.7%	17.3%

variance for boys and 65.4% for girls; the second component explained 20.1% for boys and 16.1% for girls. This offers evidence of a sexual dimorphism in body fat, probably due to body composition changes of an early onset of puberty in girls.

To look into the relationship of sex and the chosen event with the two principal component scores, a two-way ANOVA was performed. Fatness (first component) was significantly related to sex ($F (1; 264) = 44.526$, $p < 0.001$) and to the chosen event ($F (4; 264) = 20.238$, $p < 0.001$). There were significant differences in the extremity-trunk component for sex ($F (1; 264) = 30.421$, $p < 0.001$) but not for event nor interaction (Fig. 1). The differences found between sexes in the two component scores suggest physique dimorphism (body composition) due to the onset of puberty (Bailey 1982; Lieberman 1982). The chosen event also exerts a significant effect on the variation in the first component but not in the second. This suggests little difference in fat patterning among the five chosen events, which agrees with the findings of Malina et al. (1982) in Olympic athletes and Mueller, Shoup and Malina (1982) in adolescent athletes. The role of sport and presumably training is to influence the amount of subcutaneous fat and not to influence fat patterning.

Garn (1955) proposed methods for studying anthropometric fat patterning. The method applied to the anatomical distribution of fat is termed absolute and relative fat patterning. The method consists of drawing a pattern profile for an individual over several subcutaneous adipose tissue sites (fig. 2).

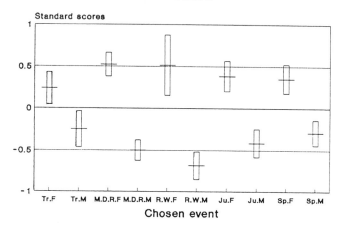

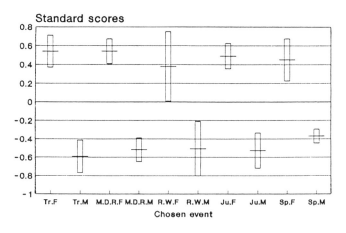

Fig. 1 Means of the two component standard scores of subcutaneous fat variation by sex and the chosen event (Tr.F, Tr.M -Throwers Female and Male; M.D.R.F, M.D.R.M -Middle Distance Runners Female and Male; R.W.F, R.W.M -Race Walkers Female and Male; Ju.F Ju.M -Jumpers Female and Male; Sp.F, Sp.M -Sprinters Female and Male).

184

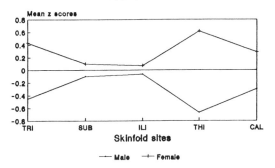

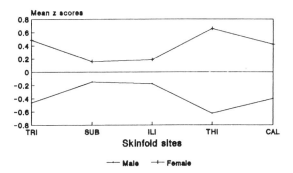

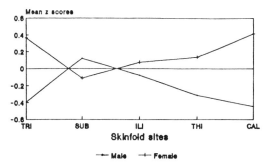

Fig. 2. Relative (z-score) profile per subcutaneous site by sex and chosen event.

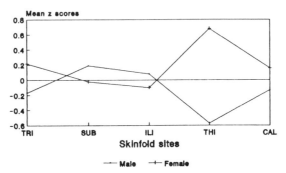

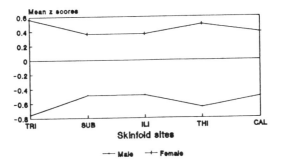

Fig. 2. Relative (z-score) profile per subcutaneous site by sex and chosen event (cont'd).

Male throwers, jumpers, middle distance runners and race walkers showed lower skinfolds at all sites than the female athletes competing in the same events. In sprinters, dimorphism is only evident for triceps, mid-thigh and medial calf skinfolds where boys show lower values. Relative profiles showed evident dimorphism in level and shape for all chosen events. These results are compatible with those of the principal component method (Fig. 1) in that the level of fatness appears to be

186

related to sex, while differences in the shape of the curves (fat patterning) are also related to chosen event.

The biological variation in fat patterning is a product of heredity and environment (Mueller 1983; Bouchard and Perousse 1988) and merits concern. Pond (1978) suggested two factors favouring a centralised fat distribution: (1) mechanical efficiency and (2) changes in sexual signalling over the life cycle. Fat patterning variation by chosen event may be related to the first factor. This means that different events require different types of mechanical efficiency. For the second factor, the suggestion is that sexual dimorphism in fat patterning at puberty may be determined by endocrine factors (Tanner 1978).

4 References

Ashwell, M. McCall, S.A. and Dixon, A.K. (1985) Fat distribution and its metabolism complications: interpretations, in **Human Body Composition and Fat Distribution** (ed N.G. Norgan), Euro-Nut report; 8, Wageningen, pp. 201-210.

Bailey, S.M. (1982) Absolute and relative sex differences in body composition, in **Sexual Dimorphism in Homo Sapiens** (ed R. Hall), Praeger, New York, pp. 263-316.

Bjorntorp, P. (1985) Fat patterning and disease: a review, in **Human Body Composition and Fat Distribution** (eds N.G. Norgan), Euro-Nut report; 8, Wageningen, pp. 201-210.

Bouchard, C. and Perousse, L. (1988) Heredity and body fat. **Am. Rev. Nutr.,** 8, 259-277.

Carter, J.E.L. (1982) Body composition of Montreal Olympic athletes, in **Physical Structure of Olympic Athletes; Part I** (ed J.E.L. Carter), Karger, Basel, pp. 107-116.

Carter, J.E.L. and Yuhasz, M.S. (1984) Skinfolds and body composition of Olympic athletes, in **Physical Structure of Olympic Athletes; Part II** (ed J.E.L. Carter), Karger, Basel, pp. 144-182.

Garn, S.M. (1955) Relative fat patterning : an individual characteristic. **Hum. Biol.,** 75-89.

Hall, R.L. (1982) **Sexual Dimorphism in Homo Sapiens - A question of Size.** Praeger, New York.

Lieberman, L.S. (1982) Normal and abnormal sexual dimorphic patterns of growth and development, in **Sexual Dimorphism in Homo Sapiens - A question of Size.** Praeger, New York, pp. 263-316.

Malina, R.M. Mueller, W.H. Bouchard, C. Shoup, R.F and Lariviere, G. (1982) Fatness and fat patterning among athletes at the Montreal Olympic Games, 1976. **Med. Sci. Sport. Exer.,**Vol. 14, 6, 445-452.

Mueller, W.H. and Reid, R.M. (1979) A multivariate analysis of fatness and relative fat patterning. **Am. J. Phys. Anthrop.,** 50, 199-208.

Mueller, W.H. and Wohleb, J.C. (1981) Anatomical destribution of subcutaneous fat and its description by multivariate methods : how valid are principal components? **Am. J. Phys. Anthrop.,** 54, 25-35.

Mueller, W.H. (1983) The genetics of human fatness. **Am. J. Phys. Anthrop.,** 26, 215-230.

Mueller, W.H. (1985) The biology of human patterning, in **Human Body Composition and Fat Distribution** (ed N.G. Norgan), Euro-Nut report, 8, Wageningen, pp. 159-174.

Pickford, M. (1986) On the origins of body size dimorphism in primates, in **Sexual Dimorphism in living and Fossil Primates** (eds M. Pickford and B. Chiarelli), Editrice "Il Sedicesimo", Firenze, pp. 77-91.

Pickford, M. and Chiarelli, B. (1986) Sexual Dimorphism in primates : where do we go from here?, in **Sexual Dimophism in Living and Fossil Primates** (eds M. Pickford and B. Chiarelli), Editrice "Il Sedicesimo", Firenze, pp. 77-91.

Pond, C.M. (1978) Morphological aspects and the ecological and mechanical consequences of fat deposition in wild vertebrates. **Annu. Rev. Ecol. Syst.,** 9, 519-570.

Ross, W.D. and Marfell-Jones, M.J. (1982) Kinanthropometry, in **Physiological Testing of the Elite Athlete** (eds J.D. MacDougall, H.A. Wenger and H.J. Green), Movement Publications, New York, pp. 99-150.

Tanner, J.M. (1962) **Growth at Adolescence**. Blackwell, Oxford.

Tanner, J.M. (1978) **Foetus into Man**. Harvard University Press, Massachussets.

Willner, L.A. and Martin, R.D. (1985) Some basic principles of mammalian sexual dimorphism, in **Human Sexual Dimorphism. Symposia of the Society for the Study of Human Biology** (eds J. Ghesquière, R.D. Martin and F. Newcombe), Taylor and Francis, London, pp. 1-42.

17

SOMATOTYPES OF FEMALE VETERAN TRACK AND FIELD ATHLETES

J. BROEKHOFF, W. PIETER, D. TAAFFE and A. NADGIR
Dept. of Physical Education & Human Movement Studies, University of Oregon, USA

Keywords: Somatotype, Veteran, Female, Track and field.

1 Introduction

Although physical characteristics are but one dimension of athletic performance, body structure may be useful in explaining differences in performance, all other things being equal (Carter 1978). Sport specific somatotypes for young and young adult (Olympic) athletes have been identified (e.g. Carter 1982, 1984, 1988; Thorland 1981). A secondary question relates to the effect of exercise on somatotype. Do outstanding athletes acquire a desirable physique type through long and intensive training or are these athletes outstanding precisely because they already possessed ideal physiques?

Somatotyping of young female athletes has been done on a wide scale and for many different sports (e.g. Bale 1981; Broekhoff, Nadgir and Pieter 1986; Carter 1982; Slaughter,Lohman, Boileau and Riner 1981). To date, however, very little information is available on the somatotypes of older female athletes. Since athletics for women at older ages is a relatively recent phenomenon, a study of these older athletes might throw some light on the questions raised above. Do their somatotypes reflect the same distribution as those of young athletic women? Do their somatotypes change with increasing age?

The purpose of this study is to describe the somatotypes of female veteran athletes competing at the 1989 World Veteran Track and Field Championships. The discussion will focus on differences in body build between these veteran athletes and younger Olympians.

2 Methods

The subjects for this study consisted of 92 female veteran track and field athletes who participated in the 1989 World Veteran Track and Field Championships in Eugene, Oregon, and who ranged in age from 35 through 79 years. The athletes were categorized in age groups of five-year increments.

Table 1. Means and Standard Deviations of Ages in Age Groups of Female Veteran Track and Field Athletes.

Age Group	n	Mean (yrs.)	SD
35 - 39	9	37.24	1.31
40 - 44	14	42.83	2.51
45 - 49	20	46.66	1.29
50 - 54	22	52.10	1.29
55 - 59	9	56.96	1.46
60 - 64	7	62.96	1.44
65 - 69	5	68.18	0.85
70 - 74	2	72.46	3.48
75 - 79	4	76.90	1.84

Table 2. Means and Standard Deviations of Ages of Female Veteran Track and Field Athletes by Event Category.

Event	n	Mean (yrs.)	SD
Field	7	50.71	4.83
Heptathlon	4	48.48	10.20
Marathon	16	48.70	8.08
M. Distance	5	58.17	15.06
L. Distance	27	53.74	11.67
Sprints	12	52.70	10.41
Walking	21	50.41	9.94

A Lange skinfold caliper was used to assess the skinfolds at the following sites: triceps, subscapula, supraspinale, abdomen, front thigh and medial calf. An anthropometric fiberglass measuring tape was used to measure the circumferences of the arm (relaxed and tensed), forearm, thigh and calf. A Harpenden steel anthropometer was used to determine the humerus and femur widths. Stature and sitting height were measured with a wooden stadiometer to the nearest 0.5 cm, while a platform balance beam scale was used to measure body weight to the nearest 0.5 kg. The somatotype of the subjects was calculated by means of the method as suggested by Carter (1980).

190

Table 3. Means and Standard Deviations of Height, Weight, and Somatotypes of Female Veteran Track and Field Athletes by Age Group.

Age Group	Height (cm)	Weight (kg)	Endo-morphy	Meso-morphy	Ecto-morphy
35 - 39	167.48	57.27	2.82	3.55	3.28
	(6.70)	(6.76)	(0.60)	(0.87)	(0.77)
40 -44	165.44	60.37	3.26	4.46	2.48
	(5.84)	(12.05)	(1.45)	(0.96)	(1.41)
45 - 49	162.56	56.17	3.43	4.41	2.64
	(6.00)	(7.21)	(1.00)	(1.05)	(1.00)
50 - 54	162.83	56.12	3.56	4.19	2.59
	(3.72)	(5.12)	(1.08)	(0.76)	(0.59)
55 - 59	163.43	58.89	3.70	4.91	2.68
	(6.66)	(12.23)	(1.18)	(1.46)	(1.51)
60 - 64	160.54	54.47	3.49	4.51	2.54
	(5.93)	(8.62)	(1.28)	(1.35)	(1.34)
65 -69	159.08	50.87	3.52	4.45	2.93
	(4.16)	(5.90)	(0.96)	(1.02)	(1.62)
70 - 74	162.00	58.80	3.66	4.30	2.08
	(9.19)	(15.70)	(0.46)	(1.09)	(1.02)
75 -79	155.80	51.05	3.43	4.68	2.16
	(7.58)	(1.90)	(0.73)	(1.19)	(1.13)

Multivariate procedures were employed to assess the differences between age groups and between classes of events. Tukey post-hoc tests were utilized to determine the exact location of significant differences.

3 Results

Table 1 shows the means and standard deviations of the various age groups. No differences were observed in any of the somatotype components between age groups.

The mean age (± SD) of the female veteran athletes in the different track and field event categories are presented in Table 2. Tables 3 and 4

Table 4. Means and Standard Deviations of Height, Weight, and Somatotypes of Female Veteran Track and Field Athletes by Event Category.

Age Group	Height cm)	Weight (kg)	Endo- morphy	Meso- morphy	Ecto- morphy
Field	165.77	72.33	4.84	5.79	1.30
	(6.45)	(12.15)	(1.15)	(1.52)	(0.95)
Heptathlon	165.70	59.05	2.79	4.69	2.60
	(7.41)	(6.26)	(0.38)	(0.86)	(1.08)
Marathon	164.32	57.06	3.18	4.08	2.71
	(4.84)	(5.86)	(0.87)	(0.71)	(0.58)
M. Distance	160.74	50.52	2.96	3.70	3.25
	(4.38)	(1.92)	(0.63)	(0.40)	(0.67)
L. Distance	162.09	53.99	3.22	4.19	2.87
	(5.63)	(5.56)	(1.03)	(0.96)	(1.12)
Sprints	160.01	53.74	3.47	4.52	2.48
	(5.98)	(4.68)	(1.00)	(0.50)	(0.75)
Walking	163.89	56.92	3.58	4.24	2.72
	(6.80)	(8.98)	(1.13)	(1.15)	(1.35)

display the means and standard deviations of height, weight, and somatotypes of the female veteran track and field athletes by age and event category, respectively.

There were significant differences in endomorphy (p <.01), mesomorphy (p <.01), and ectomorphy (p <.05) between athletes in the various event categories. Tukey's post-hoc tests showed that the field athletes were more endomorphic than the heptathletes and middle distance runners. The field athletes were more mesomorphic than the marathon runners, the middle distance runners, the long distance runners, and the walkers. The heptathletes, the marathoners, the middle distance runners, the long distance runners and the walkers were all more ectomorphic than the field athletes, while no differences existed in ectomorphy between the sprinters and the field athletes. Figures 1 and 2 depict the somatoplots of the veteran female track and field athletes by age and by event category.

4 Discussion

There is a remarkable similarity between the female veteran track and field athletes and their much younger counterparts who participated at the 1976 Olympic Games in Montreal. The Olympic athletes in the field events were more endomorphic than middle distance runners, pentathletes, and sprinters (Carter 1984), which is not unlike the field event athletes in the present study. The endomorphy rating of the veteran field athletes is close to that of Olympic shot/discus athletes (endomorphy rating: 5.3) and slightly higher than that of Olympic javelin throwers (rating: 3.4) (Carter 1984). A possible reason why no differences in endomorphy were found between the veteran field athletes and the veteran marathon and long distance runners may be related to the unique profile of the veteran athlete. Many veteran athletes participate in more than one athletic discipline as opposed to their younger colleagues at world championships and Olympic Games, who are more specialized. Similar to young athletes where the same somatotypes may be successful in different events (Carter 1978), veteran athletes may have somatotypes that allow them to compete in various activities.

While female Olympic shot putters and discus throwers were found to be more mesomorphic than sprinters, 400 to 800 m runners, and pentathletes (Carter 1984), the veteran field athletes were more mesomorphic than the veteran marathoners, middle and long distance runners, and race walkers, but no different than heptathletes and sprinters. The veteran field athletes are similar in mesomorphy to Olympic shot putters and discus throwers (mesomorphy rating: 5.3), but higher than Olympic javelin throwers (rating: 4.0) (Carter 1984). This finding is probably related to the pooling of the shot putters, discus, and javelin throwers into one category in the veteran sample.

Contrary to the veteran athletes, the Olympic sprinters were more ectomorphic than the shot putters and discus throwers (Carter 1984). Like their Olympic counterparts, however, the 400 to 800 m runners and the pentathletes were more ect omorphic than the shot putters and discus throwers. The female Olympic 800/1500 m runners recorded the highest rating in ectomorphy (3.7) (Carter 1984), which is similar to the veteran middle distance runners who were also highest in the ectomorphy component. The veteran field athletes were similar in ectomorphy to the Olympic shot putters and discus throwers (rating: 1.6); the veteran sprinters were also similar to the Olympic sprinters (rating: 3.0), and the veteran heptathletes were similar in ectomorphy to the Olympic pentathletes (rating: 3.1) (Carter 1984).

It has been well established that with increasing age in adulthood, body fat increases and lean body mass decreases (e.g. Forbes 1976; Mueller et al. 1986; Parizkova and Eiselt 1980; Stamford 1988). It was also found, however, that training had a positive effect on the age related changes in

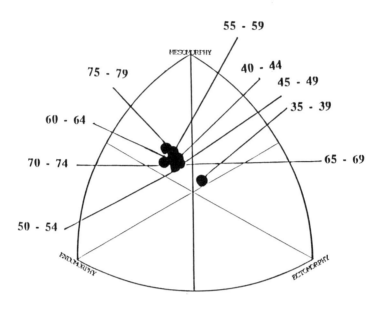

Fig. 1 Somatoplots of female veteran track and field athletes by age

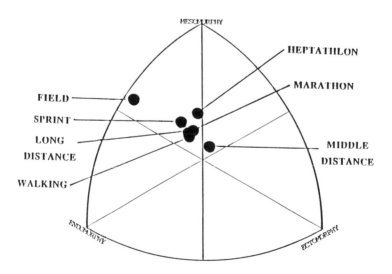

Fig. 2 Somatoplots of female veteran track and field athletes by event

body composition (Lewis, Haskell, Perry, Kovacevic et al. 1978; Shephard and Kavanagh 1978). Active middle-aged and older men and women have less fat and more lean body mass than sedentary peers (Barnard, Grimditch and Wilmore 1979; Lewis et al. 1978; Stamford 1988; Shephard and Kavanagh 1978; Wilmore and Costill 1988). Since it is known that, in sedentary women, fat increases between 40 and 70 years of age (Shimokata et al. 1989), intensive training in the present group of subjects may have helped them in maintaining a lean body type well into the sixth and seventh decades of life. This is in accordance with Stirling, Martin, Ross and Meehan (1986), who observed that moderately active older women (mean age of 68.3 years) were higher in mesomorphy and lower in endomorphy than age-matched sedentary control subjects. Increased relative body fat has been linked to coronary heart disease and adult onset of diabetes mellitus (e.g. Blair, Ludwig and Goodyear 1988). Staying physically active may go a long way in preventing these debilitating diseases of old age.

A second possibility is that the veteran athletes had lean body types to begin with, which in turn contributed to their success at this high level of competition. The present study indicates that specific somatotypes are conducive to success in certain sports events even in older adulthood. Regardless of age, the veteran athletes had the appropriate physique for success. Therefore, they may already have possessed the ideal physique for their event and training may simply have emphasized the potential of their body build.

5 References

Bale, P. (1981) Body composition and somatotype characteristics of sportswomen, in **The Female Athlete**. A Socio-Psychological and Kinanthropometric Approach (eds J. Borms, M. Hebbelinck and A. Venerando), Karger, Basel, pp. 157 - 167.

Barnard, R. I., Grinditch, G. K. and Wilmore, J. H. (1979) Physiological characteristics of sprint and endurance masters runners, **Med. Sci. Sp.**, 11, 167 - 171.

Blair, S. N., Ludwig, D. A. and Goodyear, N. N. (1988) A canonical analysis of central and peripheral subcutaneous fat distribution and coronary heart disease risk factors in men and women aged 18 - 65 years, **Hum. Biol.**, 60, 111 - 122.

Broekhoff, J., Nadgir, A. and Pieter, W. (1986) Morphological differences between young gymnasts and non-athletes matched for age and gender, in **Kinanthropometry III** (eds. T. Reilly, J. Watkins and J. Borms), E. and F. Spon, London, pp. 204 - 210.

Carter, J. E. L. (ed) (1982) **Physical Structure of Olympic Athletes. Part I**, Karger, Basel.

Carter, J. E. L. (ed) (1984) **Physical Structure of Olympic Athletes. Part II**, Karger, Basel.

Carter, J. E. L. (1978) Prediction of outstanding athletic ability: the structural perspective, in **Exercise Physiology**, Vol. 4 (eds F. Landry and W. A. R. Orban), Symposia Specialists, Miami, pp. 29 - 42.

Carter, J. E. L. (1988) Somatotypes of children in sports, in **Young Athletes. Biological, Psychological, and Educational Perspectives** (ed R. M. Malina), Human Kinetics Books, Champaign, Ill, pp. 153 - 165.

Carter, J. E. L. (1984) Somatotypes of Olympic athletes from 1948 to 1976, in **Physical Structure of Olympic Athletes. Part II** (ed J. E. L. Carter), Karger, Basel, pp. 80-109.

Carter, J. E. L. (1980) **The Heath-Carter Somatotype Method**. San Diego State University, San Diego.

Forbes, G. B. (1976) The adult decline in lean body mass, **Hum. Biol.**, 48, 161 - 173.

Lewis, S. Haskell, W. L. Perry, C. Kovacevic, C. and Wood, P. D. (1978) Body composition of middle-aged female endurance athletes, in **Biomechanics of Sports and Kinanthropometry.** Book 6 (eds F. Landry and W. A. R. Orban), Symposia Specialists Inc., Miami, pp. 321 - 328.

Mueller, W. H. Deutsch, M.I. Malina, R.M. Bailey, D.A. and Mirwald, R. L. (1986) Subcutaneous fat topography: age changes and relationship to cardiovascular fitness in Canadians, **Hum. Biol.**, 58, 955 - 973.

Parizkova, J. and Eiselt, E. (1980) Longitudinal changes in body build and skinfolds on a group of old men over a 16 year period, **Hum. Biol.**, 52, 803 - 809.

Shephard, R. J. and Kavanagh, T. (1978) The effects of training on the aging process, **Phys. Sp. Med.**, 6, 33 - 40.

Shimotaka, H. Tobin, J.D. Muller, D.C. Elahi, D. Coon, P.J. and Andres, R. (1989) Studies in the distribution of body fat: I. Effects of age, sex, and obesity, **J. Gerontol.**, 44, M 66 - 73.

Slaughter, M.H. Lohman, T.G. Boileau, R.A. and Riner, W. F. (1981) Physique of college women athletes in five sports, in **The Female Athlete. A Socio-Psychological and Kinanthropometric Approach** (eds J. Borms, M. Hebbelinck and A. Venerando), Karger, Basel, pp. 186 - 191.

Stamford, B. A. (1988) Exercise and the elderly, in **Exercise and Sport Sciences Reviews**. Vol. 16 (ed K. B. Pandolf), MacMillan Publishers Co., New York, pp. 341 - 379.

Stirling, D.R. Martin, A.D. Ross, W.D. and Meehan, S. W. (1986) Structural characteristics of active and sedentary older women, in **Kinanthropometry III** (eds T. Reilly, J. Watkins and J. Borms), E. & F. N. Spon, London, pp.185 - 190.

Thorland, W.G. Johnson, G.O. Fagot, T.G. Tharp, G.D. and Hammer, R.W. (1981) Body composition and somatotype characteristics of Junior Olympic athletes. **Med. Sci. Sport. Exer.**, 13, 332 - 338.

Wilmore, J. H. and Costill, D. L. (1988) **Training for Sport Activity**, Wm. C. Brown Publishers, Dubuque, IW.

18

RELATION OF ANTHROPOMETRIC MEASURES AND ANAEROBIC PERFORMANCE IN YOUNG BRAZILIAN SOCCER PLAYERS.

J. SOARES [1] and L.A. ANJOS [2]
[1] Centro de Performance Humana - CPH - São Paulo, Brazil
[2] Centro de Estudos da Saúde do Trabalhador e Ecologia Humana, ENSP - FIOCRUZ, Rio de Janeiro, Brazil.

Keywords: Soccer, Children, Brazil, Anaerobic Tests, Wingate Test, Anthropometry.

1 Introduction

Besides its popularity in the world, and in Brazil in particular, there has not been much research on soccer practice, especially on children. The effects of soccer training on the physical fitness characteristics of adolescent soccer players have been described in the literature (Soares and Matsudo 1980, 1982), but there have been few reports on the inter-relationship between anthropometric measures and performance in selected physical tasks used in the talent search process. Anthropometric measures have long been accepted as important factors influencing work output as measured by strength and motor tasks (Malina 1975). This study was conducted to investigate the influence of anthropometric measures used in growth research on the anaerobic performance levels of skilled young Brazilian soccer trainees.

2 Methods

The participants in this study were children involved in the sports training program at the Centro Olímpico de Treinamento e Pesquisa de São Paulo (São Paulo Olympic Training and Research Center) in Brazil. This report is based on data from 28 skilled young boys who participated in the soccer training program for an average time of 5.3 ± 1.6 years (Mean $\pm$ SD). The anthropometric data were obtained by a trained researcher and consisted of body mass (BM); stature (S); bicondylar humerus and femur width; arm, thigh, and calf circumferences; and 7 skinfolds (triceps, biceps, subscapular, mid-axillary, supra-iliac, abdominal, and calf). The skinfolds were measured with a Harpenden caliper using the techniques and sites of measurement suggested by the International Biological Program (Tanner et al. 1969). The relaxed arm circumference was measured at the

198

midpoint between the olecranon and acromion processes with a metal tape. Three measures were obtained for each variable and the mean value was used for subsequent analysis. Mid-upper arm muscle (AMA) and fat areas were calculated according to Frisancho (1981) using the triceps skinfold and the arm circumference values. Anaerobic performance tests were conducted on two consecutive days. They included the Wingate test on a cycle ergometer (peak power and mean power), vertical jump, 40 second run, and 50 m dash. Two groups of 14 boys were formed. On the first day one group performed the vertical jump and the Wingate test while the other performed the 50 m dash and the 40 second run tests. On the second day the tests were reversed. The load for the Wingate test was 0.075 kp.kg^{-1} body mass (Bar-Or 1987). The 50 m dash and the 40 second run were performed on a 400 m track. The 40 second run is an all out run in which the distance covered in 40 seconds is recorded to the nearest meter (Matsudo 1979). Statistical analysis was performed and included first order correlations between anthropometric measures and anaerobic

Table 1. Means, standard deviations (SD), Minimum (Min), and Maximum (Max) values for the anthropometric and performance measures, age, and soccer practice time.

Variable	Mean	SD	Min	Max
Age (years)	14.98	0.77	14.00	16.67
Soccer practice time (years)	5.30	1.63	1.00	8.00
Body mass (kg)	51.32	9.70	36.70	71.80
Stature (cm)	165.25	9.58	151.13	182.73
Humerus width (cm)	6.48	0.44	5.76	7.42
Femur width (cm)	9.43	0.53	8.64	10.40
Arm circumference (cm)	22.25	2.17	18.50	26.33
Thigh circumference (cm)	48.49	4.43	40.50	58.50
Calf circumference (cm)	31.59	2.51	27.50	39.00
Σ 7 skinfolds (mm)	48.68	13.52	29.86	81.53
Arm muscle area (cm^2)	31.00	6.20	20.28	43.68
Peak power (w)	558.41	125.17	346.71	823.34
Mean power (w)	473.03	110.23	301.42	726.14
40 s run (m)	249.73	17.05	210.00	279.50
50 m dash (s)	7.97	0.47	7.16	9.11
Vertical jump (cm)	38.46	5.19	26.00	49.00

performance tests. Partial correlations between anthropometric measures and anaerobic performance after controlling for body mass were also generated. Stepwise regression analysis was done with the anthropometric measures and anaerobic performance as independent and dependent variables respectively. An alpha level of 0.05 was used to determine the significance of the correlations.

Table 2. Correlation matrix for selected variables studied.

	1	2	3	4	5	6	7	8	9	10	11	12	13	14*
2	.54													
3	.54	.81												
4	.50	.74	.79											
5	.12	.64	.40	.51										
6	.54	.93	.64	.59	.54									
7	.43	.90	.60	.52	.49	.92								
8	.37	.88	.61	.67	.62	.88	.84							
9	.18	.33	.08	.10	.30	.41	.43	.40						
10	.35	.65	.28	.31	.56	.72	.72	.65	.87					
11	.52	.88	.67	.60	.46	.93	.83	.80	.04	.43				
12	.46	.94	.78	.70	.49	.91	.91	.87	.22	.54	.91			
13	.43	.66	.64	.59	.15	.60	.65	.58	-.03	.26	.67	.75		
14*	.40	.61	.61	.49	.10	.57	.57	.55	-.22	.09	.71	.75	.84	
15	.21	.56	.65	.50	.12	.53	.54	.48	-.02	.18	.58	.66	.68	.76

*The sign for the correlations with 50 m dash are reversed.

Variables are: 1) Age; 2) Body mass; 3) Stature; 4) Humerus width; 5) Femur width; 6) Arm circumference; 7) Thigh circumference; 8) Calf circumference; 9) Σ 7 skinfolds; 10) Arm muscle area; 11) Peak power; 12) 40 s run; 13) 50 m dash; 14) Vertical jump.
Correlation coefficients > 0.37 are significant ($p < 0.05$).

3 Results

Descriptive statistics of the subjects are presented in Table 1. Table 2 presents the correlation coefficient matrix for selected variables. All correlations greater than 0.37 are significant ($p < 0.05$). The sign for the correlations with 50 m dash is reversed. In general, the results of the anaerobic tests correlated more highly with body mass (variable 2) than

Table 3. Partial correlation coefficients between selected anthropometric measures and anaerobic performance tests after controlling for body mass. Symbols used: S = stature; AC = arm circumference; TC = thigh circumference; HW = humerus width; FW = femur width; Σ7SF = sum 7 skinfolds; AMA = arm muscle area.

Aerobic performance	Anthropometric Measures						
	S	AC	TC	HW	FW	Σ7SF	AMA
Peak power .	12	.27	.43	.03	-.43	-.30	.48
40 s run	.26	-.03	.19	.21	-.45	-.30	.24
50 m dash*	.25	.00	.07	.09	-.47	-.50	.46
Vertical jump	.40	.03	.11	.16	-.36	-.29	.24

*The signs for the 50 m dash are reversed.

Table 4. Stepwise regression analysis with anaerobic performance as dependent and anthropometric measures as independent variables. Symbols used : BM = body mass; AMA = arm muscle area; TC = thigh circumference.

Anaerobic performance	Variable in the model	R^2	SEE*
Peak power	BM	.89	41.77
	BM + AMA	.92	37.24
	BM + AMA + TC	.93	34.84
Mean power	BM	.91	34.51
	BM +AMA	.93	30.61
	BM +AMA + TC	.94	28.64
40 s run	AMA	.44	12.96
50 m dash	AMA	.50	.34
Vertical jump	Stature	.42	4.04

*SEE = Standard Error of Estimate.

with the other anthropometric measures. Arm circumference and its derivative, arm muscle area (variables 6 and 10), correlated similarly well with the anaerobic performance tests (variables number 11 through 14). Partial correlation coefficients were generated between selected anthropometric measures and anaerobic performance after controlling for body mass (Table 3). Most of the correlations between anthropometric measures and anaerobic performance were reduced after controlling for body mass.

Stepwise regression analysis is presented in Table 4. Together, arm muscle area and thigh circumference explained little percentagewise for the variance of the results of the Wingate test after body mass had been included in the model. The only variable in the model for the running tasks (40 s run and 50 m dash) was arm muscle area. Stature was the only variable in the model for the vertical jump.

4 Discussion

The main objective of the present study was to evaluate the relationship between anthropometric measures and anaerobic performance as measured by the Wingate test, 40 second run, 50 m dash, and vertical jump in young soccer players. The level of correlation of anthropometric measures with anaerobic performance has been shown to vary in both non-athletic (Espenschade 1963) and athletic (Meszaros et al. 1986) children depending on age and maturity level (Beunen et al. 1984). In the present study, body mass correlated moderately with the anaerobic tests (r's between 0.56 and 0.66) and highly with peak anaerobic power in the Wingate test (r = 0.94, Table 2). This high level of correlation can be easily explained by the fact that the load for the Wingate test is based on body mass. Furthermore, this is the only anaerobic performance test used in this study in which the subject remains seated and therefore, does not have to move the body. After controlling for body mass, only arm muscle area and thigh circumference contributed anything (but very little) to further explain the variance in peak power (Tables 3 and 4). The other measures of muscle mass (arm, thigh, and calf circumferences) correlated almost as highly as body mass with anaerobic performance (Table 2). However, after partialling out the effect of body mass, they contributed very little to explain the variance in anaerobic performance (Table 3). This seems to indicate that body mass is the single most important anthropometric measure to explain performance in anaerobic tasks of this sample of skilled young soccer players.

It is interesting to note that arm circumference was as important as the leg circumferences (both thigh and calf) in practically all anaerobic performance. Thus, it seems that for this sample of children involved in soccer training, arm circumference (and arm muscle area) is as good an indicator of whole-body muscle mass as the leg circumferences. This finding may have implications for the choice of anthropometric measures to assess in this population since the procedure for the estimation of muscle area in the upper limb is much easier than for the lower limb, even though these children would be thought to have developed more muscle mass in the lower limbs due to the specificity of their training.

Bone widths (humerus and femur) correlated moderately with anaerobic performance (r's between 0.10 and 0.70). However, after controlling for body mass, the level of correlations between femur width and anaerobic performance was increased and the signs reversed indicating a reduction in performance for all anaerobic performance with greater bone size.

Stature, per se, appeared to influence the performance in vertical jump. The moderate correlations between stature and the other anaerobic performance vanished after controlling for the effect of body mass.

In summary, the present data indicate that anthropometric measures correlated more highly with the results of peak anaerobic power in the Wingate test than with the other anaerobic tests. After partialling out the effect of body mass, the levels of the correlations were reduced for most variables. Thus, in this sample of young soccer players, body mass seems to be the most important determinant of anaerobic performance.

5 References

Bar-Or, O. (1987) The Wingate anaerobic test. An update on methodology, reliability, and validity. **Sports Med.**, 4, 381-394.

Beunen, G. Ostyn, M. Renson, R. Simons J. and Van Gerven, D. (1984) Anthropometric correlates of strength and motor performance in Belgian boys 12 through 18 years of age. in **Human Growth and Development** (ed J. Borms, R. Hauspie, A. Sand, C. Susanne, and M. Hebbelinck), Plenum Press, NY, pp. 503-509.

Espenschade, A. S. (1963) Restudy of relationships between physical performance of school children and age, height, and weight. **Res. Quart.**, 34, 144-153.

Frisancho, A. R. (1981) New norms of upper limb fat and muscle areas for assessment of nutritional status. **Am. J. Clin. Nut.**, 34, 2540-2545.

Malina, R. M. (1975) Anthropometric correlates of strength and motor performance. **Exercise and Sport Sciences Reviews**, 3, 249-274.

Matsudo, V. K. R. (1979) Avaliação da potência anaeróbica: Teste de corrida de 40 segundos. **Revista Brazileira de Ciências do Esporte**, 1, 8-16.

Meszaros, J. Mohacsi, J. Frenkl, R. Szabo, T. and Szmodis, I. (1986) Age dependency in the development of motor-test performance. in **Children and Exercise XII**, Human Kinetics Publ., Champaign, IL, pp. 347-353.

Soares, J. and Matsudo, V. K. R. (1980) Changes in characteristics of physical fitness in adolescents participating in soccer training. **Med. Sci. Sport. Exer.**, 12, 139.

Soares, J. and Matsudo, V. K. R. (1982) Efeitos do treinamento de futebol sobre a PWC_{170} em escolares. **Revista Brazileira de Ciências do Esporte**, 4, 7-10.

Tanner, J. M. Hiernaux, J. and Jarman, S. (1969) Growth and physique studies, in **Human biology : A guide to field methods. International biological programme, Handbook no. 9** (eds J. S. Weiner and J. A. Lourie), Blackwell Scientific Pub., Oxford, England, pp.1-71.

19

SEXUAL DIMORPHISM AND MOTOR PERFORMANCE OF FEMALE CHILDREN, WITH A REMARK ON ELITISM AND NEGATIVE SELECTION

F. SOBRAL
Faculdade de Motricidade Humana, Universidade Técnica de Lisboa, Portugal

Keywords: Children's sport, Growth, Negative selection, Sexual dimorphism.

1 Introduction

Attempts to demonstrate a consistent relationship between body type and size, and motor performance in children have led to inconclusive results, unless extreme cases are put under consideration. It seems very likely that other circumstances play an important role on motor performance and sport participation during childhood, such as parental and social encouragement towards physical activity, sound pedagogical attitudes and self-satisfaction from competitive sport involvement.

The need for an earlier start in specific training, nowadays, in many sports, is forced on coaches and sport scientists who aim to isolate some characteristics present in the outstanding child athlete. Talent spotting and guidance basically rely upon the validity of such traits in a prospective view.

Some questions arise concerning this issue, e.g. (i) are there systematic differences in body size and physique between children excelling in sport and their age peers ? (ii) how early may these differences, if any, be noted ? (iii) how much do coaches and physical educators take such differences into consideration in their selective interventions ?

With respect to girls, an additional question refers to sexual dimorphism and its association with the level of performance in a wide set of athletic events.

The purpose of the present research was to investigate whether elitism in school competitive sport, within a well confined geographical and socio-cultural setting, the Azores islands, was in some way associated to an early phenotypic selection among girls representing their schools.

2 Methods

2.1 Subjects and measures

The sample comprised 219 girls, aged 10 to 12 years, competing at the All-Azores School Tournament 1989. The girls have been primarily selected to represent their schools and, at a second stage, their islands, on the basis of a multi-sport competence (track and field, basketball, handball, volleyball, gymnastics). Chronological age, anthropometric data, order of birth and sibling number were collected. For the purpose of the present research, height, weight and sum of four skinfolds, SUMSK (triceps, subscapular, suprailiac and medial calf) were retained for analysis, as well as the best personal performances in three athletic events (long jump, hockey-ball throw and 60m run).

2.2 Indices of sexual dimorphism

Sexual dimorphism was assessed by male/female ratios. In each age group, the means of the anthropometric characteristics of the male population, according to the standards from the Azores Growth Survey (Sobral 1986), were divided by the corresponding value observed in each subject. A girl whose MF-ratio for a particular anthropometric trait is lower than 1.0 presents an absolute value above that of her average male age peer in the population. Concerning the average girl, this is expected to be the case with respect to height and weight at 11 years, weight at 12 years, and sum of skinfolds at all ages considered in the present study.

Depending on the specific trait under consideration, deviation from this pattern or the strengthening of it among girls representing their school squads may suggest the effect of a negative selection (as success of the most suitable phenotypes strongly determines sport adherence), the effect of a selective intervention by the physical educator, or both.

2.3 Statistical procedures

Linear regression equations of results in the athletic events on decimal age were derived in order to calculate residuals. Data were then handled as a single set, after the age effects had been removed. Each series of male/female ratios was, thereafter, split into two sets, one including the subjects whose ratios were equal to or greater than 1.0, the other including the subjects whose ratios were smaller than 1.0.

Furthermore, subjects were divided into four groups according to their order of birth, and into three groups according to sibling number. One-way ANOVA was employed to investigate whether significant differences existed between groups, implying an association between sexual dimorphism in girls and these biosocial variables.

3 Results

Descriptive statistics of the three anthropometric characteristics in the population of the Azores islands are summarized in Table 1. Tables 2 and 3 include descriptive statistics for the corresponding absolute values found in the sample, and for the MF-ratios, respectively.

Table 1. Means and standard deviations of three somatic characteristics in the population of the Azores.

Age	Height (cm)	Weight (kg)	SUMSK(mm)
	BOYS		
10	139.4 ± 6.3	34.5 ± 7.0	36.6 ± 20.5
11	142.6 ± 7.9	37.1 ± 8.0	39.8 ± 22.5
12	148.2 ± 8.0	39.3 ± 7.2	32.5 ± 11.9
	GIRLS		
10	137.6 ± 6.3	31.9 ± 6.0	40.9 ± 18.1
11	144.8 ± 7.2	38.0 ± 8.1	45.6 ± 21.1
12	147.7 ± 6.6	40.7 ± 8.2	47.9 ± 19.8

Table 2. Means and standard deviations of three somatic characteristics in female competitors at the all-Azores School Tournament 1989.

Age	n	Height (cm)	Weight (kg)	SUMSK(mm)
10	29	140.1 ± 6.8	32.9 ± 5.2	41.6 ± 12.9
11	114	146.3 ± 6.8	39.0 ± 7.1	49.5 ± 17.6
12	76	149.0 ± 7.1	40.7 ± 6.8	48.8 ± 15.0

Table 3. Means and standard deviations of Male/Female Ratios for three somatic characteristics in female competitors at the All-Azores School Tournament 1989.

Age	n	Height	Weight	SUMSK
10	29	.998 ± .047	1.069 ± .153	.937 ± .204
11	114	.976 ± .046	.981 ± .178	.897 ± .285
12	76	.997 ± .048	.992 ± .164	.720 ± .190

We can see from the figures that girl competitors were taller than both their male and female age peers in the population. With respect to weight, they were also above the population standards for boys (excepting the age group of 10 yrs.) and girls (excepting the age group of 12 yrs., whose arithmetic mean equals the value calculated in the population). Unexpected, indeed, was the finding that competitors presented an average sum of skinfolds above the standards for their age and sex. Since the standards have been recently established, no significant secular trend effect is likely to account for the differences in stature. Concerning skinfold measurements, observers, techniques and caliper type were kept unchanged. The fact that girls were selected also to participate in team competitions, where body bulk represents a considerable advantage, may explain the greater amount of subcutaneous fat.

The proportions of girl competitors whose MF-ratios were greater than, or smaller than 1.0 were calculated in each age group with respect to every anthropometric dimension. The hypothesis test for sample proportion against the hypothesized value of p=0.5 was employed. No evidence was found of a systematic selection in terms of sexual dimorphism, since the proportions of cases in both groups do not differ significantly. The only exception occurred with respect to standing height among 11-year old girls, where 75 % of the subjects were taller than their average male age peer in the population. This finding is not surprising, since the female standards exceed the male standards in every anthropometric characteristic at this age group.

Linear regression analysis of results in three athletic events on decimal age (X) yielded the following equations :

(i)   Dependent variable, Long Jump :
      $Y = 0.247X - 0.0126$ $(F = 21.431, df : 1; 217, p < .001)$

(ii) Dependent variable, Hockey Ball Throw :
      $Y = 3.921X - 27.475$ $(F = 31.427, df : 1; 217, p < .001)$

(iii) Dependent variable, 60m Run :
      $Y = 16.020 - 0.472X$ $(F = 17.071, df : 1; 217, p < .001)$

Calculated residuals were used to test the hypothesis of significance of differences in athletic events between groups with MF-ratios above and below unity. Results of Student's t-test are summarized in Table 5.

Sexual dimorphism in human populations is thought of as an indicator of ecological, behavioral and cultural adaptation. A number of authors have thoroughly investigated the effects of environmental stress on sexual dimorphism (e.g. Bielicki and Charzewski 1977; Stini 1979; Stinson 1985). It has also been suggested that detrimental effects on somatic measures accounted for by order of birth may act upon sexual dimorphism at two levels, say, the absolute dimensions and the bodily proportions.

In a previous research on growth and motor performance in the Azores, Sobral (1988) emphasized the need for taking into consideration order of birth and family size on the grounds of the local bio-demographic statistics. In the present research, the hypothesis of significance of differences between groups classified for birth order and sibling number was tested by means of one-way ANOVA. Subjects were assigned to four groups (1st, 2nd, 3rd, 4th child and further) and three groups (1-2 sibs, 3-4, 5 and more), respectively.

4 Discussion

The hypothesis of a birth-order effect on the measures of sexual dimorphism has to be rejected for the three anthropometric traits. Sibling number, however, happened to be significantly positively associated with height and weight MF-ratios ($F=5.041$, $p<.01$; and $F=2.945$, $p<.05$, respectively, with df : 2; 216).

Thus, in our sample, as the number of sibs increase, girls tend to be shorter and lighter in comparison with their male age peers. It is most likely that welfare and nutrition play an important role here, since the number of children is negatively correlated with education, housing quality and average income.

On the grounds of the present data, there is evidence of a selective effect on stature, as girls participating in the All-Azores School Tournament were significant taller than their counterparts of the same sex at 10 years ($t=1.972$, df=28, $p<.05$), at 11 years ($t=2.324$, df=113, $p<.01$), but not at 12 years ($p=.063$). This selective effect is still more apparent when MF-ratios are considered, as we have previously mentioned.

Despite there being only one group, where the proportion of girls with a MF-ratio for height lower than 1.0 was significantly greater (at 11 years), girls presenting such a characteristic were found to perform significantly better in long jump and 60m run, whatever the age group they were assigned to.

A similar conclusion may be drawn from skinfold data. Actually, girls whose MF-ratios for sum of 4 skinfolds (SUMSK) were equal to, or greater than unity (thus, leaner than boys of the same age), were also the best performers in 60m run, and differences were found to be highly significant.

209

Table 4. Means and standard deviations of three athletic events in female competitors at the All-Azores School Tournament 1989.

Age Groups:	10	11	12
Long Jump (m)	2.63 ± 0.47	2.81 ± 0.43	3.04 ± 0.35
Hockey Ball Throw (m)	14.90 ± 5.20	17.60 ± 5.36	20.55 ± 5.85
60m Run (sec)	10.97 ± 1.11	10.57 ± 0.90	10.22 ± 0.77

Table 5. Means of residuals (linear regression) and results of Student's t-test in the three athletic events (df=217).

5.1. Height	A : Girls with MF-ratio < 1.0, n(A) =143
	B : Girls with MF-ratio ≥ 1.0, n(B) = 76

	A	B	t	
Long Jump	0.057	-0.105	2.805	(p<0.01)
Hockey Ball Throw	0.280	-0.233	0.667	
60m Run	-0.086	0.155	1.923	(p<0.05)

5.2. Weight	A : Girls with MF-ratio < 1.0, n(A)=119
	B : Girls with MF-ratio ≥ 1.0, n(B)=100

	A	B	t
Long Jump	0.033	-0.038	1.276
Hockey Ball Throw	0.240	-0.126	0.498
60m Run	-0.038	0.041	0.652

5.3. SUMSK	A : Girls with MF-ratio < 1.0, n(A)=163
	B : Girls with MF-ratio ≥ 1.0, n(B)= 56

	A	B	t	
Long Jump	-0.019	0.057	1.187	
Hockey Ball Throw	0.172	0.494	0.350	
60m Run	0.269	-0.336	3.340	(p<0.001)

The hypothetical profile of a girl athlete whose MF-ratios are lower than unity for height and weight, and higher than unity for sum of skinfolds, is not entirely confirmed at the end of the present research. However, girls taller and leaner than the average male age peer in the population were found to be the best performers in the athletic events involving considerable body displacement.

When the Azores data are compared to the DN-JOVEM Track and Field Tournament (the most important event of elite sport in Portugal), similarities become obvious, in spite of the different levels of age, training and competitive demands. Between 12 and 14 years of age, girls participating in this event are clearly above the height and weight standards for boys of the same ages (no adiposity standards are available), and strikingly above the standards for girls between 12 and 15 years of age.

Thus, the question about phenotypical selection in early competitive sport, even in the school setting, may be put as follows : which of two agents is a determinant, negative selection (i.e. the dropping out of the unsuccessful phenotypes), or the inclination of physical educators and coaches to adopt some of the adult athlete stereotypes ? The answer demands extensive inquiry into the concepts, beliefs and paradigms prevailing in the domain of children's sport. It is also an absolute need in the countries where educational and sport authorities join their forces to promote top performance sport.

5 References

Bielicki, T. and Charzewski, J. (1977) Sex differences in the magnitude of statural gains of offspring over parents. **Hum. Biol.** , 49, 265-277.

Sobral, F. (1986) **Estatisticas e Normas Antropométricas e de Valor Fisico.** Região Autonoma dos Açores 1986. Universidade Técnica de Lisboa, Lisboa.

Sobral, F. (1988) Order of birth and variation in body size, physique and motor performance among male and female adolescents of the Azores Islands, in **Proceedings of the 5th Congress of the European Anthropological Association,** Lisboa.

Stini, W. (1979) Adaptive strategies of human populations under nutritional stress, in **Physiological and Morphological Adaptation and Evolution** (ed W. Stini), Mouton, The Hague.

Stinson, S. (1985) Sex differences in environmental sensitivity during growth and development. **Yearbook of Physical Anthropology,** (suppl. 6 to Am. J. Phys. Anthrop.), 28, 123-147.

Part Four

Growth and Performance

20

BIOLOGICAL MATURATION AND PHYSICAL PERFORMANCE [1]

G. BEUNEN
Institute of Physical Education, K.U.Leuven, Belgium

Keywords: Biological maturity, Physical performance, Physical fitness, Athletes.

[1] Manuscript revised, shortened, and updated after Beunen, G. (1989) Biological age in paediatric exercise research, in **Advances in Paediatric Sport Sciences. Volume 3, Biological Issues**. (ed O. Bar Or), Human Kinetics Books, Champaign, Ill., pp. 1-39.

1 Introduction

Chronological age seems to be a weak indicator of the individual maturity status considering the wide inter-individual variability in the physical appearance and characteristics of children of the same chronological age, especially during the pubertal years.

In the following chapter, the concept of biological maturity will be briefly discussed and an overview will be given of the relationship between biological maturity and various measures of physical performance, including the maturational characteristics of elite athletes.

2 The concept of biological maturity

Biological maturity differs in a fundamental way from a measurement of growth such as stature, in that every child finishes by reaching the same endpoint, i.e. becoming fully mature. It refers to successive tissue changes that take place until a final form is achieved. Maturation implies specialization and differentiation of cells, whereas growth can be defined as a process involving hyperplasia (increase in cell number), hypertrophy (increase in cell size) and increase in intracellular materials. As pointed out by Falkner and Tanner (1978), the processes of growth and maturation are intimately linked, since differential growth creates form.

Crampton (1908), Pryor (1905) and Rotch (1909) recognized the need for a criterion of biological maturity, and several techniques have been proposed to assess sexual, skeletal, dental and morphological maturity (see, for example: Acheson 1966; Falkner 1958; Kelly and Reynolds 1947; Marshall 1978; Milman and Bakwin 1950; Roche 1978; Reynolds and

Asakawa 1951; Sawtell 1929; Todd 1937). Sex characteristics, morphological, dental and skeletal criteria are the most commonly used characteristics to assess the biological maturity status.

In assessing sex characteristics, the criteria described by Reynolds and Wines (1948, 1951) and popularized by Tanner (1962) are most often used. For breast development, pubic hair and genital development, five discrete stages are clearly described. These stages must be assigned by visual inspection of the nude subject or by taking somatotype photographs and enlarging the specific areas. Recently, findings by Neinstein (1982) suggest that self-assessment of sexual maturation might serve as a non-invasive alternative, but further research is needed in this connection. For cross sectional data reference values can be obtained by probit or logit analysis (Finney, 1952), however, longitudinal reference values provide more accurate information (Marshall and Tanner 1969,1970). Age at menarche, defined as the first menstrual flow, can be defined retrospectively by interrogating a representative sample of women. The estimated age is then, of course, influenced by error in recall. Studies by Damon, Damon, Reed and Valadian (1969) and Damon and Bajema (1974) suggest that the retrospective technique is reasonably accurate for group comparisons. The information obtained in a longitudinal or prospective survey would be more accurate but here other problems inherent in longitudinal research are encountered. Another possibility is to interrogate representative samples of girls that are expected to experience menarche, and record whether or not periods have started at the time of investigation. For such data reference standards can be constructed using probits or logits. For all sexual criteria thus far discussed, the main problem is that the changes that occur are limited to the adolescent period. Furthermore the stages are fairly crude, discrete milestones in a continuous process.

Height age and even weight age have been used to estimate morphological age. These developmental ages can easily be found by determining the age at which the given child's actual stature equals the height of the average child. However, the measure has limited usefulness, as it confounds maturity with size. In longitudinal studies, age at peak height velocity is another very useful criterion but it has the inconvenience that children have to be followed during several years at regular intervals in order that this pubertal event should be defined accurately. An alternative technique is to estimate the percentage of adult height. This technique requires the knowledge of adult height which can be predicted. The three major techniques are those reported by Bayley (1946), Bayley and Pinneau (1952), Roche, Wainer and Thissen (1975a), and Tanner et al. (1975, 1983). The predictors in these techniques are actual height, chronological age , skeletal age and in some of them parental height and age at menarche in girls.

216

Although several attempts have been made to construct a shape development criterion no useful technique has emerged. According to Goldstein (1984), the technique developed by Bookstein (1978), with particular reference to cephalometrics rather than body shape, opens up a new perspective.

Dental age has usually been estimated from the age of eruption of deciduous and permanent teeth or from the number of teeth present at a certain age (Demirjian 1978). Eruption is only one event in the ossification process of the tooth, it has no real biological meaning and is disturbed by exogenous factors. For this reason, Demirjian et al. (1973) constructed scales for the assessment of dental maturity, based on the same principles as the Tanner-Whitehouse technique (Tanner et al. 1975) for assessing skeletal maturity of the hand and wrist.

Skeletal maturity is probably the most commonly used criterion in the assessment of biological age. What is more, it is the best single criterion (Falkner 1958; Tanner 1962; Acheson 1966).

Although there are differences in the skeletal maturation of different parts of the body, the hand and wrist area is the most valuable area for the assessment in the age range from seven to adulthood. The knee is the area of choice from birth to six years since more information is contained in the changes that take place in this area during this period (Roche 1980). Bilateral assessments are unnecessary since the differences involved are small and not of particular importance.

Three main techniques are widely used in assessing skeletal maturity: the atlas technique (Greulich and Pyle 1950, 1959), the scoring or bone-specific-approach techniques of Tanner et al. (1975, 1983) and of Roche et al. (1975b). Recently Roche, Chumlea and Thissen (1988) published the Fels-method for the hand and wrist.

The best and most extensively used standard radiographs that have been published for the hand and wrist are those of Greulich and Pyle (1959). Standards are given separately for each sex for every three-month interval from birth to two years, thereafter for every six-month interval until five years and then annually until puberty during which the standards are given semi-annually. The bone-specific methods were introduced by Acheson (1954). Tanner and Whitehouse (1959) and Tanner, Whitehouse and Healy (1962) developed a system (TW1) for the hand and wrist. Their system was revised in 1975 (TW2) (Tanner et al. 1975). In the TW2 method 7 or 8 maturity stages are identified and carefully described and illustrated. These maturity stages reflect the distance the individual has travelled along the road from complete immaturity to complete maturity. The chief concern of the authors was to construct a maturity scale. The scores allotted to the different stages of the different bones were defined in such a way as to minimize the overall disagreement between the different bones, and in combining the scores of different bones, a biological weight was assigned to the bones. The authors also developed a separate scoring

217

system on the same principles for the radius-ulna and short bones (RUS-score) and for the carpals (Carpal-score). Standards for skeletal age were then constructed for the British population.

The Roche-Wainer-Thissen method was developed for the assessment of antero-posterior radiographs of the knee (Roche et al. 1975b). The method relies on the use of maturity indicators. After retrieving all the possible maturity indicators for the knee reported in the literature, the authors of this method proceeded to grade these indicators. Thereafter, Roche et al. (1975b) selected those indicators that could be defined with a high degree of reliability. Furthermore, they checked the ability of an indicator to discriminate between children, as well as the universality, validity and completeness of each indicator. On the basis of these criteria, they selected 34 maturity indicators for the femur, tibia and fibula. The parameters used to construct the RWT-scale are the chronological age at which each indicator is present in 50% of the children in the population sample and the rate of change in each indicator's prevalence with age. These parameters are combined to give a single continuous index, using latent trait analysis. This method made it possible to estimate the sampling error, which statistic can only be calculated with the RWT-technique. A very similar approach has been used in the development of the Fels-method for the hand and wrist recently developed by Roche, Chumlea and Thissen (1988).

From the extensive studies of Nicolson and Hanley (1953), Marshall (1974), Anderson, Thompson and Popovich (1975), Bielicki (1975), and Bielicki, Koniarek and Malina (1984), it became apparent that the indices of sexual maturation, the ages at which various percentages of adult height are attained, the ages at which different stages of skeletal maturity are attained and the age of peak height velocity are fairly closely interrelated. The relationships between the maturity characteristics, however, are not strong enough to allow individual predictions from one maturity indicator to another. No single system provides a complete description of the maturation of an individual child. The above-noted interrelationships are, nevertheless, strong enough to indicate the developmental level of a group of children or populations (Malina, 1978a).

3 Biological maturity as related to physical performance

3.1 Anthropometric characteristics

Before discussing the relationship between physical performance and maturity, it would seem appropriate to review briefly the relationship between anthropometric characteristics and maturity. Maturity and body size are, indeed, confounded with reference to their effects on performance (Malina 1975) and an elucidation of the relationship between the two would lead to a better understanding of that between performance and maturity.

When the association between biological maturation and anthropometric characteristics is investigated in a given population, it is often approached in two different ways: by correlational analysis or the contrasting of maturity groups. Both approaches generally lead to the same conclusions.

From a recent review by Beunen (1989) it appears that skeletal maturity is highly related with percentage of attained adult height, in addition, age at menarche is related to height and height increments which has led some authors to predict age at menarche from height and weight (Frish 1974) or from height increments (Ellison 1981). In boys, the correlations between skeletal maturity and several anthropometric dimensions from three different studies (Bayley 1943a,1943b; Beunen et al. 1978; Clarke 1971) are strikingly similar. Highest correlations are found for height and sitting height whereas weight and especially circumferences show lower correlations. The correlations increase until 14 years and thereafter decrease for all measurements. In girls, as in boys, the highest correlations are found for height, followed by weight, widths, and cicumferences. However, in girls, the correlations reach a maximum at about 11 years, around the time of peak height velocity (Beunen 1989).

When maturity groups are contrasted, these associations are also apparent. When the mean anthropometric dimensions of 14 year old Belgian boys with advanced maturity status (skeletal age of 16 years) is contrasted with the dimensions of the retarded boys (skeletal age of 12 years), the mean height of the most retarded group (skeletal age = 12 years) is more than 2 SD's removed from the mean height of the most advanced group (skeletal age 16 years). The differences decrease somewhat for trunk widths, bone breadths and circumferences, and much smaller differences are found for skinfolds.

At all age levels between 6 and 16 years the mean somatic dimensions of average-maturing girls correspond quite closely to the means of the total sample. At all age levels, advanced girls are characterized by larger body dimensions and retarded girls by smaller dimensions. The differences are somewhat smaller at the younger ages, increase until puberty, and tend to disappear at 16 years of age. Although even at age 16 years, retarded girls still have somewhat lower weight and smaller trunk widths (Beunen 1989). The decrease in the relationships after puberty might be accounted for by the greater homogeneity for the different somatic dimensions and by the fact that upon reaching adulthood, each boy and girl attains his or her maximum skeletal maturation.

Muscle mass and size are also associated with skeletal maturity. The relationship is weak during childhood but moderately strong during puberty, especially in boys (Reynolds 1946; Johnston and Malina 1966; Malina 1978b).

As long ago as 1937 Richey demonstrated that already at 6 years of age, early-menarche girls are characterized by a superior height and weight, long before the menarche occurs. These differences between early- and late-menarche girls are also seen for chest width and biiliac diameters (Shuttleworth 1937). Clarke and Degutis (1962) and Clarke and Harrison (1962) further demonstrated that boys who were advanced in pubescent development had higher mean anthropometric dimensions.

Much discussion has centered around a proposed association between a critical body weight (Frish and Revelle 1970) and the timing of the menarche, the notion of critical body weight having been replaced by the critical fat hypothesis (Frisch, Revelle and Cook 1973). The latter investigators advanced the idea that the attainment of a certain critical weight (47 kg) or critical fat (17 % of total body weight) alters the metabolic rate, which in turn affects the hypothalamic-ovarian feedback loop, reducing the sensitivity of the hypothalamus to circulating estrogen levels. A number of severe criticisms have been made of these hypotheses: these criticsms concern the research design, the statistical analysis that has been used and the techniques for the determination of percent fat mass.

Obese children are not only fatter than their age and sex peers but are also taller, have increased skeletal size, lean body mass, and muscle status. In contrast, lean children are correspondingly smaller, and retarded in maturity status (Beunen et al. 1982, 1983; Cheek, Schultz, Parra and Reba 1970; Darn, Clarke and Guire 1974, 1975; Darn and Haskell 1959, 1960; Parizkova 1977; Quaade 1955; Seltzer and Mayer 1964; Wolff 1955). Beunen (1989) concluded that there is a slight association between biological maturation and somatotype that varies somewhat with age. It should be stressed, however, that the chronology of adolescence shows considerable independence of physique as expressed by the somatotype (Barton and Hunt 1962). In girls, the association between somatotype and maturity has not been carefully investigated. However, late-maturing girls have on the average, long legs for their stature, relatively narrow hips, less weight for height and a generally linear physique (Tanner 1962).

3.2 Physical fitness components

In analyzing the relationship between physical performance capacity and the criteria of biological age, a distinction will be made between associations found in a general population and associations observed in athletes and elite athletes.

First the association with cardiorespiratory fitness will be considered. Highly significant correlations were found between skeletal matutity and maximal oxygen uptake, however when maximal oxygen uptake was expressed per kilogram body weight the correlations became non-significant (Hollmann and Bouchard 1970; Labitzke 1971; Shephard et al.1978; Savov 1978).

Hebbelinck, Borms and Clarijs (1971), Kemper et al. (1975), Bouchard et al. (1976,1978), reported nonsignificant or rather low correlations between skeletal maturity and several indices of submaximal working, except around puberty, when substantial higher associations are reported. Bouchard et al. (1978) pointed out that in spite of the high degree of relationship between skeletal age, chronological age, height and weight, a higher association between skeletal age and submaximal working capacity was observed around puberty, although little was added by skeletal age alone. Age-specific correlations between skeletal age and submaximal working capacity in girls generally increased with age and reached a maximum at 11 to 13 years of age (see Fig. 1). The highest correlations (r^2 = .35, resp. .34) were observed between skeletal age and physical working capacity 170 (PWC170) for 11-and 13-year-old girls. The age trends in the correlations were less clear for PWC150 (Beunen 1989).

In 1940 Espenschade already demonstrated that in pubescent girls, motor performance levels off or declines with increasing skeletal maturity. Treatment of the same data as a function of age of deviation from menarche yields similar results. Conversely, pubescent boys continue to show improved motor performance with increasing skeletal age.

Since Jones (1940) demonstrated the relatively high relationship between biological maturity status at different age levels and static or isometric strength, these relationships were further documented in a number of studies (Bastos and Hegg 1986; Carron and Bailey 1974; Carron, Aitken and Bailey 1978; Clarke and Degutis 1962; Clarke and Harrison 1962; Clarke 1971).

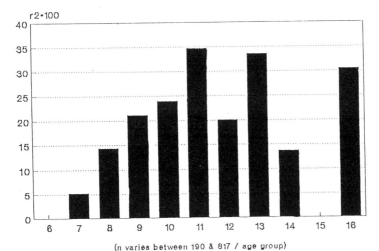

(n varies between 190 & 817 / age group)

Fig. 1. Association (coefficients of determination x 100) between skeletal maturity (TW2-system) and PWC170 in 6 to 16 years old girls (after Beunen 1989).

For prepubescent children significant associations are observed for static strength, explosive strength and running speed when a wide age range is considered. When, however, age-specific correlations are calculated, only static strength is associated with skeletal age at all age levels. During adolescence again only static strength is positively related to skeletal maturity in girls. For muscular endurance often called functional strength or dynamic strenght there is even a negative correlation at 11 through 13 years of age. In boys, static strength is positively related to biological age during adolescence. From 14 years on, however, all the gross motor abilities studied within this period are positively correlated with skeletal age. Muscular endurance tests of the upper body and lower trunk are negatively related to skeletal age in 12- and 13-year-old boys. This is not surprising, since in these tests, the subject acts against his own body weight or a part of it. As for static strength, the highest correlations for all motor items are found at 14 or 15 years of age. These findings from Beunen (1976,1978,1989), Clarke (1971), Hebbelinck et al. (1986), Rajic et al. (1979), Rarick and Oyster (1964) and Seils (1951), are confirmed by studies in which maturity groups are contrasted with respect to physical performance capacity (Beunen et al. 1974; Clarke and Harrison 1962; Ellis, Carron and Bailey 1975; Petrovcic, Medved and Horvat 1957; Savov 1978).

Several authors, however, point out that, at least in preadolescent children, the strength of the relationship between skeletal age and motor performance capacities declines considerably when height and especially weight is partialled out (Carron and Bailey 1974; Rarick and Oyster 1964; Seils 1951; Shephard et al. 1978). Beunen et al. (1979, 1981), however, demonstrated that 13-to-17-year-old boys advanced in skeletal maturity, and of the same chronological age, height and weight, perform better than their less mature peers for all gross motor items. The same authors also came to the conclusion that at each age level between 12 and 19 years, the interaction between chronological age and skeletal age as such or in combination with height and/or weight has a higher predictive value than any other single variable except for performance in muscular endurance tests (bent arm hang and leg lifts). The predictive value of body size (height and weight), skeletal maturity, and chronological age and their interactions was rather low, having varied between 0% and 17%, except for static strength (arm pull) for which the explained variance ranged from 33% to 58%. As for body dimensions, the explained variance reaches a maximum for most tests at 14-15 years of age.

Finally, Lefevre et al. (1990) have shown that the performance advantage of early maturers disappears at adult age (30 years). For most fitness components no significant differences were observed between early and late maturing boys when age at peak height velocity was taken as an indicator of their biological maturity status. Moreover late maturers tend to obtain better results at adult age for explosive and functional strength.

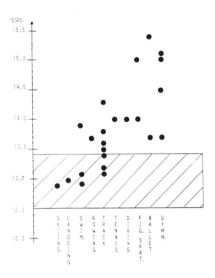

Fig. 2. Age at menarche in athletes competing in individual sports (adapted after Malina 1983). Shaded area refers to mean age at menarche in comparable non-athletic samples.

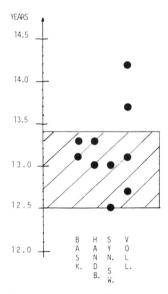

Fig. 3. Age at menarche in athletes competing in team sports (adapted after Malina 1983). Shaded area refers to mean age at menarche in comparable non-athletic samples.

223

3.3 Biological age in athletes and elite athletes

In recent years, extensive reviews of the existing data on maturity characteristics in young athletes have been published by Beunen (1989) and Malina (1978a,1978c, 1982, 1983, 1984, 1986, 1988). In the following discussion an attempt will be made to summarize the available evidence and to discuss the sex-specific maturity characteristics of athletes.

Male athletes of different competitive levels in various sports are characterized by an average or earlier biological maturity status. Whatever the criteria used or the competitive level observed, studies point to the same direction, with very few exceptions. In contrast to males, female athletes are later in their biological maturity status (see figures 2 and 3). Gymnasts, ballet dancers and figure skaters are the latest, followed by divers, tennis players and thereafter, track and field athletes, rowers and volleyball players. Canoists, alpine skiers, basketball players, handball players, swimmers and synchronized swimmers are average in their maturity status. Most recently Stager, Robertshaw and Miescher (1984) demonstrated that elite female swimmers are now also later in their age at menarche.

The marked later age at menarche in female gymnasts is further documented by Claessens et al. (1990). The age at menarche in 121 females competing in the World Championships Artistic Gymnastics (Rotterdam, The Netherlands) was 15.2 years (SD=1.4 years). Furthermore the gymnasts who scored highest had a mean age at menarche of 16.1 years as compared to 14.1 years for the girls who obtained the lowest overall scores in the competitions. As shown in Fig. 4 this later age at menarche in elite gymnasts is confirmed by their later skeletal maturation. Especially for the 16 through 18 years old gymnasts the later skeletal maturation as compared to the Belgian reference data (Beunen et al. 1990) is apparent.

Most of the literature concerning maturity characteristics in female athletes concentrates on age at menarche (see inter al. Marker 1981; Malina 1983). Consequently, several hypotheses have been proposed to explain the later maturation of female competitors in most sports. Probably one of the most popular hypotheses is that training delays menarche (see inter al. Frisch et al. 1981).

According to Malina (1986), the data dealing with intensive training and menarche are quite limited, associational, speculative, and do not control for other factors which influence the time of menarche. The conclusions arrived at by Frisch et al. (1981) are based upon a correlational analysis which does not imply a cause-effect sequence. If there is an association between training and menarche, the suggested underlying explanatory mechanism is hormonal. Presently, longitudinal data are lacking in which the cumulative effects of hormonal responses to regular training in premenarcheal girls have been studied. Furthermore, it has been suggested that a certain level of fatness, which in turn is influenced by

224

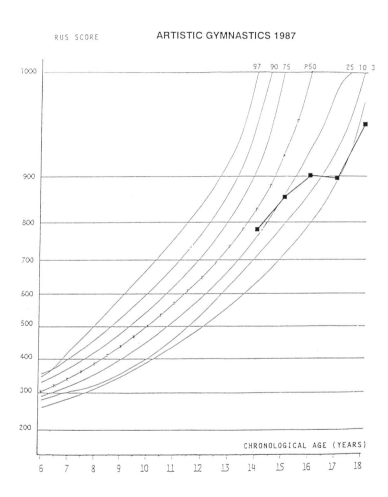

Fig. 4. Skeletal maturity score (TW2-system: RUS-score) of Caucasian female gymnasts competing at the World Championships Artistic Gymnastics, Rotterdam 1987 (Claessens et al. 1990).

225

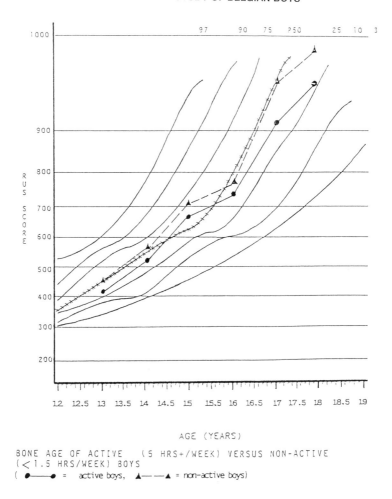

Fig. 5. Skeletal maturity score (TW2-system: RUS-score) of active (5 hours/week or more) versus non-active (less than 1.5 hours/week) boys followed longitudinally (Beunen et al., in preparation).

vigorous exercise, is needed to attain menarche (Frish et al. 1973). As discussed above, the data do not support the specificity of fatness as a critical variable for menarche. Also, the question remains unanswered of why there is a positive association between physical performance capacity and maturity status in male athletes and a negative association in female athletes, given that the underlying hormonal mechanisms of biological maturation are essentially the same. The inadequacy of the research design adopted by Frisch to demonstrate the causal relationship between age at menarche and age at onset of training has been elegantly shown by Stager, Wigglesworth and Hatler (1990). They randomly, and independently generated the age at onset of training and the age at menarche for a population of 30 000 athletes. The generated mean age at menarche was 13.4 years and the mean age at onset of training was 10.0 years. By design no correlation existed between the age at onset of training and the age at menarche. However, when premenarcheal training and post-menarcheal training groups were formed, these groups differed significantly in mean age at menarche. Moreover in each sub-group age at onset of training was significantly correlated with age at menarche although, by design, no correlation was present in the total population. These results clearly suggest that this research design results in biased estimates of statistical parameters. This bias accounts for the reported correlations between age at onset of training and age at menarche. Stager et al. therefore propose to state that the age of menarche in athletes is "LATER" rather than "DELAYED".

There is an association between age at menarche and skeletal maturation (see interrelationships) and from the few longitudinal studies on the relationship between training and skeletal age, there is no evidence that skeletal age is affected by regular physical training (Malina 1986). This hypothesis was furher tested by Beunen et al. (in preparation) on the basis of data from the Leuven Growth Study of Belgian Boys during which 588 boys were followed during six years at yearly intervals between 13 and 18 years. Two groups were selected on the basis of their participation in sports and physical education. The non-active boys were less than 1.5 hours/week active during the first three years of the follow-up, and the active boys were engaged in sports and physical education during more than 5 hours/week over the whole year during the first three years of the follow-up. The skeletal age scores (RUS-score of the TW2-system) parallel quite closely the medians of the Belgian reference population (Beunen et al. 1990) and no significant differences exist between the active and non-active groups (Fig. 5). Note that the scale is non-linear so that deviations near the end of the scale are magnified, furthermore both groups are approaching adulthood and minor differences in the maturity stadia of the bones result in marked differences in maturity scores.

Finally, as shown by Märker (1981) on the basis of 242 elite female athletes, the age of first parturition is not significantly influenced by hard training.

Among the factors which could partly explain the associations between biological age and performance capacity, the two-part hypothesis formulated by Malina (1983) is appealing and takes into account the evidence gathered so far. This hypothesis combines biological selective factors (i.e. physique and skill) and social factors. A first part of the hypothesis states that the physique characteristics associated with later maturation in girls are generally more suitable for successful athletic performance. Successful female athletes with the appropriate physique and skill are thus selected by self and/or by parents and coaches. The second part of the hypothesis relates to the socialization process. Early-maturing girls are socialized away from sports participation, while late-maturing girls are socialized into sports participation. Data on the socialization of young girls are not extensive, most of the information coming from studies on white, male, high school and college athletes or top-level amateurs (Coakley 1987). For boys, sports participation is seen as being directly linked to their development as men. In the case of girls, sports participation is seldomly associated with becoming a woman.

4 Concluding remarks

At present most of our knowledge on the maturity-performance associations is based upon correlational analyses which do not indicate any cause-effect sequences. It is plainly evident that, when skeletal age is associated with static strength, there must be an underlying mechanism which explains this link. There is thus a need for more detailed studies, in which the underlying mechanism of the associations discussed in this paper are investigated. Long-term experiments, if ethically acceptable, or long-term natural experiments, in which existing groups of children living under given circumstances, e.g. participation in an intensive training program in a specific sports discipline, would tell us more about these mechanisms. Multidisciplinary studies, in which biological, sociological and psychological factors are considered would provide the most complete information. In these studies, a large number of biological factors need to be examined: biological maturity characteristics, hormonal secretions, anthropometric dimensions, body composition, body type, physical performance components, specific sports skills, daily physical activity and training, and anthropometric and maturational characteristics of the parents and siblings.

From the above, it is clear that biological maturity status should be considered in the evaluation of the performance capacities of growing children. The point is not that the performance capacity of a youngster can be predicted from maturity status, even in combination with chronological age and size (height and weight), but rather that chronological age, maturity and size are confounded in their effects on performance, and this influence must be taken into account. In this respect, it can be argued that in youth sports, especially during adolescence, children should be classified into biological age groups instead of chronological age.

As a final conclusion, it should be stressed that biological maturity is an important biological process, which is related to growth and physical performance. Sport scientists, pediatricians, sport medical doctors, physical educators and coaches must be aware of these interrelations and should take them into account in the evaluation of the physical performance capacity of youngsters.

5 References

Acheson, R.M. (1954) A method of assessing maturity from radiographs. A report from the Oxford child health survey. **J. Anat.**, 88, 498-508.

Acheson, R.M. (1966) Maturation of the skeleton, in **Human Development** (ed F. Falkner), Saunders, Philadelphia, pp. 465-502.

Barton, W.H. and Hunt, E.E. Jr. (1962) Somatotype and adolescence in boys. **Hum. Biol.**, 34, 254-270.

Bastos, F.V. and Hegg, R.V. (1986) The relationship of chronological age, body build, and sexual maturation to handgrip strength in schoolboys ages 10 through 17 years, in **Perspectives in Kinanthropometry** (ed J.A.P. Day), Human Kinetics, Champaign, pp.45-49.

Bayley, N. (1943a) Size and body build of adolescents in relation to rate of skeletal maturity. **Child Dev.**, 14, 47-90.

Bayley, N. (1943b) Skeletal maturing in adolescence as basis for determining percentage of completed growth. **Child Dev.**, 14, 1-46.

Bayley, N. (1946) Tables for predicting adult height from skeletalage and present height. **J. Pediatr.**, 28, 49-64.

Bayley, N. and Pinneau, S.R. (1952) Tables for predicting adult height from skeletal age: revised for use with Greulich-Pyle hand standards. **J. Pediatr.**, 40, 423-411.

Beunen, G. (1989) Biological age in pediatric exercise research, in **Advances in Pediatric Sport Sciences**, Volume 3: Biological Issues (ed O. Bar-Or), Human Kinetics Books, Champaign, pp. 1-39.

Beunen, G. Lefevre, J. Ostyn, M. Renson, R. Simons, J. and Van Gerven D. (1990) Skeletal maturity in Belgian youths assessed by the Tanner-Whitehouse method (TW2). **Ann. Hum. Biol.**, 16.

Beunen, G. Malina, R.M. Ostyn, M. Renson, R. Simons, J. and Van Gerven, D. (1982) Fatness and skeletal maturity of Belgian boys 12 through 20 years of age. **Am. J. Phys. Anthropol.**, 59, 387-392.

Beunen, G. Malina, R.M. Ostyn, M. Renson, R. Simons, J. and Van Gerven, D. (1983) Fatness, growth and motor fitness of Belgian boys 12 through 20 years of age. **Hum. Biol.**, 55, 599-613.

Beunen, G. Malina, R.M. Renson, R. Lefevre J. and Claessens, A. (in preparation) Physical activity, physical growth, maturity and performance in Belgian adolescents followed longitudinally.

Beunen, G. Ostyn, M. Renson, R. Simons, J. and Van Gerven, D. (1974) Skeletal maturation and physical fitness of 12 to 15 year old boys. **Acta Paediatrica Belgica**, 28, 221-232.

Beunen, G. Ostyn, M. Renson, R. Simons, J. and Van Gerven, D. (1976) Skeletal maturation and physical fitness of girls aged 12 through 16. **Hermes**, 10, 445-457.

Beunen, G. Ostyn, M. Renson, R. Simons, J. and Van Gerven, D. (1979) Growth and maturity as related to motor ability. **S. Afr. J. Res. Sport Phys. Ed. Rec.**, 3, 9-15.

Beunen, G. Ostyn, M. Simons, J. Renson, R. and Van Gerven, D. (1981) Chronological and biological age as related to physical fitness in boys 12 to 19 years. **Ann. Hum. Biol.**, 8, 321-331.

Beunen, G. Ostyn, M. Simons, J. Van Gerven, D. Swalus, P. and De Beul, G. (1978) A correlational analysis of skeletal maturity, anthropometric measures and motor fitness of boys 12 through 16, in **Biomechanics of Sports and Kinanthropometry** (eds F. Landry and W.A.R. Orban), Symposia Specialists, Miami, pp. 343-349.

Bielicki, T. (1975) Interrelationships between various measures of maturation rate in girls during adolescence. **Studies in Physical Anthropology**, 1, 51-64.

Bielicki, T. Koniarek, J. and Malina, R.M. (1984) Interrelationships among certain measures of growth and maturation rate in boys during adolescence. **Ann. Hum. Biol.**, 11, 201-210.

Bookstein, F.C. (1978) **The measurement of biological shape and shape change**. Springer Verlag, New York.

Bouchard, C. Leblanc, C. Malina, R.M. and Hollmann, W. (1978) Skeletal age and submaximal capacity in boys. **Ann. Hum. Biol.**, 5, 75-78.

Bouchard, C. Malina, R.M. Hollmann, W. and Leblanc, C. (1976) Relationship between skeletal maturity and submaximal working capacity in boys 8 to 18 years. **Med. Sci. Sports**, 8, 186-190.

Carron, A.V. Aitken, E.J. and Bailey, D.A. (1977) The relationship of menarche to the growth and development of strength, in **Frontiers of Activity and Child Health** (eds H. Lavallée and R.J. Shephard), Editions du Pélican, Québec, pp. 139-143.

Carron, A.V. and Bailey, D.A. (1974) Strength development in boys from 10 through 16 years. **Mon. Res. Child**, 39(4, Serial N° 157).

Cheek, D.B. Schulz, R.B. Parra, A. and Reba, R.C. (1970) Overgrowth of lean and adipose tissues in adolescent obesity. **Pediatr. Res.**, 4, 268-269.

Claessens, A.L. Veer, F.M. Stijnen, V. Lefevre, J. Maes, H. Steens, G. Beunen, G. (1990) Anthropometric characteristics of outstanding male and female gymnasts. **J. Sports Sci.**, (in press).

Clarke, H.H. (1971) **Physical and Motor Tests in the Medford Boys' Growth Study**, Prentice Hall, Englewood Cliffs.

Clarke, H.H. and Degutis, E.W. (1962) Comparison of skeletal age and various physical and motor factors with pubescent development of 10, 13, and 16 year old boys. **Res. Quart.**, 33, 356-368.

Clarke, H.H. and Harrison, J.C.E. (1962) Differences in physical and motor traits between boys of advanced, normal and retarded maturity. **Res. Quart.**, 33, 13-25.

Coackley, J.J. (1987) Children and the sport socialization process, **Advances in Pediatric Sport Sciences : Vol. 2 Behavioral Issues** (eds D. Gould and M.R. Weiss), Human Kinetics, Champaign, pp. 43-60.

Crampton, C.W. (1908) Physiological age: a fundamental principle. **Am. Phys. Ed. Rev.**, 8, 3-6.

Damon, A. and Bajema, C.J. (1974) Age at menarche: accuracy of recall after thirty nine years. **Hum. Biol.**, 46, 381-384.

Damon, A. Damon, S.T. Reed, R.B. and Valadian, I. (1969) Age at menarche of mothers and daughters, with a note on accuracy of recall. **Hum. Biol.**, 41, 161-175.

Demirjian, A. (1978) Dentition, in **Human Growth: 2. Postnatal Growth** (eds F. Falkner and J.M. Tanner), Plenum, New York, pp. 413-444.

Demirjian, A. Goldstein, H. and Tanner, J.M. (1973) A new system for dental age assessment. **Hum. Biol.**, 45, 211-227.

Ellis, J.O. Carron, A.V. and Bailey, D.A. (1975) Physical performancein boys from 10 through 16 years. **Hum. Biol.**, 47, 263-281.

Ellison, P.T. (1981) Prediction of age at menarche from annual height increments. **Am. J. Phys. Anthropol.**, 56, 71-75.

Espenschade, A.S. (1940) Motor performance in adolescence including the study of relationships with measures of physical growth and maturity. **Monogr. Res. Child**, 5(1, Serial N°24).

Falkner, F. (1958) Skeletal maturation: an appraisal of concept and method. **Am. J. Phys. Anthropol.**, 16, 381-396.

Falkner, F. and Tanner, J.M. (1978) Introduction, in **Human Growth: 1. Principles and Prenatal Growth** (eds F. Falkner and J.M. Tanner), Plenum, New York, pp. IX-X.

Finney, D.J. (1952) **Probit analysis**, University Press, Cambridge.

Frisch, R. (1974) A method of prediction of age of menarche from height and weight at ages 9 through 13 years. **Pediatrics**, 53, 384-390.

Frisch, R.E. and Revelle, R. (1970) Height and weight at menarche and a hypothesis of critical body weights and adolescents. **Science**, 169, 397-399.

Frisch, R.E. Gotz-Wilberger, A.V. McArthur, J.W. Albright, R. Witschi, J. Bullen, B. Birnholz, J. Reed, R.B. and Hermann, H. (1981) Delayed menarche and amenorrhea of college athletes in relation to age of onset of training. **J. Am. Med. Assoc.**, 246, 1559-1563.

Frisch, R.E. Revelle, R. and Cook, S. (1973) Components of weight at menarche and the initiation of the adolescent growth spurt in girls: estimated total water, lean body weight and fat. **Hum. Biol.**, 45, 469-483.

Garn, S.M. and Haskell, J.A. (1959) Fat and growth during childhood. **Science**, 130, 1711-1712.

Garn, S.M. and Haskell, J.A. (1960) Fat thickness and developmental status in childhood and adolescence. **Am. J. Dis. Child.**, 99, 746-751.

Garn, S.M. Cheek, D.C. and Guire, K.E. (1974) Growth, body composition and development of obese and lean children, in **Childhood Obesity** (ed M. Winick), Wiley, New York, pp. 23-46.

Garn, S.M. Clark, D.C. and Guire, K.E. (1974) Level of fatness and size attainment. **Am. J. Phys. Anthropol.**, 40, 447-450.

Goldstein, H. (1984) Current developments in the design and analysis of growth studies, in **Human Growth and Development** (eds J. Borms, R. Hauspie, A. Sand, C. Suzanne and M. Hebbelinck), Plenum, New York, pp. 733-752.

Greulich, W.W. and Pyle, I. (1950) **Radiographic Atlas of Skeletal Development of the Hand and Wrist**, Stanford University Press, Stanford.

Hebbelinck, M. Borms, J. and Clarijs, J. (1971) La variabilité de l'age squelettique et les correlations avec la capacité de travail chez des garçons de 5me année primaire. **Kinanthropologie**, 3, 125-135.

Hebbelinck, M. Borms, J. Duquet, W. and Vanderwaeren, M. (1986) Relationships between skeletal age and physical fitness variables of 6-year-old children, in **Perspectives in Kinanthrometry** (ed J.A.P. Day), Human Kinetics, Champaign, pp. 51-56.

Hollmann, W. and Bouchard, C. (1970) Untersuchungen uber die Beziehungen zwischen chronologischem und biologischem Alter zu spiroergometrischen Messgrössen, Herzvolümen, anthropometrischen Daten and Skelettmüskelkraft bei 8-18 jährigen Jungen. **Z. Kreislauf-forsch.**, 59, 160-176.

Johnston, F.E. and Malina, R.M. (1966) Age changes in the composition of the upper arm in Philadelphia children. **Hum. Biol.**, 38, 1-21.

Jones, H.E. (1949) **Motor Performance and Growth. A Developmental Study of Static Dynamometric Strength.** University of California Press, Berkeley.

Kelly, J. and Reynolds, L. (1947) Appearance and growth of ossification centres and increase in the body dimensions. **Am. J. Roentgenol.**, 57, 477-516.

Kemper, H.C.G. Verschuur, R. Ras, K.G.A. Snel, J. Splinter, P.G. and Tavecchio, L.W.C. (1975) Biological age and habitual physical activity in relation to physical fitness in 12- and 13-year old schoolboys. **Z. Kinder-heilk.**, 119, 169-179.

Labitzke, H. (1971) Ueber Beziehungen zwischen biologischen Alter (Ossifikationsalter) und der Korperlänge, den Körpergewicht und der Korperoberflache sowie der maximalen Sauerstoffaufnahme. **Med. u. Sport**, 11, 82-86.

Lefevre, J. Beunen, G. Steens, G. Claessens, A. and Renson R. (1990) Motor performance during adolescence and adult age as related to age at peak height velocity. **Ann. Hum. Biol.**, in press.

Malina, R.M. (1975) Anthropometric correlates of strength and motor performance. **Exer. Sport Sci. Rev.**, 3, 249-274.

Malina, R.M. (1978a) Adolescent growth and maturation: selectedaspects of current research. **Y. Phys. Anthropol.**, 21, 63-94.

Malina, R.M. (1978b) Growth of muscle tissue and muscle mass, in **Human Growth, 2. Postnatal Growth** (eds F. Falkner and J.M. Tanner), Plenum, New York, pp. 273-294.

Malina, R.M. (1978c) Physical growth and maturity characteristics of young athletes, in **Children in Sport: a Contemporary Anthology** (eds R.A. Magill, M.J. Ash and F.L. Smoll), Human Kinetics, Champaign, pp. 79-101.

Malina, R.M. (1982) Physical growth and maturity characteristics of young athletes, in **Children in Sport** (2nd ed.) (eds R.A. Magill, M.J. Ash and F.L. Smoll), Human Kinetics, Champaign, pp. 79-96.

Malina, R.M. (1983) Menarche in athletes: a synthesis and hypothesis. **Ann. Hum. Biol.**, 10, 1-24.

Malina, R.M. (1984) Human growth, maturation, and regular physical activity, in **Advances in Pediatric Sport Sciences, 1. Biological Issues** (ed. R.A. Boileau), Human Kinetics, Champaign, pp. 59-83.

Malina, R.M. (1986) Maturational considerations in elite young athletes, in **Perspectives in Kinanthropometry** (ed. J. Day), Human Kinetics, Champaign, pp. 29-43.

Malina, R.M. (1988) Biological maturity status of young athletes, in **Young Athletes: Biological, Psychological and Educational Perspectives** (ed. R.M. Malina), Human Kinetics, Champaign, pp. 121-140.

Märker, K. (1981) Influence of athletic training on the maturity process of girls. **Med. Sport**, 15, 117-126.

Marshall, W.A. (1974) Interrelationships of skeletal maturation, sexual development and somatic growth in man. **Ann. Hum. Biol.**, 1, 29-40.

Marshall, W.A. (1978) Puberty, in **Human Growth: 2. Postnatal Growth** (eds. F. Falkner and J.M. Tanner), Plenum, New York, pp. 141-181.

Marshall, W.A. and Tanner, J.M. (1969) Variation in the pattern of pubertal changes in girls. **Arch. Dis. Child.**, 44, 291-303.

Marshall, W.A. and Tanner, J.M. (1970) Variation in the pattern of pubertal changes in boys. **Arch. Dis. Child.**, 45, 13-23.

Milman, D.H. and Bakwin, H. (1950) Ossification of metacarpal metatarsal centres as a measure of maturation. **J. Pediatr.**, 36, 617-620.

Neinstein, L.S. (1982) Adolescent self-assessment of sexual maturation. **Clin. Pediatr.**, 21, 482-484.

Nicholson, A.B. and Hanley, C. (1953) Indices of physiological maturity: derivation and interrelationships. **Child Dev.**, 24, 3-38.

Parizkova, J. (1977) **Body Fat and Physical Fitness**, Martinus Nijhoff, The Hague.

Petrovcic, F. Medved, R. and Horvat, V. (1957) Fixation de l'age physiologique des jeunes à l'aide de la radiographie du squelette, in **Congrès d'Etude de la Fig. Partisan de Yugoslavie** (ed. M. Mihovilovic), Fédération pour l'Education Physique, Zagreb, pp. 181-187.

Pryor, J.W. (1905) Development of the bone of the hand as shown by x-ray method. **Bulletin State College** (Kentucky), Series 2(5).

Quaade, F. (1955) **Obese Children**, Danish Science Press, Copenhagen.

Rajic, M.K. Brisson G.R. Shephard, R.J. Lavallée, H. Jéquier, J.C. Massé, R. Jéquier, S. Lussier, T. and Labarre, R. (1979) Maturité osseuse et performance physique. **Can. J. Appl. Sport Sci.**, 4, 223-225.

Rarick, G.L. and Oyster, N. (1964) Physical maturity, muscular strength, and motor performance of young school-age boys. **Res. Quart.**, 35, 523-531.

Reynolds, E.L. (1946) Sexual maturation and the growth of fat, muscle and bone in girls. **Child Dev.**, 17, 121-149.

Reynolds, E.L. and Asakawa, H. (1951) Skeletal development in infancy: standards for clinical use. **Am. J. Roentgenol.**, 65, 403-409.

Reynolds, E.L. and Wines, J.V. (1948) Individual differences in physical changes associated with adolescence in girls. **Am. J. Dis. Child.**, 75, 329-350.

Reynolds, E.L. and Wines, J.V. (1951) Physical changes associated with adolescence in boys. **Am. J. Dis. Child.**, 82, 529-547.

Richey, H.G. (1937) The relation of accelerated, normal and retarded puberty to the height and weight of school children. **Mon. Soc. Res. Child Dev.**, 2 (Serial N° 8).

Roche, A.F. (1978) Bone growth and maturation, in **Human Growth: 2. Postnatal Growth** (eds F. Falkner and J.M. Tanner), Plenum, New York, pp. 317-355.

Roche, A.F. (1980) The measurement of skeletal maturation, in **Human Physical Growth and Maturation. Methodologies and Factors** (eds F.E. Johnston, A.F. Roche and C. Suzanne), Plenum, New York, pp. 61-82.

Roche, A.F. Chumlea, W.C. and Thissen, D. (1988) **Assessing the skeletal maturity of the hand-wrist: Fels method**, Thomas, Springfield.

Roche, A.F. Wainer, H. and Thissen, D. (1975a) Predicting adult stature for individuals. **Monographs in Pediatrics**, 3, 1-114.

Roche, A.F. Wainer, H. and Thissen, D. (1975b) **Skeletal Maturity : Knee Joint as a Biological Indicator,** Plenum, New York.

Rotch, T.M. (1909) A study of the development of the bones in children by roentgen method, with the view of establishing a developmental index for the grading of and the protection of early life. **Trans. Am. Assoc. Physic.**, 24, 603-630.

Savov, S.G. (1978) Physical fitness and skeletal maturity in girls and boys 11 years of age, in **Physical Fitness assessment: Practice and Application** (eds R.J. Shephard and H. Lavallée), Thomas, Springfield, pp. 222-228.

Sawtell, R.O. (1929) Ossification and growth of children one to eight years of age. **Am. J. Dis. Child.**, 37, 61-87.

Seils, L.R.G. (1951) The relationship between measurements of physical growth and gross motor performance of primary-grade school children. **Res. Quart.**, 22, 244-260.

Seltzer, C.C. and Mayer, J. (1964) Body build and obesity. Who are the obese ?. **J. Am. Med. Assoc.**, 190, 103-110.

Shephard, R.J. Lavallée, H. Rajic, K.M. Jéquier, J.C. Brisson, G. and Beaucage, C. (1978) Radiographic age in the interpretation of physiological and anthropological data, in **Pediatric Work Physiology** (Medicine and Sport Vol. 11) (eds J. Borms and M. Hebbelinck), Karger, Basel, pp. 124-133.

Shuttleworth, F.K. (1937) Sexual maturation and the physical growth of girls age six to nineteen. **Mon. Soc. Res. Child Dev.**, 2 (Serial N° 5).

Stager, J.M. Robertshaw, D. and Miescher, E. (1984) Delayed menarche in swimming in relation to onset of training and athletic performance. **Med. Sci. Sport. Exer.**, 16, 550-555.

Stager, J.M. Wigglesworth, J.K. and Hatler, L.K. (1990) Interpreting the relationship between age of menarche and prepubertal training. **Med. Sci. Sport. Exer.**, 22, 54-58.

Tanner, J.M. (1962) **Growth at Adolescence**, Blackwell Scientific Publications, Oxford.

Tanner, J.M. and Whitehouse, R.H. (1959) **Standards for Skeletal Maturity: Part 1.**, International Children's Centre, Paris.

Tanner, J.M. Whitehouse, R.H. and Healy, M.J.R. (1962) **A new System for Estimating Skeletal Maturity from the Hand and Wrist, with Standards derived from a Study of 2600 Healthy British Children: Part 2: The Scoring System**, International Children's Centre, Paris.

Tanner, J.M. Whitehouse, R.H. Cameron, N. Marshall, W.A. Healy, M.J.R. and Goldstein, H. (1983) **Assessment of Skeletal Maturity and Prediction of Adult Height (TW2 Method)**, Academic Press, London.

Tanner, J.M. Whitehouse, R.H. Marshall, W.A. Healy, M.J.R. and Goldstein, H. (1975) **Assessment of Skeletal Maturity and Prediction of Adult Height (TW2 Method)**, Academic Press, London.

Todd, J.W. (1937) **Atlas of Skeletal Maturation: Part 1. Hand**, Mosby, London.

Wolff, O.H. (1955) Obesity in children: a study of the birth weight, the height, and the onset of puberty. **Q. J. Med.**, 24, 109-123.

21

A COMPARISON OF OXYGEN UPTAKE DURING RUNNING IN CHILDREN AND ADULTS

R.G. ESTON, S. ROBSON and E. WINTER
Dept. of Movement Science and Physical Education, University of
Liverpool, England

Keywords: Oxygen uptake, VO_2max, Running, Children, Adults.

1 Introduction

A number of studies have compared the oxygen demands of running in children and adults (Astrand 1952; Rowland et al. 1987; Rowland and Green 1988; Unnithan and Eston 1990). These studies observed a higher oxygen uptake in children, expressed relative to body mass, at any given running speed. It has also been observed that the fractional utilisation of maximal oxygen uptake ($\%VO_2$max) is also greater at any given speed (see Figs. 1 and 2). These differences have been attributed to a variety of biomechanical, ventilatory and cellular factors.

Practical and statistical use of the ratio oxygen uptake : body mass (O_2:kg) for correlational analyses has been subject to some criticism (Katch 1973; Katch and Katch 1974). Furthermore, intergroup comparisons of the energy cost of subjects who differ greatly in body mass and stature, has also been criticised (Tanner 1949). Traditional methods of analysis (analysis of variance) indicate that subjects with a higher mass : height ratio (e.g. adults) have a lower oxygen uptake when this is expressed relative to body weight ($ml\,kg^{-1}.min^{-1}$). Conversely subjects with a lower mass : height ratio tend to have a higher relative oxygen uptake.

Thus, as the ratio of body mass : stature decreases, the ratio of oxygen consumption : body mass is seen to increase. This phenomenon was observed in a recent study (Unnithan and Eston 1990) which compared a group of aerobically fit boys (aged 9-10 years) to a similar group of young men (aged 18-25 years). The ratio of mass : height expressed in the form of Quetelets Index (mass (kg) : height $(m)^2$), was significantly higher ($p<0.01$) in the men (23.2 ± 2.4 cf 16.4 ± 1.5). As expected, the oxygen uptake in the men's group was lower ($p<0.01$), at all submaximal speeds although there was no difference in maximal oxygen uptake values. These inter group comparisons were determined by analysis of variance.

It has been suggested (Tanner 1949) that when large differences in stature and body mass exist, an alternative analytical procedure (analysis

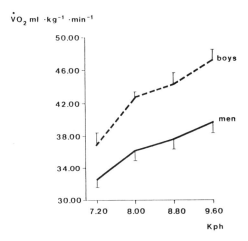

Fig. 1. Submaximal running economy in men and boys.

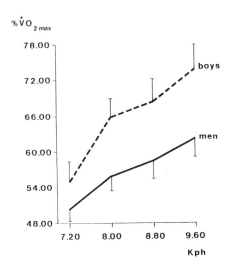

Fig. 2. Percent maximal oxygen uptake at submaximal running speeds in men and boys.

of covariance), should be used to compare the regression lines of oxygen uptake : mass between groups. This principle has been illustrated recently (Winter et al. 1990). Analysis of covariance is primarily used as a procedure for the statistical control of an uncontrolled variable, such as body mass. If, for example, differences between treatment effects disappear or are negligible when the effects of the uncontrolled variable are removed, this may mean that differences in the dependent variable (oxygen in take) are a consequence of the uncontrolled variable (body mass) (Ferguson 1981).

The purpose of this study was to apply the analysis of covariance technique to compare the regression lines of mass: oxygen uptake at each submaximal running speed (7.2, 8.0, 8.8 and 9.6 kph) in men and boys, on data that were originally presented by Unnithan and Eston (1990).

2 Methods

Ten healthy prepubertal boys, who were regular members of the school cross-country team (mean age 10.4 ± 0.5 yrs) and 10 healthy and trained male university students (mean age 20.8 ± 1.2 yrs) volunteered for this study. Informed consent was obtained from the children, their parents, and the adults. The mean height and mass for the boys was 138.4 ± 7.9 cm and 31.3 ± 3.7 kg; for the men it was 178.5 ± 8.8 cm and 73.9 ± 11.2 kg.

The treadmill protocol of Rowland et al. (1987) was replicated in this study. All subjects performed a continuous submaximal treadmill running protocol. Following an initial period of getting used to the treadmill, the subjects had a 3 minute warm-up at 4.8 km.h^{-1} and 0% grade, followed by an increase to 7.2 km.h^{-1} for a period of 3 minutes. Subsequent increments of 0.8 km.h^{-1} were implemented every 3 minutes up to a speed of 9.6 km.h^{-1}.

Open circuit spirometry was used to measure oxygen consumption, as recommended by the British Association of Sports Sciences (1989). A Mijnhardt Oxycon was used to measure oxygen and carbon dioxide fractions. The analyzer was calibrated with 0% CO_2, 14.6% and 4.9% CO_2. Expired gas was collected by the Douglas Bag technique in the final minute of each submaximal running phase.

3 Results

Individual within-group relationships and inter group comparisons at each speed are shown in Table 1. As expected, there were positive correlations ranging from 0.74 to 0.95 for body mass: oxygen consumption for both groups at all speeds. Thus, heavier individuals in both groups

Table 1. Relationships (r) of mass : oxygen uptake, standard error of estimate (See), Coefficient of variation (V%) in both groups and intergroup comparisons by analysis of covariance.

Treadmill speed (kph) :	7.2			8.0			8.8			9.6		
	r	See	V%	r	See	V%	r	See	V%	r	See	V%
Boys	0.80	0.15	5.0	0.95	0.06	6.7	0.88	0.12	5.6	0.87	0.12	6.2
Men	0.82	0.23	6.3	0.74	0.25	7.2	0.78	0.31	5.7	0.74	0.31	6.5
Comparison of Slope (1,16df)	F =	1.56		F =	2.39			1.43			1.36	
Comparison of Elevation (1,17df)	F =	0.02		F =	0.58			0.17			0.03	

$F_{cv\,0.05}$ (1,16df) = 4.49 (All intergroup differences are non-significant)

were characterised by a higher oxygen uptake at all speeds. Analysis of covariance revealed no difference in the gradient of the regression lines of mass : oxygen uptake at each speed and no difference in the elevation of the regression lines between groups. These results are exemplified in Fig. 3 which compares the typical response of the two groups at 8 kph.

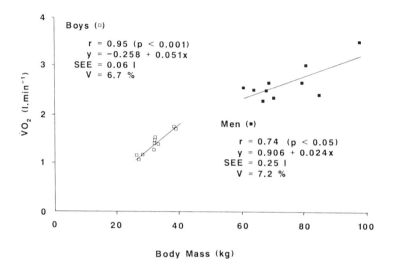

Fig. 3. VO$_2$ versus Body Mass at 8 kph.

4 Discussion

The results of analysis of covariance indicated that there was no real difference in the dynamics of oxygen uptake for men and boys in this study. It is questionable whether the hyperaerobic response in children is real, or whether it is really attributable to the confounding and uncontrollable factor of body size and the latter's relationships to the body mass: oxygen uptake ratio. The traditional method of analysis by analysis of variance does not take this into account. The analysis of covariance technique controlled for body mass. It indicates that any apparent difference in oxygen uptake between groups may be attributable to innappropriate analysis rather than inherent physiological differences. It would be interesting to apply the same procedures to compare groups of very small and very large individuals (e.g. pygmies v American footballers). This may have implications for studies which have used ratio standards.

5 References

Astrand, P.O. (1952) Experimental Studies of Physical Working Capacity in Relation to Sex and Age, Ejnar Munksgaard, Copenhagen.

British Association of Sports Sciences. (1989) **Position Statement on the Physiological Assessment of the Elite Competitor**. White Line Press, Leeds.

Ferguson, G.A. (1981) **Statistical Analysis in Psychology and Education**. McGraw-Hill, New York.

Katch, V.L. (1973) Use of the oxygen/body weight ratio in correlational analyses : spurious correlations and statistical considerations. **Med. Sci. Sports**, 5, 253-257.

Katch, V.L. and Katch, F. (1974) Use of weight-adjusted oxygen uptake scores that avoid spurious correlations. **Res. Quart.**, 45, 447-451.

Rowland, T.W. and Green, G.M. (1988) Physiological responses to treadmill exercise in females: adult-child differences. **Med. Sci. Sports. Exer.,** 20, 474-488.

Rowland, T.W. Auchinachie, J.A. Keenan, T.J. and Green, G.M. (1987) Physiologic responses to treadmill running in adult and pre-pubertal males. **Int. J. Sport. Med.,** 8, 292-297.

Tanner, J.M. (1949) Fallacy of per-weight and per-surface area standards and their relation to spurious correlation. **J. Appl. Physiol.,** 2, 1-15.

Unnithan, V. and Eston, R.G. (1990) Stride frequency and submaximal treadmill running economy in adults and children. **Pediatr. Exer. Sci.,** 2, 149-155.

Winter E.M., Brookes, F.B.C. and Hamley, E.J. (1990) Maximal exercise performance and lean leg volume in men and women. **J. Sport. Sci.,** 9 : 1, 3-13.

22

PHYSICAL PERFORMANCE DECLINE OR IMPROVEMENT OF GIRLS AT THE TIME OF PHV AND LATER MAXIMAL PERFORMANCE

J. BORMS, W. DUQUET, M. HEBBELINCK, J.A.P. DAY* and
A. HENDERIX
Vrije Universiteit Brussel, HILOK, Brussel, Belgium
*University of Lethbridge, Canada

Keywords: PHV, Decliners, Improvers, Physical performance,
Anthropometry

1 Introduction

The period of the adolescent growth spurt is remarkable in many respects. As early as 1922 (Homburger, in Beunen and Malina 1988) it was described as a period of a temporary disruption between physical growth and motor coordination. Terms such as 'adolescent awkwardness', clumsiness, or 'outgrowing his strength' are often used to describe this period. Much of the data dealing with this topic are derived, however, from cross-sectional studies or from longitudinal data analyzed cross-sectionally. Beunen and Malina (1988) compared two groups of boys from a longitudinal sample, who showed respectively negative and positive velocities for six motor performance tasks during the interval of peak height velocity (PHV). They were compared on several anthropometric dimensions at the beginning of the PHV interval and at young adulthood. They found that the groups did not differ significantly in strength and motor performance around the age of 18. They also found that there were no consistent trends in anthropometric dimensions, both at the beginning of the PHV interval and in young adulthood, in boys who showed negative velocities in the performance of motor tasks at the time of PHV. They concluded that the concept of adolescent awkwardness is a very complex one.

Corresponding longitudinal data on girls during the adolescent spurt are generally lacking. The purpose of this study therefore was to find out if there were girls in the Belgian LEGS study who demonstrated negative velocities in motor performance tests during their growth spurt and, if so, to find out if these girls would show different growth and performance patterns from girls who demonstrated positive velocities during their growth spurts.

2 Methods

The data were taken from a longitudinal study of the growth, maturity and physical performance capacity of a sample of over 500 boys and girls, 5 to 18 years of age, from the Longitudinal Experimental Growth Study (LEGS) carried out by the Vrije Universiteit Brussel. Data on these Belgian school children were collected from 1970 to 1986. A detailed description of the sampling and measurement procedures of LEGS is given in Hebbelinck et al. (1980).

Subjects were measured at least once each year, and twice during the years of the adolescent growth spurt. Many subjects were measured on more than 15 different occasions. A high degree of intra-observer reliability was guaranteed by the many years of measuring experience of the kinanthropometrists, prior to the start of the LEGS project. The leadership and the measurement staff of the undertaking were constant throughout the study. The latter observation implies that the investigation of the inter-observer reliability becomes superfluous. It is generally known from the literature on comparable variables, that possible learning effects are strongest in the first years of a longitudinal study and tend to level off later. The period of the PHV interval coincides more or less with the sixth measurement period. Therefore, should some results be influenced by learning effects, these influences will occur less frequently.

Secondly, as far as the anthropometric variables are concerned, we have chosen the age of 17 years as the second point of comparison, meaning that all subjects were in the project an equally long time. Therefore, if there is a learning effect, we expect it to be similar for all subjects.

The anthropometric dimensions used in this study include weight, height, sitting height, leg length, tibia length, bicondylar humerus breadth, bicondylar femur breadth, upper arm girth and calf girth.

In the battery of six physical performance capacity tests, the following factors were measured: static strength (hand grip strength with dynamometer), explosive strength (standing long jump and medicine ball push), local muscular endurance (30 sec sit up), coordination (hockey ball throw) and speed (25m sprint). Skeletal maturity was estimated using the TW2 scoring system (Tanner et al. 1975).

Curve fitting procedures, using the Preece-Baines model 1 function (Preece and Baines 1978) were used to fit each subject's serial measurements of body height in order to characterize the individual growth patterns. PHV and age at PHV were used as experimental variables.

Furthermore, skeletal age at PHV, height at PHV, velocity at PHV and age at PHV minus age at take-off were calculated. The fitting could only be performed in subjects with sufficient measuring points. The time of PHV could be identified for 130 girls in the total LEGS sample. Some results of the application of the Preece-Baines model to these data have been published elsewhere (Hebbelinck et al. 1991).

Growth curves of each motor performance test were drawn for each subject. An interval consisting of a period of six months before and six months after the age at PHV, was plotted over each individual curve. Girls who showed a decrease, even the smallest, in performance during that interval were designated as 'decliners'. The others were designated as 'improvers'.

Descriptive statistics, including a normality check, were calculated for each anthropometric variable at the beginning of the interval of PHV and at age 17 years. For the motor performance variables, only the maximum performance after PHV, was taken into consideration. Differences between the means of decliners and improvers were tested for statistical significance (t-test and Mann-Whitney U-test). AN OVA tests were performed, partialing out weight, height, and weight and height.

3 Results and discussion

The number and percentage of girls showing a decrease in six motor performance tests during the interval of PHV, are given in Table 1. Only 26 (21.7%) and 35 (28.0%) girls respectively showed a decrease in the medicine ball push and hand grip strength during the interval of PHV, while 60 (50.8%) showed a decrease in hockey ball throw. More than 48% showed decreases in three other tests (sit up, standing long jump, 25m sprint). The three latter tests require the subject to move her own body with vigor and speed. The two former tests challenge her ability to apply force or power to an object external to her own body. This also applies for the hockeyball throw, but to a lesser extent, since success in the hockey ball throw depends on a complex of attributes other than force or power. Normally, it is hypothesized that the performance curves of medicine ball push and hand grip strength show a smooth evolution with a small chance to show negative velocities. This is confirmed by the low number of decliners for these items.

The growth, maturity and motor performance characteristics of the decliners and improvers were contrasted for each of the six motor performance tests. For the anthropometric variables, the comparisons were done at the beginning of the interval of PHV (Table 2) and at the age of 17 (Table 3). For the motor performance tests, the comparisons were done relative to the maximal performance after PHV (Table 3).

From Table 2, it appears that of a total of 54 comparisons of group means, only four are significantly (p<.05) different from each other. Girls who declined in medicine ball push were heavier, with a larger mean humerus breadth, and a larger mean calf girth. Girls who declined in the 25 m sprint had a larger mean humerus breadth.

244

Table 1. Number and percentage of girls showing a negative velocity in six motor performance tests during the interval of PHV

Test	Total number observed	Girls with negative velocities	
		Number	Percent.
Sit up 30 sec	123	77	62.6
Medicineball push	120	26	21.7
Standing long jump	126	61	48.4
Handgrip strength	125	35	28.0
25 m sprint	118	61	51.7
Hockeyball throw	118	60	50.8

Table 2. Mean somatic and maturity characteristics at the beginning of the interval of PHV in girls who declined or improved in specific motor performance tests during the interval of PHV*

Somatic variable	Medicine ball push		25 m sprint	
	Decl.	Impr.	Decl.	Impr.
Weight (kg)	38.9	35.6		
Humerus width (cm)	5.7	5.5	5.6	5.4
Calf girth (cm)	30.5	28.9		

* Means are reported only when a significant difference between decliners and improvers was observed (t- and Mann-Whitney U-tests, $\alpha = .05$).

Decliners and improvers in performance during the interval of PHV did not differ significantly in anthropometric dimensions and maximum motor performance, with some 5 exceptions out of the 90 comparisons (Table 3). These exceptions are : a greater mean tibia length for improvers in the 30 sec sit up, a greater weight and a smaller number of sit ups for the decliners in medicine ball push, a better maximum performance in medicine ball push and hand grip strength for the improvers in hand grip strength. Taking into account the number of comparisons performed (54 + 90) and the probability level selected(p <.05), the few observed significant differences may be attributable to chance.

Although Tables 2 and 3 also suggest the comparison of maturity characteristics of decliners and improvers, these are not shown since they were only reported when a significant difference between the two groups was observed.

The phenomenon of decline or improvement in one performance item did not necessarily occur for the other items in the same girl. The percentage of those who declined varied from 8.5 to 57.7%. The latter high percentage occurred for the 30 sec sit up, a test that requires a vertical lifting of the body with vigor. Girls who declined in performance during the interval of PHV generally attained the same levels of maximal motor performance (after PHV) as girls who were in the 'improver' group. The decline in performance during the interval of PHV was temporary and apparently did not influence maximum performance (after PHV), which is usually but not necessarily around the age of young adulthood. Of course the question still remains why some girls decline and others improve. Do they differ in skeletal age so that the decreases in performance can be ascribed to an individual maturity variation? Or are there differences in the timing of PHV? Or are there differences in the intensity of the growth spurt?

In an attempt to answer these questions, skeletal ages of the two groups, at the beginning of the PHV interval were compared, as well as the following variables at the age of PHV: skeletal age, chronological age, height and height spurt velocity. In addition, the difference between age at PHV and age at growth spurt take-off was compared between the improvers and the decliners (Table 4). Only two comparisons, out of 36, produced significant differences (velocity at PHV and time between age at PHV minus age at take-off, both for medicine ball push).

Perhaps not one, but a number of factors are responsible for the phenomenon of declining and improving. For one, the operationalization and definition of the 'decliners' and 'improvers' could be a reason for not finding many differences. Indeed even the smallest decline in performance during the interval of PHV was classified as a decline.

There is also the general observation that the motor performance of girls reaches a plateau during adolescence, and/or a decline, as was observed but not reported in this study. This decline is not necessarily due to internal factors alone but also to external ones. In other words the decline may be multifactorial. In order to avoid confounding factors, we decided to use as reference mark the maximal performance after PHV, whatever the time of occurence was.

Table 3. Mean somatic characteristics at 17 yrs of age and maximal motor performance (after age at PHV) in girls who declined or improved in performance during the interval of PHV*

Measure	30 sec sit up		Medicine ball		Handgrip	
	Decl.	Impr.	Decl.	Impr.	Decl.	Impr.
Weight (kg)			61.0	55.3		
Tibia length (cm)	36.5	37.4				
Sit up (number)			19.2	21.4		
Medicine ball push (m)					6.39	6.96
Hand grip (kg)					35.0	38.9

* Means are reported only when a significant difference between decliners and improvers was observed (t- and Mann-Whitney U-tests, α = .05).

Table 4. Mean growth and maturity characteristics at PHV in girls who declined or improved in performance of specific motor tests during the interval of PHV*

Growth and maturity variables	Medicine ball push	
	Decliners	Improvers
Velocity at PHV (cm/yrs)	7.31	7.96
Age at PHV minus age at T. O. (cm/yrs)	2.70	3.01

* Means are reported only when a significant difference between decliners and improvers was observed (t- and Mann-Whitney U-test, α = .05).

Our results seem to be comparable with those on boys obtained by Beunen and Malina (1988). The final conclusion is that girls who demonstrate a decline in motor performance at the age of PHV, seem to catch it up when they grow older.

4 Acknowledgement

This investigation was supported in part by the Nationaal Fonds voor Wetenschappelijk Onderzoek (NFWO) of Belgium, by the Fonds voor Kollektief Fundamenteel Onderzoek (FKFO), contract number 935, as well as by the Research Council (OZR) of the Vrije Universiteit Brussel.

5 References

Beunen, G. and Malina R. M. (1988) Growth and Physical Performance relative to the timing of the adolescent spurt. **Exer. Sport Sci. Rev.**, 16, 503-539.

Hebbelinck, M. Blommaert, M. Borms, J. Duquet, W. Vajda, A. and Vandermeer J. (1980) A multidisciplinary longitudinal growth study - Introduction of the project 'Legs', in **Kinanthropometry II**. (eds M. Ostyn, G. Beunen and J. Simons), University Park Press, Baltimore, pp. 317-325.

Hebbelinck, M. Duquet W. Day J. Borms, J. and Hauspie, R. (1990). Application of the Preece-Baines longitudinal growth fitting procedure to other anthropometric measures than standing height, in **Children and Exercise, Pediatric Work Physiology XV** (eds R. Frankl and I. Szmodis), National Institute for Health Promotion (NEVI), Budapest, Hungary, 1991, pp. 303-308.

Homburger, A. (1922) Ueber die Entwicklung der menschlichen Motorik und ihrer Beziehung zu den Bewegungsstörungen der Schizophrenen, Z. Neurol. Psychiatr., 78 : 561-570, cit. in Beunen, G. and Malina R.M., Growth and Physical Performance relative to the timing of the adolescent spurt, **Exer. Sport Sci. Rev.**, 16, 1988, pp. 503-539.

Preece, M. A. and Baines, M. J. (1978) A new family of mathematical models describing the human growth curve, **Ann. Hum. Biol.**, 5 : 1-24.

Tanner, J.M. Whitehouse, R.H. Marshall, W.A. Healy, M.J.R. and Goldstein, H. (1975) **Assessment of skeletal maturity and prediction of adult height (TW2 method)** Academic Press, London.

23

TRACKING AT THE EXTREMES IN HEALTH-AND PERFORMANCE RELATED FITNESS FROM ADOLESCENCE THROUGH ADULTHOOD

J. LEFEVRE, G. BEUNEN, A. CLAESSENS , R. LYSENS, H. MAES, R. RENSON, J. SIMONS, B. VANDEN EYNDE and B. VANREUSEL
Institute of Physical Education, K.U.Leuven, Belgium

Keywords: Tracking, Stability, Health-related fitness, Performance-related fitness.

1 Introduction

The concept of tracking concerns the maintenance of relative rankings within the distribution among a group of peers over time (Foulkes and Davis 1981) and quantifies the degree of stability exhibited by each individual's set of measurements (Goldstein 1981). To analyze the consistency in a measurement or performance task over time, longitudinal data are required. Correlations, or more specifically, interage correlations between measurements made at one stage of growth with outcomes later in growth or in adulthood are used most often in tracking research. Bloom (1964) suggested a correlation of +0.50 as a criterion for a minimum level of consistency over at least a one year interval.

From the literature, it can be concluded that the stability of fitness during adolescence is generally moderate to low (Malina 1990). Until now, little is known about the stability of fitness from late adolescence into adulthood, at the extremes of distributions.

This paper thus considers the tracking or stability of fitness components in a longitudinal sample of boys and men, 12 to 30 years of age. Data for weight, health-related fitness (fatness, flexibility, trunk strength, functional strength) and performance-related fitness (speed of limb movement, explosive strength, static strength, running speed) are evaluated.

2 Materials and methods

The data are part of the follow-up study of Flemish boys who were followed from 12 through 18 years and subsequently remeasured at 30 years of age. The first part of the study, the "Leuven Growth Study of Belgian Boys" consisted of a mixed longitudinal study of the growth and the physical fitness of a nationally representative sample of Belgian schoolboys (Ostyn et al. 1980). In this study 588 boys were followed longitudinally at yearly intervals over 6 years (between 1969 and 1974) from ±12.5 to ± 18.5 years. A number of subjects in the original study were followed in adulthood (in 1986) at the age of ±30 years. Only Dutch speaking subjects were selected and 278 volunteered. For this paper, complete data are available for about 145 subjects.

The data in the annual observations included, among others, body weight and four skinfolds: triceps skinfold, subscapular skinfold, supra-iliac skinfold, and medial calf skinfold, and several motor tests, each representing an independent motor factor: sit and reach (flexibility), leg lifts (trunk strength), bent arm hang (functional strength), plate tapping (speed of limb movement), vertical jump (explosive strength), arm pull (static strength), shuttle run 50m (running speed). For a description of the measurements and tests, reference is made to Ostyn et al. (1980). Tracking was studied in two ways. First, interage correlations were calculated between status during late adolescence and status at 30 years. In addition, a longitudinal principal component analysis was carried out for each variable on the six successive measures during adolescence. The first component can be interpreted as a 'magnitude' or 'average percentile level' component, or as an 'indication of relative size' (Lefevre et al. 1989). This means that the first component characterizes the general position of an individual distance curve relative to the average distance curve during the period analyzed. Boys with high positive scores on component 1 have a pattern of high distance values (high percentile levels) across adolescence, while boys with high negative scores have a pattern of low distance values (low percentile levels). Boys with an average score (± 0) have performance values (for the different motor tests) which approximate the average performance of the group at each age (average percentile levels). Correlations were calculated between the individual scores on the first component and status at 30 years of age.

In a second analysis, tracking at the extremes was considered. For each variable or test, those boys who were at or below the 10th percentile and those boys who were at or above the 90th percentile at the age of 18 were included and the tendency to remain (expressed by percentages) in the first or last decile at the age of 30 was considered.

3 Results

The most important results of the first analysis are given in Table 1. Between the age of 18 and 30, young men have, on average, gained 8.2 kg in body weight and have increased in all skinfold measurements. Mean performances for most motor characteristics at 30 years of age are better than those at 18 years of age. Only for flexibility (sit and reach) and for running speed (shuttle run 50m) did the mean performance decrease during the third decade of live.

Table 1. Statistics (means and standard deviations) at the age of 18 and at the age of 30, percent of variation explained by the first component (%EV); coefficients of correlation between status at the age of 18 with status at the age of 30; coefficient of correlation between individual component scores with status at the age of 30.

	X ± SD (18 ys)	X ± SD (30 ys)	% EV	r (18 - 30)	r (C1 - 30)
Weight (kg)	66.10 6.97	74.30 8.40	86.7	0.74	0.59
Triceps sk. (mm)	7.23 3.41	10.36 3.87	74.7	0.50	0.60
Subsc. sk. (mm)	9.17 2.27	12.94 4.55	83.6	0.57	0.53
Supra-il. sk. (mm)	7.91 3.66	13.34 7.57	83.1	0.53	0.52
Calf sk. (mm)	4.71 1.44	5.76 2.10	68.2	0.37	0.55
Sit and reach (cm)	26.70 7.47	24.70 8.09	85.1	0.83	0.81
Leg lifts (N)	17.54 2.04	18.04 1.92	60.1	0.53	0.62
Bent arm hang (sec)	32.70 17.90	34.44 15.94	72.7	0.55	0.55
Plate tapping (N)	97.14 9.45	100.0 8.42	75.5	0.54	0.60
Vertical jump (cm)	49.60 7.15	51.20 6.70	74.4	0.69	0.66
Arm pull (kg)	76.00 12.70	85.50 14.40	79.2	0.66	0.51
Shuttle run (sec)	20.50 1.25	20.82 1.34	63.0	0.52	0.58

The first longitudinal principal component explains between 60.1% (leg lifts) and 86.7% (weight) of the variance.

Correlations for variable at the age of 18 with status at 30 years vary between 0.37 (calf skinfold) and 0.83 (sit and reach). Correlations between the individual scores on the first longitudinal principal component and status at the age of 30 are of the same magnitude.

The percentages of the boys who were at or below the 10th and who were at or above the 90th percentiles at the age of 18 as well as at the age of 30 are given in Table 2. For weight, about 50% of the boys remained at the extreme deciles. For the skinfolds about 30% of those who were initially low/high remained low/high at the age of 30. For the motor characteristics, the percentages vary between 29% (shuttle run <P10) and 74% (sit and reach >P90).

4 Discussion

Fatness is a component of health-related fitness. Several studies (Parizkova 1977; Roche et al. 1982; Beunen et al. 1986; Kaplowitz et al. 1988) indicate that during adolescence the stability of fatness is moderate to high. A similar trend is observed in this study. The amount of variance explained by the first component indicates to what extent the

Table 2. Percentage of males who remain in the same extreme decile ($\leq$ 10th and $\geq$ 90th) at 18 and 30 years of age.

	$\leq$ P10	$\geq$ P90
Weight	47%	50%
Triceps skinfold	30%	31%
Subsc skinfold	29%	29%
Supra-iliac. skinfold	29%	25%
Calf skinfold	29%	27%
Sit and reach	50%	74%
Leg lifts	48%	63%
Bent arm hang	29%	35%
Plate tapping	33%	33%
Vertical jump	56%	28%
Arm pull	35%	50%
Shuttle run	29%	59%

variable is stable over time. If the first component explains a great amount of the observed variance, subjects tend to remain at approximately the same channel. In other words, if the first component explains a great amount of the observed variance, one can conclude that there is not much intraindividual variability in percentile position during adolescence. Results of this analysis (table 1) indicate a reasonably stable course for subcutaneous fat during adolescence since the first component explains between 68.2% of the total observed variance for the calf skinfold and 83.6% for the subscapular skinfold. While subcutaneous fat declines gradually during adolescence (Lefevre et al. 1990), there is a considerable increase in subcutaneous adiposity during the third decade of life. Furthermore, all correlations, except that between the score for calf skinfold at 18 and 30 years of age reach .50, Bloom's (1964) suggested criterion for a stable trait. However, only 25 to 31% of the men in the 90th or 'fattest decile' at 18 years of age remain at the 90th decile at the age of 30. This means that at the extremes there is only a moderate stability in subcutaneous fatness between late adolescence and adulthood. Since a lot of subjects shift away from the 'fattest decile', due to internal and/or external factors, this suggests that the third decade of life may be a sensitive time to control the development of (increase or decrease) adiposity (diet, active life style, ...).

Flexibility of the lower back, trunk strength and functional strength are also indicated as components of health-related fitness. The percentages of explained variance of the first component suggest that these health-related characteristics track well across adolescence. Between late adolescence and 30 years of age, trunk strength and functional strength, on average, increase, while flexibility decreases. Flexibility however is a very stable trait since the interage correlations are higher than .80. Also 50% of men in the lowest decile ($\leq$ 10th percentile) and 74% of men in the highest decile ($\geq$ 90th percentile) remain at these extreme levels 12 years later. Between-age correlations are moderately high for leg lifts and the bent arm hang. However, more than 50% of the men who were at or below P10 at 18 years shifted away from this extreme profile. These results indicate that for an accurate individual prediction of adult performance, other factors than the performance at late adolescence are needed.

Speed of limb movement, explosive strength, static strength and running speed are components of performance-related fitness. Percentages of explained variance of the first component suggest that these characteristics also track well across adolescence. At 30 years of age, mean performances are, on average, better (especially in static strength) than at 18 years of age for all motor items with the exception of shuttle run (running speed) where an average decrease of 0.32 sec is noted. All between-age correlations are higher than .50 and vary from .51 to .69. The correlations are of the same magnitude as those reported by Rarick and Smoll (1967). By studying the stability of motor performance in boys during adolescence (12-17 years of age), Rarick and Smoll noted correlations of, respectively, .73 and .52 for the standing long jump (explosive strength) and for the 30-yard dash (running speed). In the present analysis (table 2), a reasonable percentage of the boys shifted away from the extreme percentile positions, both in negative and positive directions.

In conclusion, interage correlations between status at late adolescence (18 years) and at adulthood (30 years) suggest that the stability of indicators of health- and performance-related fitness is generally moderate. Correlation, however, is a group statistic and some individuals may be more or less stable than indicated by the magnitude of the correlation. This is clearly illustrated by the percentages in table 2. Many boys (more than 50%) who were at the extremes at 18 years shifted away from the extremes during the third decade of their life. It would seem logical, therefore, to now consider the life styles of those who shifted in extreme positions. To what extent are health-related fitness and performance-related fitness influenced during the third decade of life by factors such as daily physical activity, diet, sport participation, leisure time activities, and so on? Note, however, that growth continues into the mid-20 s in some characteristics. Also internal genetic factors can explain the decile shifting of some subjects. For example, late maturers can show a relatively large increase in some variables as compared with a relatively low increase or no increase for early maturers.

5 Acknowledgments

The authors are grateful to Prof. Dr. R.M. Malina for the editorial assistance in the preparation of the manuscript.
The "Leuven Growth Study of Belgian Boys" received support grants from the Ministries of Dutch and French Culture, the Administration of Physical Education, Sport and Open Air activities, the Ministry of Public Health and the Family, and the National Medical Research Fund.

6 References

Beunen, G. Claessens, A. Ostyn, M. Renson, R. Simons, J. Lefevre, J. and Van Gerven, D. (1986) **Stability of subcutaneous fat patterning in adolescent boys**. Paper presented at the 5th Congress of the European Anthropological Association, Lisbon, October.
Bloom, B.S. (1964) **Stability and change in human characteristics**. Wiley, New York.

Foulkes, M.A. and Davis, C.E. (1981) An index of tracking for longitudinal data. **Biometrics, 37**, 439-446.

Goldstein, H. (1981) Measuring the stability of individual growth patterns. **Ann. Hum. Biol.,** 8, 549-557.

Kaplowitz, H.J. Wild, K.A. Mueller, W.H. Decker, M. and Tanner, J.M. (1988) Serial and parent-child changes in components of body fat distribution and fatness in children from the London Longitudinal Growth Study, ages two to eighteen years. **Hum. Biol.,** 60, 739-758.

Lefevre, J. Beunen, G. Claessens, A. Lysens, R. Maes, H. Renson, R. Simons, J. Steens, G. Vanden Eynde, B. and Vanreusel, B. (1990) Stability in level of subcutaneous fat between adolescence and adulthood, in **Children and Exercise XIV** (eds G. Beunen, J. Ghesquière, T. Reybrouck and A.L. Claessens), Band 4 Schriftenreihe der Hamburg-Mannheimer-Stiftung, Enke Verlag, Stuttgart, pp. 20-26.

Lefevre, J. Beunen, G. and Simons, J. (1989) Longitudinal Principal Component Analysis of Somatic and Motor Characteristics. **Am. J. Hum. Biol.,** 1, 757-769.

Malina, R.M. (1990) Tracking of physical fitness and performance during growth, in **Children and Exercise XIV** (eds G. Beunen, J. Ghesquiere, T. Reybrouck and A.L. Claessens), Band 4 Schriftenreihe der Hamburg Mannheimer-Stiftung, Enke Verlag, Stuttgart, pp. 1-10.

Ostyn, M. Simons, J. Beunen, G. Renson, R. and Van Gerven D. (1980) **Somatic and Motor Development of Belgian Secondary Schoolboys: Norms and Standards.** Leuven University Press, Leuven.

Parizkova, J. (1977) **Body fat and physical fitness.** Martinus Nijhoff, The Hague.

Rarick, G.L. and Smoll, R.M. (1967) Stability of growth in strength and motor performance from childhood to adolescence. **Hum. Biol.,** 39, 295-306.

Roche, A.F. Siervogel, R.M. Chumlea, W.C. Reed, R.B. Valadian, I. Eichorn, D. and McCammon, R.W. (1982) **Serial changes in subcutaneous fat thicknesses of children and adults.** Karger, Basel.

24

GROWTH, PHYSICAL PERFORMANCE AND PSYCHOLOGICAL CHARACTERISTICS OF DISADVANTAGED BRAZILIAN PRESCHOOL CHILDREN *

M. B. ROCHA FERREIRA [1] and L. L. ROCHA [2]
[1] State University of Campinas - UNICAMP - Campinas, Brazil
[2] State University of São Paulo, São Paulo, Brazil

Keywords: Growth, Physical performance, Psychological development, Disadvantaged preschool children.

1 Introduction

Protein energy malnutrition (PEM) is an important factor affecting physical growth and performance, and psychological development. From the western point of view, malnutrition is defined as dietary inadequacy of energy and or protein. The contributing causes of the imbalance of protein and energy intakes of the population are economic, social and cultural. The PEM effects range from mild to severe, depending on the intensity, duration and timing of the stress. The mild-to-moderate effects on health are more difficult to specify compared to clinical manifestation of the severe forms. Moreover, the great variety of the methodologies used in various studies and ambiguity in terminology, and the general unfamiliarity with the ethiology of the disease make it difficult to obtain a consensus among scholars on the specifics of PEM and its effects.

The most common consequences of PEM, when it occurs during the first years of life, are stunted physical growth, reduced muscle mass, decreased maximal oxygen consumption, delayed maturation of the nervous system, delayed or impaired learning ability, increased susceptibility to infectious diseases, and elevated mortality rates (Jelliffe 1959; Habicht et al. 1974; Malina 1981, 1984, 1985, 1986; Malina and Buschang 1985; Spurr et al. 1982,1983,1984).

Malnutrition can also affect motor performance. Malnourished children generally present low levels of physical performance in tests of speed, strength, long distance runs, and throwing (Spurr 1983; Rocha Ferreira 1979, 1987; Malina 1981, 1984, 1986; Ghesquiere and Eeckels 1984; Malina and Buschang 1985; Rocha Ferreira et al. 1990, 1991).

The study of malnutrition and psychological development is generally

----
* This research was sponsored by Conselho Nacional de Pesquisa Cientifica e Tecnologica - Brazil

related to morphological and functional brain development. Many authors have suggested that severe undernutrition during infancy can have an irreversible effect on growth and development of the brain. Retardation of intellectual capacity is, therefore, a likely consequence (Stoch and Smythe 1963; Cabak and Najdanvic 1965; Edwards and Craddock 1973; Freeman et al. 1977). However, there are also other socio-cultural influences on intellectual development which can increase the complexity of the problem. It is difficult, therefore, to isolate the variables determining the delay of mental development.

The purpose of this research is to study the growth, physical performance and psychological development of Brazilian preschoolers, five to seven year old, both sexes, attending two different preschools, living in conditions of chronic mild to moderate undernutrition.

2 Method

The children attended two public schools from different neighbourhoods considered "periferia", i.e of a low socioeconomic class in the city of São Jose dos Campos, State of São Paulo, Brazil. The schools were studied in two consecutive years. In 1988, the sample of 47 girls and 49 boys was taken from two different preschools; and in 1989, the sample of 21 girls and 25 boys was from one of the schools studied in the previous year. Only 11 girls and 12 boys participated in both years; the longitudinal data will not be analysed in this paper.

The anthropometric dimensions included weight, height, circumferences (arm and calf), skinfold thickness (biceps, triceps, subscapular, supracristailiac, abdominal and medial calf) and breadths (bicondylar and biepicondylar). The physical performance tests included standing long jump, shuttle run, 20 meters dash, and 30 seconds sit-up. The psychological development status of the child was viewed in terms of intellectual development assessed by the Terman-Merril Stanford-Binet scale, form M (Terman Merril 1966), visuo-motor perception estimated using Bender's graphic test of perceptive organization as revised by Santucci and Galifret-Franjon (1963), and body image with Goodenough's "Draw a Man" test (Goodenough 1951). Food intake at home and school and socioeconomic information were collected through interviews with the adult responsible for each child (Rocha Ferreira 1987). To estimate food intake over a 24-hour-period, the recall method was used. The Brazilian tables elaborated by Tudisco et al. (1978) were used to transform the food intake into grams. The tables of FIBGE (1977) were used to estimate the energy content and protein value of the food consumed.

Table 1. Means, standard deviations for anthropometric and performance variables in 47 (1988) and 21 (1989) Brazilian and 25 Czechoslovakian girls.

Variables	1988 Brazil		1989 Brazil		Czechoslovakia	
	mean	sd	mean	sd	mean	sd
Age	6.5	0.56	6.9	0.31	6.3	0.23
Weight (kg)	21.1	3.36	21.8	1.89	21.6	2.81
Height (cm)	117.0	5.14	120.8	5.46	118.7	2.8
Sitting ht (cm)	63.7	2.64	65.6	2.51	64.7	2.8
Circumferences (cm)						
Arm relaxed	17.7	1.50	17.0	1.05	17.8	1.2
Arm tensed	18.2	1.44	18.1	1.25	-	-
Calf	23.7	1.66	23.9	1.88	-	-
Skinfolds (mm)						
Biceps	6.1	1.63	6.2	1.50	4.2	1.2
Triceps	8.8	2.30	9.4	1.83	9.4	2.4
Subscapular	5.8	2.62	6.0	1.91	5.6	2.3
Suprailliac	4.9	3.44	4.7	1.15	4.9	3.2
Calf	10.0	3.50	10.6	1.77	5.0	1.8
Skinfolds (mm)						
Trunk	10.8	6.00	10.7	2.70	-	-
Extremity	18.8	5.50	20.0	3.20	-	-
Total	35.7	12.30	36.9	6.40	-	-
Breadths (cm)						
Biepicondylar humerus	4.4	0.26	4.6	0.27	4.6	0.2
Biepicondylar femur	6.9	0.37	7.0	0.30	6.9	0.5
Performance						
St. l. jump (cm)	96.0	14.20	102.9	25.80	96.2	16.5
20m dash (sec)	5.8	0.50	6.1	0.63	5.1	0.2
Shuttle run (sec)	15.7	1.62	15.9	1.26	-	-
Sit up (30sec)	5.8	3.91	5.9	4.24	-	-

Skinfold trunk = sum of subscapular and suprailiac
Skinfold extremity = sum of triceps and calf

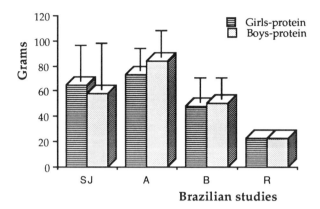

Fig. 1 Estimated mean (standard deviation) protein intake in children from different Brazilian studies and recommended dietary allowances (WHO/FAO), (SJ=SJ Campos; A= Alphaville; B= Barueri; R= Recommended).

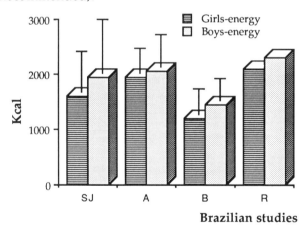

Fig. 2 Estimated mean (standard deviation) energy intake in children from different Brazilian studies and recommended dietary allowances (WHO/FAO), (SJ=SJ Campos; A= Alphaville; B= Barueri; R= Recommended).

259

3 Results

The majority of the families made three to four times the minimum monthly salary (one minimum monthly income is equivalent to $ 36). The majority of the fathers worked for multinationals, and the mothers stayed at home. The topography of one neighbourhood was flat, and the other was slightly hilly. There was no recreational center in the area. The water supply, garbage collection and electricity were under the aegis of public companies. Residences were constructed of bricks. There were no houses from scraps of wood, therefore, no slums. The "merenda escolar", a state wide meal program was served daily, based on 300 kcal and 8 grams of protein per meal.

The mothers report about the children's physical activity showed that they did not participate in any kind of organized exercise program. The school had only a good educational program focusing mainly on fine motor development. The children were not allowed to play where they wanted without permission. They played mainly at home or at the neighbour's house. Boys tended to practice more active games than girls.

The children presented a large variation of estimated protein and energy intake (figures 1 and 2). Boys tended to have higher estimated protein and energy intake than girls. Means and standard deviations for anthropometric and physical performance of the children are shown in Tables 1 and 2. The average age of the children in 1988 was older than those in studied 1987, consequently all the results of the anthropometric measurements, performance and psychological tests were higher.

The differences between sexes were small. Boys tended to have slightly higher values for overall body size, sitting height, circumferences and breadths, and lower values for skinfold thickness than girls. Boys performed slightly better on the physical performance tests. The majority of the children studied performed well in the psychological tests. There was a slight tendency for the girls to have higher scores in those tests (Table 3).

Body weight tended to have a low-to-moderate negative correlation with jumping (except for boys in 1988) and running tasks, and stature tended to have a low-to-moderate negative correlation with motor performance tests in both sexes (Table 4). The signs of the coefficients for dash and shuttle run were inverted since a lower time reflects a better performance. The second order partial correlations between body size and performance, controlling for age and stature or weight can better explain the relationship (Table 4). The correlation range runs from low to moderate. When age and stature are controlled, heavier children tend to have lower scores on motor performance tests. Stature, when age and weight were controlled, tended to have a higher correlation with motor performance tests. The differences between sexes in the correlation direction were bigger between weight and motor performance than stature and motor

Table 2. Means, standard deviations for anthropometric and performance variables in 50 (1988) and 24 (1989) Brazilian and 25 Czechoslovakian boys.

Variables	1988 Brazil		1989 Brazil		Czechoslovakia	
	mean	sd	mean	sd	mean	sd
Age	6.5	0.64	6.8	0.29	6.6	0.3
Weight (kg)	21.7	3.49	22.2	3.82	22.1	2.7
Height (cm)	118.0	5.20	120.7	6.90	119.3	4.1
Sitting ht (cm)	64.9	3.06	65.4	3.56	65.5	2.6
Circumferences (cm)						
Arm relaxed	17.1	1.62	17.2	1.25	17.7	1.1
Arm tensed	18.2	1.71	18.7	1.48	-	-
Calf	23.6	1.90	24.2	2.08	-	-
Skinfolds (mm)						
Biceps	5.3	1.78	6.4	2.32	2.9	0.6
Triceps	7.9	2.27	8.8	2.99	7.2	1.7
Subscapular	5.3	1.55	5.6	1.80	4.0	0.4
Suprailliac	4.1	1.89	4.3	1.43	3.0	0.6
Calf	8.8	3.61	9.3	3.76	4.0	1.0
Skinfolds (mm)						
Trunk	9.3	3.30	9.9	3.00	-	-
Extremity	16.7	5.50	18.8	5.50	-	-
Total	31.4	9.60	34.5	11.40	-	-
Breadths (cm) Biepicondylar humerus	4.6	0.37	4.8	0.32	4.8	0.3
Biepicondylar femur	7.2	0.42	7.4	0.32	7.5	0.3
Performance						
St. l. jump (cm)	97.3	16.60	104.4	28.90	103.5	18.7
20m dash (sec)	5.7	0.52	5.9	0.44	4.9	0.2
Shuttle run (sec)	15.6	1.57	14.9	1.19	-	-
Sit up (30sec)	6.0	4.26	8.1	4.32	-	-

Skinfold trunk = sum of subscapular and suprailiac
Skinfold extremity = sum of triceps and calf

Table 3. Frequencies and percentages of the psychological developmental level (intelligence, motor perception and body image) in Brazilian girls and boys.

Developm. level	Year	Signif. immature		Immature		Normal		Above normal		Tot.
	IQ:	50 -70		70 - 80		80 - 110		110 - 120		
		n	%	n	%	n	%	n	%	n
Intelligence										
Girls	1988	0	0.0	2	4.3	43	91.4	2	4.3	47
	1989	1	4.7	1	4.7	20	95.2	0	0.0	21
Boys	1988	4	8.0	5	10.1	42	84.0	0	0.0	50
	1989	1	4.0	0	0.0	24	96.0	0	0.0	25
Motor Perception										
Girls	1988	1	2.1	5	10.6	41	87.2	-	-	47
	1989	1	4.7	2	9.5	18	85.7	-	-	21
Boys	1988	9	18.0	7	14.0	34	68.0	-	-	50
	1989	3	12.0	4	16.0	18	72.0	-	-	25
Body Image										
Girls	1988	1	2.1	11	23.4	35	74.5	-	-	47
	1989	0	0.0	4	19.0	17	80.9	-	-	21
Boys	1988	8	16.0	14	28.0	28	56.0	-	-	50
	1989	2	8.0	9	36.0	14	56.0	-	-	25

The differential response of muscle tissue to environmental factor is reasonably well documented (Jelliffe 1959). Arm and calf circumferences are commonly used as an indicator of relative muscularity. The sample studied is similar to other low socioeconomic samples in Brazil.

The anthropometric and physical performance data from the present study are compared to corresponding data for children in Czechoslovakia, adapted from Parizkova et al. (1977). The mean values from different body size and the standing long jump are simi lar to Czechoslovakian preschool children. The 20 meters dash scores are lower than th ,se.

Body size and proportions have low to moderate positive correlations with motor performance, which is consistent with the literature (Seils 1951; Rarick and Oyster 1964; Malina 1975). Zero order correlations from different Brazilian studies are presented in Table 4. The pattern of the correlations between stature and weight and physical performance is generally similar in magnitude and direction to the other samples.

Low to moderate correlations like those noted above suggest that performance is not highly dependent on body weight and stature. There are other variables affecting body dimensions and motor performance. The low correlations and the differences in the direction can probably be explained by the different backgrounds of the children, previous physical activity, nutritional status, and stimulation at home.

To better explain the relationship between morphological aspects and performance, second order correlations, controlling for age and either stature or weight, were calculated. Data from different Brazilian studies are presented in Table 4. Children with higher weight tend to have lower motor performance scores. This is consistent with the observation that movements in which the body is projected (such as standing long jump and dashes) tend to have low negative correlations with body weight (Malina 1975).

Stature, when age and weight are controlled, has a significant positive correlation with jumping, agility, sit-up, and speed. These findings are similar to other studies done in different geographic areas (Seils 1951; Rarick and Oyster 1964; Malina and Buschang 1985; Malina et al. 1987; Rocha Ferreira 1987).

The intellectual development of the children was better than other samples from low socioeconomic status in São Paulo area (Silva Carmo 1986; Rocha Ferreira 1987). In the present study, only 4.29% had low scores in the intellectual level (IQ >50 <70) which data have been found in the general population (Silva Carmo 1986, 1989; Rocha Ferreira 1987). The largest frequencies were within the normal range. The mean score of the intellectual level, i.e. IQ=90 was found, while Rocha Ferreira (1987) found the mean IQ score of 80 in 8-year-old children from a low socioeconomic background in the São Paulo area. This fact suggests that there are positive factors influencing the mental development of the children studied.

The low perceptive visuo-motor scores found were within expectation for the age group studied. At this age the visuo-psychological process is still in development, and is expected to mature at the age of 11 to 12 years Perceptual immaturity, however, should be followed carefully because it might influence the process of learning at school.

5 Conclusions

Estimated protein intake of the children studied meets the recommended daily allowance, but the estimated energy intake is below. The children present a large variation in protein and energy intake.

The growth, performance, and psychological status of the preschool children studied is consistent with the marginal economic circumstances of their families. Their growth status and physical performance scores

263

performance, in both the zero order correlation and the second order partial correlations.

4 Discussion

The estimated food intake data suggest that on average the children may be under energy deficiencies. However, the values are still above those found in the 8-year-old lower socioeconomic status children from Barueri, and they are almost equivalent to the upper socioeconomic status children from Alphaville (Rocha Ferreira 1987). Given the shortcomings of the 24-hours recall procedures, the estimated protein and energy intake in this study is only used to give an overview of the food intake of the population studied.

The large standard deviations of the estimated protein-energy intakes show an important variation of the group, which is consistent with different studies (Rocha Ferreira 1979, 1987; Rocha Ferreira et al. 1990). The wide variation of the food consumption suggests individual metabolic demand. In addition, males tended to have higher food consumption than females.

The sexual di morphism is already present in this early age, although the variation is not significant. Boys tended to be taller and bigger than girls, except for fatness.

Skinfold thicknesses are more easily affected by measurement variation, and therefore, comparisons among studies should be done with caution. The low skinfold thickness values found in the present study are consistent with other studies from low socioeconomic backgrounds (Parizkova, 1976, 1979; Parizkova et al. 1974, 1977; Rocha Ferreira 1979, 1987; Malina 1981, 1984, 1985, 1986). Boys have smaller skinfolds than girls in all samples. The smaller skinfold thicknesses of lower SES children suggest either a deficit of energy intake and/or greater energy expenditure. Ethnic background, however, may be a confounding factor, given ethnic variation in subcutaneous fat distribution.

Differences in the distribution of extremity versus central fat between groups of widely different nutritional status may be affected by genetic differences in relative distribution of body fat (Mueller 1986). It is also possible that extremity fat is more sensitive to environmental factors than central fat (Bogin and MacVean 1981), which has been questioned by Mueller (1986). The present sample show a higher concentration of fat in the calf, followed by triceps. The values of the extremity skinfold sum are higher than those from the 8-year-old Brazilian children from a low socioeconomic background (Rocha Ferreira 1987). In general, the children of the present study seem to be in better condition than the children in the above mentioned study. There is, thus, a possible indicator that the extremity fat is more sensitive to environmental factors.

compare with other lower socioeconomic class Brazilian children, and the Czechoslovak children, except for 20 meter dash. Their intellectual, perceptual motor organization and body image scores are within the average population. Some of the low scores observed in the group might reflect the limited stimulation of their home environment.

6 References

Anjos, L.A. (1989) Indices antropométricos e estado nutricional de escolares de baixa renda de um municipio do estado do Rio de Janeiro (Brazil) : um estudo piloto. **Revista de Saude Publica, São Paulo,** 23, 221-229.

Bogin, B. and MacVean R.B. (1981) Nutritional and biological determinants of body fat patterning in urban Guatemalan children. **Hum. Biol.,** 53, 259-268.

Buschang, P.H. (1980) Growth status and rate of school children 6 to 13 years of age in a rural Zapotec speaking community in the Valley of Oaxaca, Mexico. Doctoral Dissertation, University of Texas at Austin.

Cabak, V. and Najdanvic R. (1965) Effect of undernutrition in early life on physical and mental development. **Arch. Dis. Child.,** 40, 532-539.

Cassidy, C.M. (1982) Protein-energy malnutrition as a culture-bound syndrome. Culture, **Med. Psychiat.,** 6, 325-345.

Cravioto, J. De Licardie, E.R. and H.G. Birch (1966) Nutrition, growth, and neurointegrative development: an experimental and ecologic study. **Pediatrics,** 38, 319-372.

Edwards, L.D., and Craddock L.J. (1973) Malnutrition and intellectual development: a study in school-age aboriginal children at Walgett, N.S.W. **Med. J. Australia** 1, 880-884.

Freeman, H.E., Klein R.E. Kagan J. and Yarbrough C. (1977) Relations between nutrition and cognition in rural Guatemala. **Am. J. Public Health,** 67, 233-239.

Fundação Instituto Brazileiro de Geografia e Estatistica (1977) **Estudo Nacional da Despesa Familiar - ENDEF - Tabelas de Composição dos Alimentos.** Secretaria de Planejamento da Presidencia da Republica. Rio de Janeiro.

Ghesquiere, J. and Eeckels R. (1984) Health, physical development and fitness of primary school children in Kinshasa, in **Children and sport** (eds J. Ilmarinen and L. Valimaki), Springer-Verlag, Berlin, pp. 18-30.

Goodenough, F.L. (1951) **Test de inteligencia infantil por medio del debujo de la figura humana.** Traduccion Cabanera, M.L.F., ed Paidos, Buenos Aires, Argentina.

Habicht, J.P. Martorell, R. Yarbrough, C. Malina, R.M. and Klein R.E. (1974) Height and weight standards for preschool children: how relevant are ethnic differences in growth potential. **Lancet,** 1, 611-615.

265

Jelliffe, D.B. (1959) Protein-calorie malnutrition in tropical preschool children, a review of recent knowledge. **J. Pediatr.**, 54, 227-256.

Malina, R.M. (1975) Anthropometric correlates of strength and motor performance. **Exer. Sport Sci. Rev.**, 3, 249-274.

Malina, R.M. (1981) **Growth and performance of Latin American children.** Prepared for the Kinanthropometry section of the PanAmerican Congress of Sports Medicine and Exercise, Miami, May 23-26.

Malina, R.M. (1984) Physical activity and motor development / performance in populations nutritionally at risk, in **Energy intake and activity** (eds E. Pollitt and P. Amante), Alan R. Liss, New York, pp. 285-302.

Malina, R.M. (1985) Growth and physical performance of Latin American children and youth: socioeconomic and nutritional contrasts. **Collegium Anthropologicum**, 9, 9-331.

Malina, R.M. (1986) Motor development and performance of children and youth in undernourished populations, in **Sport Health and Nutrition** (ed F.L. Katch), Human Kinetics Publishers, Champaign, Illinois, pp. 31-226.

Malina, R.M. and Buschang P.H. (1985) Growth, strength and motor performance of Zapotec children, Oaxaca, Mexico. **Hum. Biol.**, 57, 163-181.

Malina, R.M. Little, B.B. Shoup, R.F. and Buschang P.H. (1987) Adaptative significance of small body size: strength and motor performance of school children in Mexico and Papua New Guinea. **Am. J. Phys. Anthropol..** In Press.

Mueller, W.H. (1986) Environmental sensitivity of different skinfold sites. **Hum. Biol.**, 58, 499-506.

Parizkova, J. (1974) Nutritional status, somatic and funcional development in preschool children as related to ecological factors and exercise. **Acta Facultatis Medical Universitatis Brunensis**, 57,333-340.

Parizkova, J. and Kabele, J. (1988) Longitudinal study of somatic motor and psychological development in preschool boys and girls. **Collegium Anthropologicum**, 1, 67-73.

Parizkova, J.; Cermak, J. and Homa, J. (1977) Sex differences in somatic and functional characteristics of preschool children. **Hum. Biol.**, 49, 437-451.

Rarick, G.L. and Oyster N. (1964) Physical maturity, muscular strength, and motor performance of young school-age boys. **Res. Quart.**, 35, 523-531.

Rocha Ferreira, M.B. (1979) Estado nutricional e aptidao fisica em pré-escolares. Tese de mestrado apresentada na Escola de Edução Fisica da Universidade de São Paulo.

Rocha Ferreira, M.B. (1987) **Growth, physical performance and psychological characteristics of eight year old Brazilian children from low socioeconomic background.** Dissertation presented to the Faculty of the Graduate School of the University of Texas at Austin.

Rocha Ferreira, M.B. Malina R.M. and Rocha L.L. (1990) **Anthropometric, functional and psychological characteristics of eight-year-old Brazilian children from low socioeconomic status**. Medicine Sport Science, Basel, Karger, 31 (printing).

Rocha Ferreira, M.B. Malina, R.M. Zucas, S.M. Little, B. (1990) **Nutritional status and physical performance of Brazilian prescholars from low socioeconomic background**. In preparation.

Santucci, H., and N. Galifret-Granjon (1963) **Prova gràfica de organizacion perceptiva, in Manual para el examen psicològico del nino.** (ed R. Zazzo), Editorial Kapelusz, Buenos Aires, pp. 177-208.

Seils, L.G. (1951) The relationship between measures of physical growth and gross motor performance of primary-grade school children. **Res. Quart.**, 22, 244-260.

Silva C᠎ ᠎o, H.M. (1986) **O problema dos repetentes da la série primaria nos grupos escolares de São Paulo**. Report, Instituto de Psicologia, Universidade de São Paulo.

Silva Carmo, H.M. (1989) **Reflexoes sobre psico-diagnostico : analise e critica de estudos de caso tendo em vista a organizaçao posterior de modelos abreviados de psico-diagnostico.** Tese de doutorado apresentada no Instituto de Psicologia da Universidada de São Paulo.

Spurr, G.B. (1983) Nutritional status and physical work capacity. **Yearbook of Physical Anthropology,** 26, 1-35.

Spurr, G.B. Reina, J.C. and Barac-Nieto M. (1983) Marginal malnutrition in school aged Colombian boys, anthropometry and maturation. **Am. J. Clin. Nutr.**, 37, 119-132.

Spurr, G.B. Reina, J.C. Barac-Nieto M. and Maksudo M.G. (1982) Maximum oxygen consumption of nutritionally normal white, mestizo and black Colombian boys 6-16 years of age. **Hum. Biol.**, 5, 553-557.

Spurr, G.B. Reina, J.C. Barac-Nieto, M. and Ramirez R. (1984) Marginal malnutrition in school-aged Colombian boys: efficiency of treadmill walking in submaximal exercise. **Am. J. Clin. Nutr.**, 39, 452-459.

Stoch, M.B. and P.M. Smythe (1963) Does undernutrition during infancy inhibit brain growth and subsequent intellectual development? **Arch. Dis. Child.**, 38, 546-552.

Terman, L.M. and Merrill M.A. (1966) **Medida de la inteligencia, metodo para el empleo de las pruevas de Stanford-Binet nuevamente revisadas.** Espasa-Calpe, Madrid.

Tudisco, E.S., N.J. Manoel, and D.M., Sigulem (1978) **Guia para avaliçao da dieta do paciente em consulta ambulatoria.** Resumos do Congresso Internacional de Nutrição. Rio de Janeiro, pp. 272.

World Health Organization (1973) **Energy and protein requirements**. Report of a Joint FAO/WHO ad hoc expert committee. Technical Report Series n. 552, World Health Organization.

25

CHANGES IN RUNNING SPEED AND ENDURANCE AMONG GIRLS DURING PUBERTY

S. SZCZESNY [1] and J. COUDERT [2]
[1] INSEP, Laboratoire de Mesures, Paris, France
[2] Faculté de Médecine, Univ. de Clermont-Ferrand, France

Keywords: Running speed, Endurance, Girls, Puberty.

1 Introduction

The physical capacities of an individual can be determined by series of field tests suggested by different groups of scientific experts. Being reliable, sound and accurate (Simri 1974; Alderman and Howell 1974; Simons et al. 1969) the series drawn up by AAHPERD (1980), CAHPER (1980), ICSPFT (1974), EUROFIT (1987) now seem suited to a practical use.

Analysis of the tests making up these series brings out the fact that we systematically find in each one both a short-duration run and a long run called endurance which both express in an indirect way the manner of carrying out a performance of the bioenergetic systems.

Following the suggestions of several authors, we suppose that a performance over a short distance is likely to call upon the alactic anaerobic system (Fox and Mathews 1983; Crielaard and Pirnay 1985). Margaria et al. (1966) consider that the duration of the test bringing into play the alactic anaerobic system is from 4 to 6 seconds.

It is equally permissible to think that a long-duration test such as the 12 minute run for example, expresses endurance on the field. According to Cooper (1968), 12 minutes represents the duration limit during which a subject can maintain an activity at an intensity close to the maximal aerobic power (MAP). This type of effort is principally limited by VO_2 max and a relation between the performance during the run and the maximal oxygen consumption has been found by different authors.

Amongst adults Cooper finds a correlation of 0.90 between the performance and VO_2 max (n=115). For children, Maksoud and Coutts (1971), Jackson and Coleman (1976) observe significant correlations between the average performance for a 12 minute run and VO_2 max. estimated in the laboratory. The same authors, as well as Rassmussen (1981), record higher and significant correlations - above 0.90 between the test and the retest. It is for these reasons that, even if the forecast of VO_2 max. based on the performance is put into question (Lacour, Flandrois et al. 1981), performance over a 12 minute run is considered as a sound and accurate field test.

Moreover it is known that puberty, which is not completed until a few years later, appears on average around 12-13 years for girls. Puberty, an important transition period between "late childhood" and the beginning of "youth" when growth accelerates, leads adolescents towards the acquisition of the morphological sexual and functional characteristics of adults (Vandervael 1980). For all girls who develop normally, after the peak of statural growth comes the peak of weight gain and the arrival of the menstrual cycle. Synthesis of different studies concerning this subject shows that the range of this phenomenon varies from 10 to 16.5 years. This large variability of the ages when puberty begins and finishes leads us to give chronological age - taken as a reference criterion for classing individual performances - only a relative value.

For girls, puberty is also accompanied by an increase in fat tissue, representing a sizable fraction of their body mass (Parizkova 1961; Tanner 1962; Crenier 1977). Adipose tissue, estimated to be roughly 50% of the body's total fat, is practically inert metabolically. Also its prevalence in the body mass has repercussions on the capacity for effort (von Döbeln 1956; Parizkova 1977; Rutenfrantz et al. 1981). Indeed it has been proven that individuals with an increased percentage of adipose tissue are less active in daily life and have poorer performance than subjects who are active and not laden with fat tissue (Parizkova 1963; Gleeson et al. 1989).

In so far as performances over a short or long distance can be considered as reflecting the development of maximal speed and endurance, the object of the present study is to see if the passage from one stage of puberty to another influences the level of performance and if the development of these two motor qualities follows a linear course or on the contrary is marked with accelerations and decelerations.

2 Material and method

The study concerns 230 girls from the Paris region whose only sports involvement is the physical activity at school. The information compiled includes chronological age, puberty stages, the age at menarche, distance covered in a 12 minute run and the timed performance over 40 meters. The age is calculated in months. Those students whose age is between 138 and 149 months are considered to be 12 and following the same principle the other girls are placed in the different age groups.

The puberty stages were estimated directly from the observation of secondary sexual characteristics by the school doctor. The classification used is that described by Tanner (1962). The date of menarche was provided by the same doctor who questioned the girls. The height and weight were obtained using the method put forward by Sempé et al.

269

(1979). The four cutaneous folds were measured in the areas recommended by Durnin and Rahaman (1967), using Holtain type calipers with constant pressure. In order to avoid relative errors in the determination of the percentage of total fat, using the given equation the sub-cutaneous fat was expressed as the sum of the four folds. Indeed, the use of an equation to predict density based on the fat mass is only valid on those subjects whose measures have been taken (Heyters 1987).

The 12 minute run took place on a flat circular track. The subjects ran in groups of 10. The recorded performance is the distance covered measured in meters.

The running speed is calculated from the formula s = d/t (s = speed, d = distance, t = time) based on a 40 meter run along a straight flat track. The start was individual, the subject stood in a half-crouched position, feet apart. The two timers were set off manually when the back foot left the ground. The recorded performance is the average of the two results obtained correct to within 0.1 second.

3 Results and analysis

Table 1 presents the distribution of the number of subjects involved according to two criteria : puberty stage and chronological age. It is observed that for each age, different stages are possible.

Analysis of Table 1 shows, with the calculations carried out on all ages and all stages (n=230), that there is a relation (r = 0.63; p<0.01) during puberty between age and puberty stages.

Table 2 shows the averages of the studied variables when the results are regrouped according to age. Compared to the values based on a longitudinal study of the French population by Sempé et al. (1979), the statural growth and weight increase of the girls in question here appears "normal", the t test being non-significant, except at 12 or 13 years old when the weight of the examined girls is significantly heavier than that mentioned by Sempé.

We suppose that the arrival of the menstrual cycle is an obvious indicator of puberty. In the sample of girls questioned, 142 had reached the menstrual cycle, that is 61.74 %. The average age for the arrival of the menstrual cycle was 12.57 ± 1.02 years old. This value is slightly less than that recorded by Ducros et al. (1978), 12.8 ± 1.3 years old, based on a survey carried out in 1974.

Figure 1 shows that during puberty, the number of post-menarcheal girls increases stage by stage and that of the pre-menarcheal girls drops. This indicates a normal occurrence of the phenomenon. A decrease in the age of menarche - attributed to the improvement in living conditions -

Table 1. Distribution of subjects according to puberty stage and age

Puberty	AGE (YEARS)					Total
Stage	12	13	14	15	16	
5		12	19	24	16	71
4	10	36	26	13	6	91
3	14	17	7	1		39
2	21	6	2			29
Total	45	71	54	38	22	230

Table 2. Average value of studied variables according to age

		12 years n = 45	13 years n = 71	14 years n = 54	15 years n = 38	16 years n = 22
Puberty stage	M	2.75	3.76	4.15	4.60	4.73
	SD	0.80	0.84	0.79	0.55	0.43
Weight (kg)	M	41.55	46.75	48.93	53.06	55.25
	SD	6.73	7.54	6.92	9.11	8.19
Height (cm)	M	148.78	154.89	158.77	158.26	161.93
	SD	6.34	5.33	5.97	5.69	5.35
Sum of 4 skin-	M	44.04	44.45	44.73	51.76	49.79
folds (mm)	SD	18.94	17.91	18.29	18.35	15.77
40 m run	M	5.48	5.64	5.74	5.84	6.05
(m.sec $^{-1}$)	SD	0.37	0.41	0.37	0.53	0.53
12 min run	M	1779	1851	1757	1930	1977
(m)	SD	211	245	346	321	401

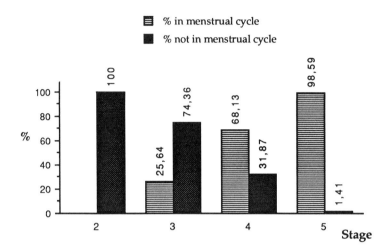

Fig. 1. Proportion of girls in menstrual cycle and not in menstrual cycle as a percentage of the number in each puberty stage.

has been observed over several decades in different countries (Eveleth and Tanner 1976). In France this same tendancy has been evident for over a century. Thus in terms of stature, weight and age at menarche, the girls of our sample were growing normally.

4 Study of the correlations

The results given in Table 3 show that the correlation (Pearson's r) between the subjects' age and their puberty stage is only significant at 12 years old (r = 0.30; p<0.05). For the following ages, it stays nonsignificant. This shows that there is no relation between the criteria "age" and "puberty stage". For the girls between 12 and 15 years, the correlations between the morphological characteristics and the puberty stages are significant and greater than those established between the same characteristics and chronological age. Thus as a criterion for growth determination, the puberty stages seem more pertinent than age and confirm the suggestions of Olivier (1971) to the effect that, during puberty "... the chronological age is no longer useful, the physiological age must be determined by observing the puberty stages. The child's physical aptitude - his work capacity - depends on the state of his biological growth much more than his civil age..."

Table 3. Correlation coefficients of studied characteristics based on two criteria of classifying, on one hand age and the other puberty stage.

	class. by	12 years	13 years	14 years	15 years	16 years
Puberty Stage	Age	0.30*	0.21	-0.00	0.19	-0.02
	Stage					
Weight (kg)	Age	0.17	0.08	0.24	0.03	-0.23
	Stage	0.40**	0.49**	0.56**	0.39*	0.22
Height (cm)	Age	0.38**	0.11	0.17	0.02	-0.27
	Stage	0.45**	0.45**	0.10	-0.03	-0.05
Sum of 4 skin-folds (mm)	Age	-0.09	-0.03	-0.00	0.06	-0.16
	Stage	0.10	0.25*	0.51**	0.44**	0.30
40 m run (m.sec⁻¹)	Age	0.20	0.18	0.23	-0.00	-0.11
	Stage	0.05	0.34*	0.08	-0.08	-0.21
12 min run (m)	Age	-0.11	-0.00	0.14	0.13	-0.18
	Stage	-0.11	-0.18	-0.14	0.02	-0.32
12 min/Weight (m.kg⁻¹)	Age	-0.08	-0.07	-0.03	-0.03	0.03
	Stage	-0.39**	-0.49**	-0.48**	-0.25	-0.38

$*$ $p < 0.05$
$**$ $p < 0.01$

Running speed is independant of both age and puberty stages, except at the age of 13 when it is significantly related to the value of the stage ($r = 0.34$; $p<0.05$).

Performances over a 12 minute run expressed without adjustment are independent of both age and puberty stages.

It should be stressed that if each child successively goes through all the puberty stages, it is obviously impossible to analyse individual puberty evolution in a transversal study.

Moreover, puberty stages are considered as one of the qualitative biological criteria, whereas age is considered as a quantitative criterion.

Since in the study the determination criterion is precisely the puberty stage which emphasizes the progression of the sexual maturation, the average values from each stage characterizing the morphological growth and the physical capacities of the girls can be compared. To establish this comparison a distribution of the values of the performances and the biological indications is carried out in terms of the puberty stages (Table 4). The significance of the Student t values is shown in Table 5.

4.1 Analysis of the evolution of running speed

We recall that the calculations of the correlation coefficient showed a significant correlation between speed and the puberty stage at 13 years of age (Table 3). However at this age the four stages are possible -allowing a comparison of the differences in the average speeds in terms of puberty stages.

The results grouped in Table 6 show that the average speeds of the girls aged 13 in the 3rd or 4th stage differ significantly ($p<0.01$) in favour of the girls in the 4th stage. This is confirmed when the comparison of the average speeds is carried out (Table 5) on all the girls ($n=230$; $p<0.001$).

It thus seems that only the passage between the 3rd and 4th stage corresponds to a significant increase in the speed recorded over the 40 meter distance. It could even be said that arrival in the 4th puberty stage marks the end of maximal speed development for non-sportive girls. Similarly at this moment there is also (Table 5) a large increase in stature ($p<0.001$) and above all in weight ($p<0.001$).

4.2 An approach to the evolution of endurance

By comparing the differences in the averages of the girls' performances - divided up by puberty stages (Table 5) we are trying to work out the influence of sexual maturation - expressed by the puberty stages - on performances in the 12 minute run.

It seems that there are no significant differences ($p>0.05$) between the average performances of girls classed by puberty stages. This lack of difference can be attributed to the weight gain of the subjects which increases in a significant manner ($p<0.001$) from one stage to the next.

To make the sample of girls more homogeneous, at least in part, relative to the weight gain, we created the ratio "number of meters covered/ weight" ($m.kg^{-1}$). The average values of this ratio appear in Table 4 and show their decrease in absolute value throughout puberty. However the significant differences (Table 5) only appear between the 2nd and 3rd stages ($p<0.01$) and between the 4th and 5th stages ($p<0.001$). This decrease in the ratio $m.kg^{-1}$ is confirmed when the comparison is carried out on the differences of the averages of the ratio $m.kg^{-1}$ for girls of the same age classed by their puberty stage (Table 7). Up till 14 years old, whatever the age, significant differences in the ratio $m.kg^{-1}$ appear between the 2nd and 3rd and then between the 4th and 5th puberty stages.

Table 4. Average value of studied variables following puberty stages.

		Stage 2 n = 29	Stage 3 n = 39	Stage 4 n = 91	Stage 5 n = 71
Age (months)	M	146.55	153.46	163.56	174.85
	SD	7.71	9.17	12.79	13.04
Height (cm)	M	146.33	153.46	157.62	158.73
	SD	5.74	6.03	5.64	5.81
Weight (kg)	M	38.76	42.93	48.42	54.35
	SD	6.63	5.70	6.25	8.29
Sum of 4 skin-folds (mm)	M	39.22	39.24	43.16	55.88
	SD	20.27	13.41	16.28	18.07
40 m run ($m.sec^{-1}$)	M	5.45	5.51	5.79	5.82
	SD	0.30	0.37	0.48	0.45
12 min run (m)	M	1858	1777	1868	1829
	SD	252	312	309	311
12 min/weight ($m.kg^{-1}$)	M	49.74	42.11	39.26	34.31
	SD	10.92	9.26	8.60	7.22

4.3 Correlation between the physical capacities and the subcutaneous fat of girls at puberty.

During puberty, girls have an increase in the quantity of adipose tissue before and especially after the arrival of the menstrual cycle (Young et al. 1968). Among the girls of our sample, the fat tissue increases in absolute value between the 2nd stage, where no girl is yet in the menstrual cycle, and the 5th stage when almost all are (Table 4, Fig.1). This increase in adipose tissue is especially visible between the 4th and 5th stages, the t test being significant (p<0.001) in favour of the girls classed in the 5th stage (Table 5). There are significant correlations between body mass and subcutaneous fat tissue (Table 8). This relationship - absolutely normal since subcutaneous tissue is part of the body mass - gives correlation coefficients going

Table 5. Significance of student t after comparison of averages of studied parameters, grouped in terms of puberty stages.

Puberty Stage	3 - 2	4 - 3	5 - 4
Height	5.20***	3.67***	1.22
Weight	2.91**	4.88***	5.01***
Skinfolds	0.004	1.43	4.64***
40 m (m.sec^{-1})	0.46	3.45***	0.77
12 min (m)	1.18	1.53	0.81
12 min Weight (m.kg^{-1})	3.04**	1.64	3.98***
df ($= n_1 + n_2 - 2$)	66	128	160

** $p < 0.01$ *** $p < 0.001$

Table 6. Comparison of differences between averages in running speed (m.sec^{-1}) of girls classed in different puberty stages, all of age 13.

Stage	Numbers	Average	Variation	t
2	$n_1 = 6$	5.31	0.39	
3	$n_2 = 17$	5.48	0.20	-1.29^{ns}
3	$n_1 = 17$	5.48	0.20	
4	$n_2 = 36$	5.74	0.45	-2.91**
4	$n_1 = 36$	5.74	0.45	
5	$n_2 = 12$	5.76	0.40	-0.14^{ns}

ns = non-significant

** = $p<0.01$

from 0.75 to 0.62 ($p<0.01$) for girls in puberty. The determination coefficient (r^2) shows that in the 2nd stage, 56% of the common variance is accounted for by the relationship between the sum of the cutaneous folds and the weight. This percentage drops slightly in the following stages but at the end of puberty, in the 5th stage, it accounts for 39% of the common variance. This shows that knowledge of the total weight alone doesn't allow evaluation of its influence on the level of performances without knowing the degree of its fat component.

Knowing the puberty stage, the value of relative endurance (m.kg^{-1}) and the developed speed over 40 meters for each girl, we tried to find out if a

Table 7. Comparison of differences of averages (t test) from the ratio m.kg^{-1} of girls classed at the same age according to their puberty stage.

Age	Puberty stage	Numbers	Average m.kg^{-1}	Variation	t
12	2	$n_1 = 21$	47.54	7.97	
	3	$n_2 = 14$	41.39	8.09	2.16*
12	3	$n_1 = 14$	41.39	8.09	
	4	$n_2 = 10$	39.90	8.84	0.41^{ns}
13	2	$n_1 = 6$	54.58	15.14	
	3	$n_2 = 17$	42.88	9.52	2.09*
13	3	$n_1 = 17$	42.88	9.52	
	4	$n_2 = 36$	39.93	7.69	1.18^{ns}
13	4	$n_1 = 36$	39.93	7.69	
	5	$n_2 = 12$	33.96	5.80	2.41**
14	3	$n_1 = 7$	39.79	11.07	
	4	$n_2 = 26$	37.50	6.58	0.67^{ns}
14	4	$n_1 = 26$	37.50	6.58	
	5	$n_2 = 19$	32.01	6.31	2.75***
15	4	$n_1 = 13$	39.03	12.75	
	5	$n_2 = 24$	36.17	8.13	0.81^{ns}
16	4	$n_1 = 6$	42.27	11.72	
	5	$n_2 = 16$	34.50	7.54	1.74^{ns}

ns = non-significant   ** $p < 0.02$

* $p < 0.05$ *** $p < 0.01$

relation existed between the physical capacities and the sum of the four cutaneous folds.

The relations of the two variables are determined from four equation models ($y = a+bx$; $y = ae^{bx}$; $y = a + b \log x$; $y = ax^b$). The choice of the adjustment model favours the one where the r coefficient is the highest and the standard error of estimate (SEE) is the smallest. The r coefficient is significant at p = 0.01.

Tables 9 and 10 present the values of the coefficients a and b of the exponential model ($y=ae^{bx}$). We see that the values of the correlation coefficients are negative at each stage, which shows that the adipose tissue doesn't help performance achievement. This is evident in the short duration exercise - at the end of puberty, that is at the 4th or 5th stage - and especially so in the long duration exercise, throughout puberty. The determination coefficient (r^2) shows that at the second stage, 54% of the common variance is accounted for by the relation between the ratio m.kg^{-1} and the sum of the folds. For the following stages this percentage is not as high. At the end of puberty, at the 5th stage, 30% of the common variance is accounted for by the relation between these two variables. It therefore appears that the more advanced a girl's puberty, the more her endurance decreases and this decrease is, in part, dependent on the increase of the adipose layer.

5 Discussion and conclusion

Different authors (Beunen et al. 1978; Savov 1985; Pineau 1987; Havlicek 1989) have studied the influence of growth, based on biological criteria, on the development of the physical capacities, among non active children as well as those who regularly play sport. The quoted authors conclude that the part played by age in the motor development of the subjects is sometimes smaller than that played by physiological age. By providing precise details on the evolution of endurance and speed, our research

Table 8. Correlation between body mass and sum of 4 cutaneous folds for girls divided up by puberty stage.

Puberty stage	r	r^2	df
2	0.75**	0.56	27
3	0.62**	0.38	37
4	0.68**	0.46	89
5	0.63**	0.39	69

** p<0.01

Table 9. Value of regression coefficients a and b between the speed (y) and the sum of the four folds (x) of girls classed according to puberty stage.

Puberty stage	a	b	r	r^2	SEE	p	df
2 $y=ae^{bx}$	5.5583	-0.0004	-0.16	0.0267	0.0547	ns	27
3 $y=ax^b$	6.7500	-0.0568	-0.27	0.0760	0.0657	ns	37
4 $y=ax^b$	7.3414	-0.0651	-0.28	0.0774	0.0778	0.01	89
5 $y=ax^b$	9.0345	-0.1113	-0.45	0.2076	0.0695	0.01	69

Table 10. Value of regression coefficients a and b in power $y=ax^b$ between the ratio $m.kg^{-1}$ (y) and the sum of four folds (x) of girls divided up by puberty stage.

Puberty stage	a	b	r	r^2	SEE	p	df
2 $y=ae^{bx}$	190.555	-0.3810	-0.7375	0.5440	0.1565	0.01	27
3 $y=ax^b$	110.669	-0.2742	-0.3851	0.1483	0.2184	0.01	37
4 $y=ax^b$	121.036	-0.3103	-0.4898	0.2399	0.1913	0.01	89
5 $y=ax^b$	160.717	-0.3951	-0.5495	0.3020	0.1897	0.01	69

confirms these conclusions for pubescent girls based on field tests.

Thus the estimation of the level of adolescents' performance needs to be done very carefully, when referring to estimation tables set up in terms of age, and the establishment of estimation Tables based on performance, taking only age as a criterion to differentiate between subjects, can thus be challenged. All these estimation Tables allow only an approximate evaluation of the motor efficiency. They disadvantage above all those children whose growth is called physiologically "late" and favour those whose growth is "advanced". Estimation of the value of an individual performance can be made comparative by taking account of the puberty stage - one of the quantitative biological criteria.

Moreover, the determination of endurance in terms of age based on the bare performance is not very accurate for girls undergoing puberty. This estimation seems more reasonable when the ratio "number of meters covered/ weight" ($m.kg^{-1}$), which evolves with the puberty stage, is considered.

Finally, during puberty, girls undergo a decrease in endurance and an increase in speed over 40 meters. This decrease in endurance can be attributed to the increase in the amount of adipose tissue.

This decrease in endurance - a conclusion which can be challenged since the data have been compiled cross-sectionally - is nevertheless comparable to that noted by Bar-Or (1987). The research carried out by this author relative to the development of the VO_2 max expressed in ml min^{-1} kg^{-1}, shows its rapid decrease for girls from the age of 10. Bar-Or (1987) attributes this decrease in the VO_2 max to an increase of fat tissue, also noted in our research.

The longitudinal study of Bailey (1973) concerning children (n=250) aged 8 to 15 shows up a slight decrease in the VO_2 max from the age of 9. This decrease is larger between the ages of 12 and 15.

Shephard et al. (1977) in their longitudinal study (n=546) concerning Canadian children aged between 6 and 12, note that the VO_2 max of the girls remains stable from ages 6 to 12 and then decreases.

The evolution of running speed over a short distance, which we have noted here, is equally comparable to that noted in a study where the number of girls was greater : Denisiuk et al. (1969) analysing the performances of over 9000 girls aged from 8 to 18, also concluded that performances over 60 meters improve up until 13-14 years of age.

The conclusion can also be obtained from the results of the research carried out by Kurowski (1977). The author notes that the maximal anaerobic power (kg/cal/kgh) - based on 294 girls and boys, aged between 9 and 16, using the Margaria test, increases for girls until the age of 14-15, and then decreases.

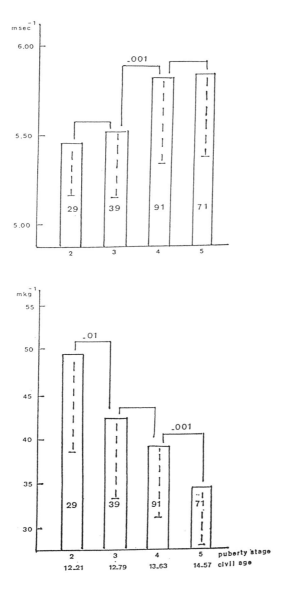

Fig. 2 Difference in the averages (Student t) in endurance (m.kg^{-1}) and in speed (m.sec^{-1}) of girls classed according to puberty stage.

In conclusion, the decrease in the relative endurance (m.kg^{-1}) and the increase in speed, being in relation with the degree of sexual maturation, show up in alternate ways. This is illustrated in Fig. 2. When the endurance drops significantly, the speed does not increase and, inversely, when the endurance drops a non-significant amount, the speed increases greatly. The motor development is thus characterised by periods of slowing down and of acceleration in the physical capacities relative to the maximal effort of short and long duration.

Determining the puberty stage allows us to account for variations for the same age, due to sexual maturation - something which chronological age does not bring out.

6 Acknowledgements

We thank Mrs. Jeanneret, school doctor, for the determinations of puberty stages and Mrs. F. Moreaux, PE teacher, for carrying out the field tests.

7 References

A.A.H.P.E.R. (1980) Lifetime Health related physical fitness,Test manual.

Alderman, R.B. and Howell M.L. (1974) Validity of Human Performance Assessments, in **Fitness, Health and Work Capacity. International Standards for Assessment** (ed A. Larson), Macmillan, New York, pp. 380-391.

Bailey, D.A. (1973) Exercise, fitness and physical education for the growing child. **Canad. J. Publ. Health**, 6, 421-430.

Bar-Or, O. (1987) Réponse métabolique a l'exercice chez l'enfant, in **Médecine du Sport chez l'enfant,** Masson, Paris, pp. 2-37, Appendice I, pp 303-316.

Beunen, G. De Beul G. Ostyn, M. Renson, R. Simons, J. and Van Gerven D. (1978) Age of menarche and motor performance in girls aged 11 through 18. **Med. Sport**, 11, 118-123.

CAHPER (1980) **Fitness-performance test manual for boys and girls 7 to 17 years of age**. Cahper.

Chrominski, Z. (1985) The level of biological development and physical fitness in school children aged 10-15 years. **Biol. Sport**, 2, 2, 141-150.

Cooper, K.H. (1968) A means of assessing maximal oxygen intake. **J. Am. Med. Assoc.**, 203, 201-204.

Crenier, E.J. (1977) Prédiction de la masse maigre et du pourcentage de graisse des enfants de 10 à 12 ans. **Biométrie Humaine**, 12, 59-67.

Crielaard, J.M. and Pirnay, F. (1985) Etude longitudinale des puissances aérobie et anaérobie alactique. **Méd. du Sport**, 59, 4-6.

Denisiuk, L. and Milicer, H. (1969) **Développement moteur des enfants et des adolescents.**, Ed. Nationale, Varsovie.

Ducros, A. and Pasquet P. (1978) Evolution de l'age d'apparition des premières règles (menarche) en France. **Biométrie Humaine**, 13, 35-43.

Durnin, J.V.G. and Rahaman M.M. (1967) The assessment of the amount of fat in the human body from measurements of skinfold thickness. **Br. J. Nutr.**, 21. 681-688.

EUROFIT, **Manuel pour les tests d'aptitude physique**, Conseil de l'Europe, Strasbourg, 1987.

Eveleth, P.B. and Tanner J.M. (1976) **Worldwide variation in human growth**. Cambridge University Press.

Fox, E.L. and Mathews, D.K. (1983) **Bases physiologiques de l'activité physique**. Vigot, Paris.

Gleeson, N. Tancred, B. and Banks, M. (1989) Psycho-biological factors influencing habitual activity in male and female adolescents. **Phys. Educ. Rev.**, 2, 110-124.

Havlicek, I. Seligerova, M. and Ramacsay L. (1989) Zavislost Motorickej Vykonnosti na biologickom veku. **Teoric a Praxe Telesne Vychovy**, 12, 757-761.

Heyters, C. (1987) Validité de l'évaluation de la graisse corporelle totale d'un individu par l'utilisation d'équations anthropométriques existantes. **Sci. et Sports**, 2, 109-117.

ICSPFT (1974) International Committee for standardisation of Physical Fitness Tests in **Fitness, Health and Work capacity** (ed L.H. Larson), Macmillan, New York, London, pp. 382.

Jackson, A.S., and Coleman A.E. (1976) Validation of distance run tests for elementary school children. **Res. Quart.**, 47, 1.

Kurowski, T. and Smith D.P. (1977) Maximal anaerobic power of children: development trends. **Med. Sci. Sport**, 1, 54.

Lacour, J.R., Flandrois, R. and Denis, C. (1981) Les tests d'effort, in **Sports et Sci.** (ed Vigot), Paris, 235-266.

Maksoud, M.G. and Coutts, K.D. (1971) Application of the Cooper twelve minutes run-walk test to young males. **Res. Quart.**, 42, 2.

Margaria, R. Aghemo, P. and Rovelli E. (1966) Measurement of muscular power (anaerobic) in man. **J. Appl. Physiol.**, 21. 1662-1664.

Olivier, G. (1971) La croissance, in **Morphologie et types humains**, Vigot, Paris, pp. 94-113.

Parizkova, J. (1961) Total body fat and skinfold thickness in children. **Metabolism**, 10, 794-807.

Parizkova, J. (1963) Impact of age, diet and exercice on man's body composition. **Ann. N.Y. Acad. Sci.**, 110, 661-674.

Parizkova, J. (1977) **Body fat and physical fitness**. M. Nijhoff, The Hague.

Pineau, J.C. (1987) Importance de la puberté sur les résultats aux tests physiques chez les jeunes sportifs garçons et filles. **Cah. Anthrop. Biom. Hum.**, 1-2. 91-111.

Rassmussen, B. (1981) Influence éventuelle de la variation de la technique de course sur les resultats d'un test de Cooper, **Conseil de l'Europe, Strasbourg,** 12-20.

Rutenfranz, J. Andersen, K.L. Seliger, V. Klimmer, F. Berndt, I. and Ruppel , M. (1981) Maximum Aerobic Power and Body Composition During the Puberty Growth Period : Similarities and Differences Between Children of Two European Countries. **Eur. J. Pediatr.,** 136, 123-133.

Savov, S.G. (1978) Physical fitness and skeletal maturity in girls and boys 11 years of age in **Physical Fitness Assessment,** C. Thomas, pp. 222-228.

Sempé, M. Pedron, G. and Roy-Pernot, M.P. (1979) **Auxologie, méthodes et séquences,** Theraplix, Lyon.

Shephard, R.J. Lavallée, H. Rajic, M. Jéquier, J.C. Beugage, C. and Labare, B. (1977) Influence of added activity classes upon the working capacity of Québec school children, in **Limites de la capacité physique chez l'enfant** (eds H. Lavallée and R.J. Shephard), Ed. du Pelican, pp. 237-245.

Simons, J. Beunen, G. Ostyn, M. Renson, R. Swalus, P. Van Gerven, D. and Willems, E. (1969) Construction d'une batterie de tests d'aptitude motrice pour garçons et filles de 12 à 19 ans, par la méthode factorielle. **Kinanthropologie,** 1, 323-362.

Simri, U. (1974) Assessment Procedures for Human Performance, in **Fitness, Health and Work Capacity, International Standards for Assessment,** (ed A. Larson), Macmillan, New York, pp. 362-379.

Tanner, J. M. (1962) **Growth at adolescence,** Blackwell Scientific Publ., London.

Vandervael, F. (1980) **Biométrie humaine.** Ed. Masson, Paris.

von Döbeln, W. (1956) Human standard and maximal metabolism rate in relation to fat-free body mass. **Acta Physiol. Scand.,** 37 (Suppl. 126).

Young, C.M. Sipin, S.S. and Roe, D.A. (1968) Body composition of preadolescent and adolescent girls. **J. Dietetic Assoc.,** 53, 25-31.

26

YOUTH SPORTS: READINESS, SELECTION AND TRAINABILITY

R.M. MALINA
Dept. of Kinesiology and Health Education, Univ. of Texas, Austin, Texas, USA

Keywords: Readiness, Selection for sport, Trainability, Youth sports, Maturity-matching.

1 Introduction

The concept of readiness has applicability to a variety of disciplines. As ordinarily used, readiness relates to the ability of the individual to successfully handle the demands of an instructional and learning situation, e.g., school, learning to read, specific instruction in motor skills, and so on. Readiness is occasionally used in the context of identifying talented youngsters, as in some visual and performing arts, who might benefit from early experiences in these domains. Both facets of readiness are applicable to sport, i.e., readiness of a child to handle the demands of a competitive sport, and identification of talented youngsters for early training in specific sports.

Many issues come to mind when individual readiness for a sport is considered, and there are no simple answers. For example, what are the criteria of readiness for a given sport, and are the criteria applicable to other sports? All too often, the physical (size, biological maturity), motor (skill) and perhaps aerobic components are emphasized. A more comprehensive approach might include social, emotional and cognitive readiness. Is there a best time for entrance into competitive sports? Given the broad range of individual variation in growth, maturation and development, i.e., in readiness, there is clearly no single answer. The subsequent discussion considers several biological issues related to readiness for sport. Note, however, that these cannot be treated in isolation from issues related to cognitive, social and emotional readiness. The latter are just as important and interact with biological concerns (see Malina 1986, 1980).

2 The readiness equation

Readiness is a functional concept which emphasizes the relationship between the ability of an individual and the demands of a specific activity or task. Using the theoretical framework developed by Brenner (1957) for school readiness, readiness for sport is defined as the match between a child's ability and the task demands presented in a sport. Readiness occurs when a child's ability is commensurate with or exceeds the task demands of a sport; unreadiness occurs when a child's ability is exceeded by the demands of a sport (Table 1). Thus, success or failure in sport can be viewed as dependent upon the balance between the child's ability and the task demands of a sport.

The readiness equation includes two components, the ability of the child and the demands of a sport. Ability is viewed as the biosocial matrix of growth, maturational and developmental characteristics of the individual (Table 2). Growth refers to measurable changes in size, physique and body composition, and various systems such as the cardiovascular which influences aerobic power. Maturity refers to the tempo and timing of progress towards the mature biological state. Development is a broader concept which relates to competence in a variety of interrelated domains as the individual adjusts to his/her cultural milieu, the amalgam of symbols, values and behaviours that characterize the population.

Table 1. The readiness equation - readiness and unreadiness for sport.

READINESS		
ABILITY	$\geq$	DEMANDS OF A SPORT
UNREADINESS		
ABILITY	$<$	DEMANDS OF A SPORT

Table 2. Ability, the biosocial matrix of growth, maturational and developmental characteristics.

ABILITY		
BIOSOCIAL MATRIX OF CHARACTERISTICS		
GROWTH	MATURATION	DEVELOPMENT
Size	Skeletal	Cognitive
Physique	Sexual	Emotional
Composition	Somatic	Social
Systemic	Neuromuscular	Motor

SELF-CONCEPT

PERCEIVED READINES FOR SPORT

Note that the motor domain is included in both maturation and development. The development of basic movement patterns is dependent to a large extent upon the individual's genotypically mediated pattern of neuromuscular maturation; once basic movement patterns are established, experience, learning and practice are significant factors affecting motor competence.

Growth and maturation are essentially biological processes, while development is a broader concept involving primarily behavioural domains, of course within a cultural context. Thus, the ability of a child is a biocultural entity. It is a product of the interaction of the child's genotype with the multiple environments in which he/she was reared and presently lives. It logically follows, therefore, that readiness of a child is a bicultural concept. The child in sport should be approached neither in a purely biological nor in a purely behavioral manner. Rather, both the biological and cultural characteristics of the child must be incorporated into the readiness equation.

Growth, maturation and development interact to mould selfconcept, which in turn influences the child's perceived readiness for sport. The child's perception of his/her readiness for sport has not been systematically studied and merits equal concern with other issues in youth sports research.

The other half of readiness equation is the demands of a sport, which are ordinarily described in technical manuals. They can be divided into three components: objectives, tasks, and rules (Table 3). The tasks of a sport can be subdivided into techniques, i.e., skills, and tactics, i.e., strategy, position play, and so on. Obviously, the decision making required to implement specific strategies with the tasks of a sport is an ongoing process that varies during the course of a contest. Applicability of sport specific rules, techniques and tactics to children and/or youth is more complex, since the rules of most sports have been developed for and by adults. Children, of course, are not miniature adults. How can tasks and rules be adjusted to meet the changing needs of growing, maturing and developing individuals? This has been done for a variety of sports, most notably Little League baseball, youth soccer and youth basketball.

Table 3. Demands of a sport.

DEMANDS OF A SPORT

        OBJECTIVES

        RULES

        TASKS: SKILLS & TACTICS

Readiness also has both temporary and permanent features. It is temporary in the context of a child's readiness for a specific task at a given point in time, e.g., is the child ready to learn the skills needed to participate in a sport at five or six years of age? On the other hand, it is permanent in the context of the individual's continuous readiness to meet the demands of tasks throughout his/her sporting career. Readiness is thus not only functional, but is also dynamic. Factors which influence ability and in turn readiness change, first, as the child grows, matures and develops, and second, as he/she adapts to the demands of a sport.

It should be emphasized that readiness for sport is not entirely a child-sport issue. The readiness of parents for their child in sport, and of coaches to instruct and train children in the context of sport are important considerations which are beyond the scope of this presentation (see Malina 1986, 1988).

3 Readiness and critical periods

Readiness is related to the theory of critical periods. These are specific times during which the child is maximally sensitive to environmental influences, both positive and negative, during growth and maturation and during the development of skills and behaviors. The theory of critical periods assumes that the changes underlying growth, maturation and development occur rapidly during a specific period of time and that organizational processes can be modified most easily at this time (see Scott 1986; Bornstein 1989). Critical periods, if they can be established with certainty, may thus represent times of maximal readiness.

The concept of critical periods is particularly related to the issue of specialization in sport and its corrollaries, selection and trainability. Should children and youth be permitted to specialize in a specific sport, or an event or position within a sport at an early age? If so, when should they be permitted, i.e., when are they ready, to specialize? On what criteria is a child selected for specialization? Who selects the child for specialization, i.e., who makes the decision, the child, parent, coach, or perhaps society? Specialization, it turn, requires a more demanding training program. What are the effects of early sport specialization and more rigorous training programs on the child? They should, presumably, be beneficial. Is this in fact the case? Can early specialized training have a negative effect on the growth, maturation and development of the individual?

4 Selection

Selection criteria and practices for a particular sport vary with the objectives of the program. Most programs emphasize mass participation, e.g., Little League baseball, youth soccer, kickball, and so on. Age and willingness to participate are the primary criteria. On the other hand, some programs emphasize the elite and have as their objective the identification and training of athletes with potential for success in the national and/or international arena, i.e., high performance sports. In the context of the latter, much discussion has focused on the success of sport systems in several Eastern European countries, which has been based in part on systematic selection at relatively young ages. Note, however, that recent changes in these political systems and re-evaluation of the role of sports, specifically high performance sports, in national agenda has apparently placed some elaborate sport systems in jeopardy. Nevertheless, selection practices developed in Eastern European countries have influenced those currently in use for some sports in Western countries.

Selection can thus be an important factor in youth sports, especially if the identification of potentially elite young athletes is an objective. However, in the context youth sports programs at the local level, should tests of readiness be used in the selection process for participation? Should such programs adopt a policy of competency based eligibility? Given the premium placed upon motor skills in sports, should perceptual- motor, performance and skill tests be used in assessing a child's readiness or competence for sports with such demands? Some sports such as running and swimming place heavy demands on the developing cardiovascular and respiratory systems. Should the status and trainability of the aerobic system be assessed to evaluate a child's readiness for such sports? Size and physique requirements of some sports are also selection criteria. Similar questions can be raised concerning social readiness for group participation, or for social interaction with peers and adults in the context of sport.

4.1 High Performance Sports

If gold medals in the future or success in high performance sport are objectives, the selection process begins early and is rather systematic. For example, the Soviet Union and German Democratic Republic had reasonably similar selection criteria and practices for gymnastics. According to Hartley (1988, p. 50), "Priority is given to selection of those children and young people thought most likely to benefit from intensive sports training and to produce top-class results in national and international competition." The process began at about five years of age with intial observation of school children by coaches (Table 4). In addition to general health status, children with a suitable build were subsequently invited for a more systematic trial. The latter included tests of strength, speed and coordination. Children with good results were invited to trial training sessions during which coaches evaluated behavioural characteristics. A smaller select group was then invited, i.e., selected, for systematic training in gymnastics in special schools.

The general pattern of initial evaluation of anthropometric, motor and behavioural characteristics is applied in other Eastern European countries as well (see, for example, Karacsony (1988) for Hungary and Bompa (1985) for Roumania). It has also been incorporated to a large extent into the Talent Identification Program of the Canadian Gymnastics Federation (Bajin 1987). The program recommends pre-selection of female gymnasts and initiation of formal training at about 6-7 years of age. In addition to interest, body composition and constitution and a battery of ability tests emphasizing flexibility, strength, speed and power are used (Table 5). The United States also has a program for elite gymnasts, the Junior Elite Development Program National Training Camps of the United States Association of Independent Gymnastics Clubs (Feigley 1987).

Anthropometric, motor and behavioral characteristics of children and youth are also used as selection criteria in other sports, but the timing of evaluation varies somewhat. For example, potential rowers, basketball players and weight lifters are not selected until after puberty in the Soviet Union and the German Democratic Republic (Hartley 1988). A primary selection phase for talent identification in Roumania occurs between 3 and 8 years of age, but the more important secondary phase varies by sport: 9-10 years for gymnastics, figure skating and swimming, 10-15 years for girls and 10-17 years for boys in other sports (Bompa 1985).

Table 4. Selection criteria for gymnastics in the Soviet Union and German Democratic Republic*

---

1. General health status
2. "Suitable build" - based on stature-weight relationships, proportions and posture
3. Tests of strength, speed and coordination:
   a. USSR - 20 m run, standing long jump, chin-ups, L-hang
   b. GDR - obstacle course, running backwards, speed and orientation running, standing long jump, leg lifts, chin-ups
4. Children with good results - invited to trial training sessions; coaches focus on behavior

---

*Adapted from Hartley (1988).

Table 5. Components of the selection criteria used in the Canadian Talent Identification Program for female gymnasts*

---

1. Age - 6 to 7

2. Medical evaluation

3. Body composition and constitution evaluation

4. Interest

5. Physical ability:

a.	glide kips	f. vertical jump
b.	20 m run	g. push-ups (dips)
c.	leg lifts	h. hip pull over
d.	standing long jump	i. rope climb
e.	chin-ups	

---

*Adapted from Bajin (1987).

Physical and motor requisites for selection also vary among sports. Anthropometric and motor criteria for potential throwers (shot and discus) among 12-13 year old girls in the Soviet Union are summarized in Table 6. The selection process for female throwers continues for about two years, during which time the girls are evaluated for improvement in motor performance, especially power tasks, ease with which technical elements of throwing events are learned, and ability to adapt to the training regimen (Komarova and Rashimshanova 1980).
Ballet, though considered primarily as an art form, has rather rigorous anatomical criteria that rival those of some sports (Table 7). The highly selective nature of ballet is described by Hamilton (1986, p. 61):

"Beginning with the first ballet class, a constant natural selection process is at work weeding out those aspiring dancers with the wrong bodies and those who lack either the talent or the tenacity to persevere."

4.2 Agency Sponsored Sports
In sharp contrast to programs concerned with elite athletes, youth sports programs in many parts of the world are generally aimed at mass participation. Agency sponsored programs in North America have at least 20 stated objectives. These can be summarized into six categories that are not necessarily mutually exclusive: learning motor skills, physical fitness, participation and belonging, learning socially acceptable values and behaviours, long term skills for leisure, and enhancing child-adult relationships (Seefeldt 1987). When asked why they participate in sports responses of children conform, in general, with the stated objectives: to have fun, to improve skills and to learn new skills, to be with friends or

to make new friends, for thrills and excitement, to become physically fit, and to succeed or win (Smith et al. 1983).

Within the context of such a diverse array of objectives of sports programs and participants, willingness to participate and access to programs are major considerations, and the criterion for selection is ordinarily age or grade in school. Thus, selection of a sport at this level is most likely a child-parent decision. This is not selection for sport.

Table 6. Selection criteria for potential throwers (shotput and discus) among 12-13 year old girls in the Soviet Union*

---

1. Stature - at least 168 to 170 cm
2. Weight - not specified, but must be restricted
3. Biological maturity status - apparently to eliminate size advantage of early maturers
4. Motor performance:
    a. standing long jump - 200 to 210 cm
    b. vertical jump - 40 to 42 cm
    c. 3 kg medicine ball throw - 8 to 10 m
    d. 30 m sprint - 4.8 to 5.0 sec
    e. auditory reaction time - 160 to 180 msec

---

*Adapted from Komarova and Rashimshanova (1980).

Table 7. Anatomical criteria for ballet*

---

1. Body proportions - "She should be thin ... long trunks, short legs, large buttocks, swayback, round shoulders, spinal curvatures, large heads, and short necks are all considered unesthetic."
2. Ligamentous laxity
3. Turnout of the hip - "The most important anatomic feature . . . . This is the cornerstone of proper ballet technique . . . . It is the sum total of the entire leg's external rotation."
4. Leg alignment - "Most dancers tend to be slightly bowlegged."
5. Hyperextension of the knee
6. Ankle-instep flexibility

---

*Adapted from Hamilton (1986).

Maturity-matching, i.e., classification of children by maturity status, is occasionally used to equalize competition in an attempt to enhance chance of success and to reduce injury associated with side mismatches. Maturity-matching is thus a form of selection. There is, however, more to equalizing than biological maturity status; some indication of skill and fitness level should be incorporated.

The Selection/Classification Program of the New York State Public High School Athletic Association is a good example of a systematic procedure to determine the readiness of 7th and 8th grade youth (about 13-14 years) for interscholastic high school (grades 9-12) competition (Hafner et al. 1982; Willie 1982). In addition to approval of the local board of education and the child's parents, the procedure includes assessment of (1) medical status, (2) sexual maturity status, pubic hair development in boys and years past menarche in girls, (3) stature and weight, (4) previous experience in sports, (5) physical fitness based on tests of agility, strength, speed and endurance, (6) a placement decision that permits the child to try out for a team, and (7) coach's rating of skill proficiency relative to the demands of the sport (Willie 1982).

Applicability of maturity-matching to younger ages presents a major logistical problem for agency sponsored sports, e.g., large numbers, who will examine the children, and so on. There is also the practical problem of change in maturity status and in turn size and strength during the season. Using Little League baseball, which has a chronological age limit of 12 years, as an example, teams in Texas are selected in March, the season starts in April and continues into July. By early June, some early maturing boys will have experienced their adolescent spurts, so that relatively small size differences are now magnified. Thus, should matching be an ongoing process during the season? This obviously is not practical.

Age, stature and weight will probably match the majority of children under 12 years of age, given the association among age, body size and maturity status. In addition, many agency sponsored youth sports programs have various competitive levels based on age and skill, and "try outs" permit coaches to assess the skill levels of each child.

Identifying and selecting the potentially elite athlete and subsequently perfecting his/her talent is not an objective of most youth sports programs in North America. This does not imply that potentially elite athletes will not be identified in such programs. The method of selecting most high performance athletes in North American countries is often described by Eastern European sport specialists as "natural selection":
"an athlete enrols in a sport as a result of local influence (school tradition, parents' wishes, or peers). However, the performance evolution of athletes determined by natural selection depends, among other factors, on whether the individual, by coincidence, happened or

didn't happen to take part in a sport for which he/she had talent" (Bompa 1985, p. 2).

(Needless to say, the use of the term "natural selection" above and in the preceding discussion of ballet has no relevance to natural selection in the Darwinian sense (see Malina 1990).

The identification and selection of the potentially elite athlete is, to a large extent, a by-product of specific sport programs and local interest, particularly as levels of skill and competition increase. Youngsters participating in local sport programs are routinely observed by adults with varying degrees of interest and expertise in coaching. It is in this context that skill, size and physique characteristics of children and youth become important selective factors, among others. Success in sport associated with skill and size often facilitates the acquisition of expert coaching, which in turn builds upon the youngster's talent. The interaction of the individual's physical and motor characteristics with social circumstances, i.e., being noticed, is an essential component of the selection process. Individuals so identified generally have access to better coaching and competition, and in turn have greater opportunity for further success in sport, heightened motivation, and so on, all of which may lead to persistence in sport and perhaps perfection of talent.

However, not all talented children and youth benefit from such favorable biosocial or biocultural interactions. Economic resources are often a limiting factor in securing access to facilities, expert coaching, and related requisites for success. Exploitation of youngsters, especially those from minority and impoverished backgrounds, is an additional factor as level of competition and selection in some sports becomes more intense, e.g., agency and/or school sponsored basketball in many American cities.

Selection may also occur to some extent by default. Some individuals may choose not to participate, although they may have the skill, physical and behavioural requisites which are conducive to success in sport. Changing social interests, parental and coaching pressures, overemphasis on winning, and so on are often reasons given for dropping out of sport. In addition, normal growth and maturation may influence a youngster's decision. These biological processes do not occur in a social vacuum, and associated changes in size, body composition, performance and behavior are the backdrop against which youth evaluate and interpret their own status among peers. Participation in sports is an important component of the evaluative process. Thus, changing relationships with peers, parents and coaches which accompany the adolescent growth spurt and sexual maturation may influence participation in sport, and there are most likely sex differences in the process.

5 Trainability

The trainability of children, i.e., how responsive are developing individuals at different stages of growth and maturation to a training stimulus, is related to readiness and selection. The issue of trainability has been related primarily to the effects of regular training on the development of aerobic power. It has been suggested, for example, that youngsters are more susceptible to the beneficial effects of training during periods of rapid growth (a critical period?), with an emphasis on adolescence. It has been applied more recently to muscular strength and is also applicable to the effects of instruction and practice on motor skill.

Figure 1 summarises a paradigm that attempts to incorporate potential causal factors associated with differential responses to instruction and/or training. Sensitivity to instruction and/or training depends on a variety of factors including age, perhaps sex, prior experiences, pre-instruction or pre-training level of skill, strength and aerobic power (i.e., current phenotype), and possibly specific genetic variations (genotype). With the exception of studies of responses of sedentary young adults to aerobic training (Bouchard 1986; Malina and Bouchard, in press), these factors are not ordinarily controlled in studies of instruction and training.

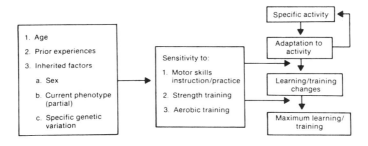

Fig. 1 A simplified model of factors associated with variation in responses to instruction/practice of motor skills and to training of strength or aerobic power (modified after Bouchard and Malina (1983) and Bouchard (1986).

5.1 Motor Skills

There is rapid progress in the development of fundamental movement skills during early childhood and the interaction of genotype, movement experiences and rearing environment is paramount in the process. By 6-8 years of age, basic movement patterns are, on average, reasonably well developed, although the mature patterns of some skills do not develop until later (Branta et al. 1984; Haubenstricker and Seefeldt 1986). It is also at these ages that many children enter organized sport programs and are probably ready for specific instruction and practice in more specialized skills, including sports skills. Casual observation of progress made by children during the course of a season in a sport would seem to verify this expectation since the skills utilised in many sports are combinations and/or modifications of fundamental movement patterns. What is of interest, however, is that many coaches of youth sports are not specialists in the area of teaching motor skills; rather, most are volunteers. Although practice sessions in youth sports are often reasonably planned instructional programs, whether they include appropriate motor task sequences and adequate time for practice, i.e., essential elements of successful instruction, is another matter. In contrast to local programs, children involved in more elite programs spend more time in systematic instruction and practice under the supervision of specialists in the particular sport.

On the other hand, many 6-8 year old children have not yet developed sufficient motor control to successfully accomplish mature patterns of some fundamental motor skills. Although entry into youth sports may result in negative experiences, regular instruction and practice may facilitate the development of basic skills.

Proficiency in sport skills improves considerably during middle childhood and adolescence, so that it is difficult to partition practice and learning effects from those associated with growth and maturation. Motor performance improves more or less linearly with age during middle childhood. It continues to improve during adolescence in males, but tends to reach a plateau in females at about 14 or 15 years of age. Maturity-associated variation in size and performance is an additional factor which may influence the response to instruction and practice, and is often associated with success in youth sports. Boys advanced in biological maturity status tend to perform better than those who are delayed. On the other hand, differences in the performances of girls of contrasting maturity status are not marked, and in some tasks better performances are attained by girls delayed in maturity status (Malina and Bouchard, in press).

5.2 Muscular Strength

Historically, resistance training for the development of strength was not recommended for prepubescent children. It was assumed that the lack of sufficient quantities of circulating androgenic hormones in prepubescent boys precluded strength improvement with such training. A secondary factor was the risk of injury in unsupervised resistance training programs. Thus, the 1983 statement of the American Academy of Paediatrics (1983, p. 161) offered the following conclusion: "Maximal benefits are obtained from appropriate weight training in the postpubertal athlete, and minimal benefits are obtained from weight training in the prepubertal athlete."

The statement suggests that prepubertal children are not as trainable with resistance programs involving weights or special machines as pubertal or postpubertal youth. Several recent studies, however, indicate significant gains in strength with resistance programs in both prepubertal and pubertal boys (Pfeiffer and Francis 1986; Weltman et al. 1986). It is important to note that increases in strength are not necessarily accompanied by muscular hypertrophy, which emphasizes the role of the neuromuscular system in the physiological increases in strength associated with resistance training. Prepubertal boys generally made the largest relative gains in strength, followed by pubertal and then postpubertal boys (Pfeiffer and Francis 1986). Among prepubertal boys, control subjects also improved in several strength measurements but not to the extent observed in trained boys (Weltman et al. 1986). Gains experienced by control subjects reflect the combined effects of learning, i.e., how to perform the tests, normal day-to-day physical activity, and growth-associated changes in strength during the program.

Corresponding data are not extensive for girls, but the evidence indicates increases in both static and functional strength in girls in response to several training programs (Nielsen et al. 1980). Further, younger girls (<13.5 years) made greater gains than older girls.

Training programs which emphasize muscular endurance also suggest differential responses of strength and endurance that depend on age. In the study of Ikai (1966), for example, small samples of 8-14 year old boys trained for 5 weeks, working to exhaustion at one-third of maximum strength on an arm ergometer (Table 8). As expected, trained boys made significant gains while control subjects had more variable changes. Among the trained subjects, younger boys made greater relative gains in maximal strength, while older boys made greater relative gains in muscular endurance.

5.3 Aerobic Power

A summary of training-associated relative changes in VO_2 max per unit body weight (ml/min/kg) in children and youth reported in specific studies is given in Table 9. Samples are arbitrarily grouped into three age categories, < 10, 10-13, and 14+, and studies in which children were grouped across a broad age range, e.g., 8-13 or 10-15, are excluded.

Table 8 Relative changes in muscular strength and endurance after five weeks of training on an arm ergometer in boys*

Age	Maximal Trained	Strength Control	Muscular Trained	Endurance Control
8	34.2%	0 %	34.3 %	2.6 %
10	29.6 %	13.5 %	45.6 %	3.5 %
12	23.3 %	-3.9 %	44.8 %	-3.9 %
14	6.5 %	-4.0 %	60.0 %	6.1 %

* Adapted from Ikai (1966)

Table 9. Relative changes in VO_2 max (ml/min/kg) associated with training in children and youth*

		Relati ve Changes in VO_2 max in Specific Studies				
Age	N	< 0%	+1 to +5%	+6 to +10%	+11 to +15%	>15%
< 10	13	4	8			1
10-13	12	1	2	3	2	4
14 +	3			1		2

* Based on reviews of Mocellin (1975), Rowland (1985) and Pate and Ward (1990). N refers to the number of training studies in the indicated age range.

Numbers of children vary among studies as do the intensity and duration of training.

The available data indicate relatively little trainability of maximal aerobic power in children under 10 years of age. With one exception, changes in maximal aerobic power per kg of body weight in children under 10 years of age are less than 5%, and in several studies negative changes are apparent. It is not certain whether the results derived from young children are a consequence of low trainability, i.e., a low adaptive potential to aerobic training, or are due to inadequacies of training programs. For example, if it can be assumed that young children are habitually more physically active than adolescents and adults, a more intensive aerobic training program may be required to induce significant changes in maximal aerobic power. On the other hand, most activities of young children proceed at submaximal work rates, so that maximal aerobic power may not be the appropriate measure. It may be more appropriate to consider changes in submaximal work efficiency in response to training (Malina and Bouchard, in press).

Among older children and adolescents, on the other hand, responses of aerobic power to training are clearly apparent, but results are variable across studies. Among early adolescents 10-13 years, relative gains associated with training range from 1% to 19%, and there are no negative values. In addition, there does not appear to be a sex difference. Among adolescents 14 years and older, data are less extensive and overlap those of 10-13 year old youth. The variability among studies probably relates to sampling and methodological variation. Some studies have used young athletes as subjects, while others have used reasonably active or sedentary youth. Training programs vary and outside activity is difficult to control. Hence, it is no wonder that results are variable. Nevertheless, when older children and adolescents are rather sedentary at the start of the program, short-term training studies generally yield improvements in maximal aerobic power that are similar to those observed in young adults (Pate and Ward 1990; Malina and Bouchard, in press).

8 References

American Academy of Pediatrics (1983) Weight training and weight lifting: information for the pediatrician. **Physician Sportsmed.**, 11, 157-161

Bajin, B. (1987) Talent identification program for Canadian female gymnasts, in **World Identification for Gymnastic Talent** (eds B. Petiot, J.H. Salmela and T.B. Hoshizaki), Sport Psyche Editions, Montreal, pp. 34-44.

Bompa, T.O. (1985) Talent identification. **Sports: Science Periodical on Research and Technology in Sport, Physical Testing G1**. Coaching Association of Canada, Ottawa.

Bornstein, M.H. (1989) Sensitive periods in development: Structural characteristics and causal interpretations. **Psychol. Bull.**, 105, 1-19.

Bouchard, C. (1986) Genetics of aerobic power and capacity, in **Sport and Human Genetics** (eds R.M. Malina and C. Bouchard), Human Kinetics, Champaign, Illinois, pp. 59-08.

Bouchard, C. and Malina, R.M. (1983) Genetics for the sport scientist: Selected methodological considerations. **Exer. Sport. Sci. Rev.**, 11, 275-305.

Branta, C. Haubenstricker, J. and Seefeldt, V. (1984) Age changes in motor skills during childhood and adolescence. **Exer. Sport. Sci. Rev.**, 12, pp. 467-520.

Brenner, A. (1957) Nature and meaning of readiness for school. **Merrill-Palmer Q.**, 3, 114-135.

Feigley, D.A. (1987) Characteristics of young elite gymnasts, in **World Identification for Gymnastic Talent** (eds B. Petiot, J.H. Salmela and T.B. Hoshizaki), Sport Psyche Editions, Montreal, pp. 94-112.

Hafner, J.K. Scott, S.E. Veras, G. Goldberg, B. Nicholas, J.A. and Shaffer, T.E. (1982) Interscholastic athletics: Method for selection and classification of athletes. **New York State J. Med.**, 82, 1449-1459.

Hamilton, W.G. (1986) Physical prerequisites for ballet dancers : Selectivity that can enhance (or nullify) a career. **J. Musculoskel. Med.**, 3, 61-66.

Hartley, G. (1908) A comparative view of talent selection for sport in two socialist states - The USSR and the GDR - with particular reference to gymnastics, in **The Growing Child in Competitive Sport**, The National Coaching Foundation, Leeds, pp. 50-56.

Haubenstricker, J. and Seefeldt V. (1986) Acquisition of motor skills during childhood, in **Physical activity and Well-Being** (ed V. Seefeldt), American Alliance for Health, Physical Education, Recreation and Dance, Reston, Vinirgina, pp. 41-101.

Ikai, M. (1966) The effects of training on muscular endurance, in **Proceedings of International Congress of Sport Sciences**, 1964 (ed K. Kato), University of Tokyo Press, Tokyo, pp.145-150.

Karacsony, I. (1988) The discovery and selection of talented athletes and talent management in Hungary, in **The Growing Child in Competitive Sport,** The National Coaching Foundation, Leeds, pp. 34-49.

Komarova, A. and Rashimshanova, K. (1980) Identification of female throwing talent, in **The Throws** (ed J. Jarver), Tafnews, Book Division of Track & Field News, Los Altos, California, pp. 55-56.

Malina, R.M. (1986) Readiness for competitive sport, in **Sport for Children and Youths** (eds M.R. Weiss and D. Gould), Human Kinetics, Champaign, Illinois, pp. 45-50.

Malina, R.M. (1988) Readiness for competitive sports, in **The Growing Child in Competitive Sport**, The National Coaching Foundation, Leeds, pp. 67-77.

Malina, R.M. (1990) Darwinian fitness, physical fitness, and physical activity, in **Applications of Biological Anthropology to Human Affairs** (eds G. Lasker and N. Mascie-Taylor), Cambridge University Press, Cambridge (in press).

Malina, R.M. and Bouchard, C. (1991) **Growth, Maturation, and Physical Activity**. Human Kinetics, Champaign, Ill.

Mocellin, R. (1975) Jugend und sport. **Med. Klin.**, 70, 1443-1457.

Nielsen, B. Nielsen, K. Behrendt Hansen, M. and Asmussen, E. (1980) Training of "functional muscular strength" in girls 7-19 years old, in **Children and Exercise IX** (eds K. Berg and B.O. Eriksson), University Park Press, Baltimore, Maryland, pp. 69-78.

Pate, R.R. and Ward, D.S. (1990) Endurance exercise trainability in children and youth. **Adv. Sports Med. Fit.**, 3, 37-55.

Pfeiffer, R.D. and Francis, R.S. (1986) Effects of strength training on muscle development in prepubescent, pubescent, and postpubescent males. **Physician Sportsmed.**, 14, 134-143 (Sept.).

Rowland, T.W. (1985) Aerobic response to endurance training in prepubescent children: a critical analysis. **Med. Sci. Sport. Exer.**, 17, 493-497.

Scott, J.P. (1986) Critical periods in organizational processes, in **Human Growth. Vol. 1. Developmental Biology, Prenatal Growth** (eds F. Falkner and J.M. Tanner), Plenum Press, New York, pp. 181-196.

Seefeldt, V. (1987) **Handbook for Youth Sport Coaches**. American Alliance for Health, Physical Education, Recreation, and Dance, Reston, Virginia.

Smith, N.J. Smith, R.E. and Smoll, F.L. (1983) **Kidsports: A Survival Guide for Parents**. Addison-Wesley, Reading, Massachusetts.

Weltman, A. Janney, C. Rians, C.B. Strand, K. Berg, B. Tippitt, S. Wise, J. Cahill, B.R. and Katch, F.I. (1986) The effects of hydraulic resistance strength training in pre-pubertal males. **Med. Sci. Sport Exer.**, 18, 629-638.

Willie, M.C. (1982) **Revised maturity and physical fitness standards for the selection/classification screening procedures.** Division of Physical Education, Fitness, Health, Nutrition and Safety Services, The University of the State of New York, The State Education Department, Albany.

Index

This index uses keywords assigned to the individual chapters as its basis. The numbers are the page numbers of the first page of the relevant chapter.